Medical
Problem
Solving

Medical Problem Solving

An Analysis of Clinical Reasoning

Arthur S. Elstein
Lee S. Shulman
Sarah A. Sprafka

with

Linda Allal
Michael Gordon
Hilliard Jason
Norman Kagan
Michael J. Loupe
Ronald D. Jordan

Harvard University Press
Cambridge, Massachusetts
and
London, England
1978

Copyright © 1978 by the President and Fellows of Harvard College
All rights reserved
Printed in the United States of America

Library of Congress Cataloging in Publication Data
Elstein, Arthur Shirle, 1935–
    Medical problem solving.

   Bibliography: p.
   Includes index.
   1. Medical logic. 2. Medicine—Decision making.
3. Problem solving. 4. Diagnosis. I. Shulman,
Lee S., joint author. II. Sprafka, Sarah A., 1941–
joint author. III. Title. [DNLM: 1. Problem solving.
2. Decision making. 3. Medicine. WB100 E486m]
R723.E47   616.07′5′019   77-21505
ISBN 0-674-56125-2

*To the memory of
Aaron and Rae E. Elstein*

Foreword

What are the characteristics of effective physicians? What are the components of clinical competence? Are the enormous costs of creating and sustaining physicians justified by either the uniqueness or the high quality of their skills?

Such questions are being asked with growing frequency (and intensity) by people both inside and outside the medical profession, and we are still some distance from any widely accepted answers. We do know that there is more to being a physician than merely possessing a large body of information. But what are the other abilities required? Surely they include, at least under some conditions, the capacity to deal with high levels of uncertainty and ambiguity; the capability for self-initiated, independent learning; effectiveness in establishing trust-based, empathic relationships; and the ability to identify and solve complex clinical problems. The significance of any of these competencies cannot be denied. There is considerable dispute, however, over whether they are present among current physicians to the extent that society deserves. A root concern is whether these characteristics are adequately understood; until they are, they cannot be dependably taught or evaluated.

The investigations reported in this volume were prompted largely by practical concern with finding ways to improve our capacities to teach and measure one of the important physician characteristics noted above: the skill of problem solving and reasoning.

Problem solving in medicine has been aptly, if somewhat cynically, described as "the process of making adequate decisions with inadequate information." With a few words the anonymous originator of that observation captured several of the essential features of a set of intellectual/emotional events that are both critical and perplexing.

The need for medical decisions that are at least adequate is vital (in the root sense of that word), both for the people directly affected and for the national economy. U.S. Secretary of Health, Education, and Welfare Joseph A. Califano observed in a June 1977 address to the American Medical Association that in 1976 health costs in this country totaled 139 billion dollars and that by 1980 they will probably reach 230 billion dollars, or 10 percent of the country's gross national product. He added that "the physician is the central decision maker for more than 70 percent of health care services," including the decision for (and length of) hospitalization, types of medication ordered, and diagnostic tests used. These observations provide substantial justification for improving our understanding of the decision-making process of physicians.

It has taken until this decade for the leading contributors to the licensure and certification of physicians in North America, the National Board of Medical Examiners and the American Board of Internal Medicine, to begin a research program aimed at enhancing our understanding of clinical decision making. A report on progress to date (John R. Senior, "Toward the Measurement of Competence in Medicine," November 1976) is available from Dr. Senior at the Graduate Hospital of the University of Pennsylvania in Philadelphia. Both the designers and the users of the influential evaluation instruments of these bodies recognize the need to move beyond our traditional dependence on measuring the information possessed by physicians, without due consideration of the ways in which information is utilized to identify and resolve clinical problems. The studies reported here should move us several steps toward the fulfillment of this need.

Complementing the pragmatic concerns just noted as a stimulus for the studies reported in this book were the theoretical challenges of achieving fuller understanding of a set of cognitive processes that continue to perplex and confound a growing group of devoted researchers. The intellectual heritage of the present studies is thoroughly summarized in Chapter 2. The duality of the origins and consequences of this work—the practical and the theoretical—has presented the authors with a dilemma: how to do justice to both sides of the issues so as to be equally communicative with the two rather different potential audiences that these matters concern, the clinicians/teachers and the psychologists/educators. The two groups bring substantially different backgrounds, interests, and vocabularies to any exchange on the matters at hand. It is difficult to imagine any one book that would be equally responsive to both groups. This book is not. It is weighted in the direction of the psychologists/educators—as well it should be. Given that the present work is a series of steps forward in a continuing sequence, not a set of definitive conclusions, the main communication should be with those most likely to utilize present findings in pursuit of future research.

Still, this book is not without practical consequences for the teaching, evaluation, and conduct of clinical inquiry. Partly because of the importance of those consequences, and partly because they are scattered throughout the book, the most striking are summarized here:

(a) *Hypotheses are generated early.* As experienced clinicians know (although most of our clinical teaching has not yet acknowledged), problem solving begins with the formulation of tentative hypotheses, which serve to guide further inquiry. In direct contrast to our conventional instructional strategy of urging students to defer all hypotheses until the history taking and physical examination have been concluded, competent physicians begin generating hypotheses in the earliest moments of their encounters with patients. Indeed, they never use the student-oriented approach. In addition to this important finding, some preliminary experiences are reported with new approaches to the teaching of problem solving based on this information.

(b) *The hypotheses considered are limited in number.* In confirmation of the findings for people in general, from problem-solving research in other fields, clinicians are found to have a distinctly limited capacity for simultaneously considering multiple hypotheses, regardless of the complexity of the problem. Rarely does the number exceed five, and virtually never will an individual be entertaining more than seven. Given that further investigation of a patient's problems often will be limited to those hypotheses that survive the revision process taking place during the initial inquiries, it is important to understand that any of three things may go wrong as a consequence of the mind's apparent need for parsimony: (1) hypotheses may be retained that are excessively general (for example, "abdominal infection" rather than "mesenteric adenitis"), as a way of embracing inconsistent findings; (2) selected findings may be disregarded (to avoid having to generate new hypotheses, even if they could account for the findings more effectively than currently held hypotheses); and (3) some findings may be assigned exaggerated importance, to justify retention of existing hypotheses. Both these processes and these risks need to be understood for effective instruction and evaluation in the area of clinical problem solving.

(c) *The most common interpretive error is that of overinterpretation.* As noted above, the human intellect apparently needs to perceive problems as having limited degrees of complexity. The consequent tendency to simplify appears to be most commonly expressed by assigning new information to existing hypotheses— rather than creating new hypotheses or remembering the new information separately. The error (here called overinterpretation) of regarding noncontributory information as confirmation of an existing hypothesis was far more common than either disregarding new information or regarding it as disconfirming when it was not. If this is the highest risk error, it is the one deserving most attention in teaching.

(d) *Competence may be case related.* Both physicians and medical students were found to vary considerably in their diagnostic effectiveness, according to the nature of the problem at hand. These findings are contrary to the widely held assumption that there is a clear (although not yet demonstrated) distinction between physicians who are "competent" and those who are not. Put another way, we may have to abandon our hope that competence, even in the subsidiary area of ability as a clinical problem solver, is a general characteristic. A more likely conclusion will probably be that the issue of physician competence (like the medical care process to which it applies) is more complex than we have wanted to acknowledge. Individuals will have to be evaluated by far more thorough procedures than is possible with a few formal examinations or clinical cases. We will need to think in terms of *profiles* of competence, in which individuals are regarded as being effective with particular types of problems, in particular situations.

(e) *Information and experience appear to be basic to competence.* While we have much to do to complete our understanding of competence in clinical problem solving, these studies do increase our assurance that two of its foundation components are the possession of relevant bodies of information and a sufficiently broad experience with related problems to permit the determination of which information is pertinent, which clinical findings are significant, and how these findings are to be integrated into appropriate hypotheses and conclusions. As a minimum, the effective clinician has knowledge of (1) the relation of findings to conditions (for the problems at hand), (2) the relative frequencies of different possible conditions (their population base-rates), and (3) the particular characteristics of those conditions which carry severe risk, even if their rate of occurrence is low. The capacity to retain this information, and to mobilize it when needed, appears to be an outcome of repetitive practice. The implications for education appear clear: learning information is important, but far from sufficient. Repetitive practice in application of information to solution of the same range of problems that will be confronted later is probably mandatory.

These five generalizations provide a glimpse, not a summary, of the richness of this book. Beyond contributing a set of specific practicalities, as suggested by the brief list above, the work embodied here achieves the important general purpose of demonstrating that a fundamental component of physician competence can by systematically studied. This demonstration should encourage others to continue the overdue pursuit of these intriguing, vital issues to the point where our depth of understanding will be sufficient to assure regular and effective instruction, evaluation, and performance of this central component of medical care.

HILLIARD JASON, M.D., ED.D.
Association of American
Medical Colleges

Acknowledgments

This book is the product of the imagination and effort of many people in the Office of Medical Education Research and Development (OMERAD) at Michigan State University. We wish to take this opportunity to thank, all too briefly, those who helped us and to identify the contributions of each associate.

Arthur Elstein guided the day-to-day operations of the project laboratory, supervised construction of the materials used to study the reasoning processes of the panel of experienced physicians, and was co–project director responsible for the observational research involving this panel. He is senior author of Chapters 3, 4, 5, 6, and 11.

Lee Shulman was co–project director responsible for the experimental studies that were designed to test significant portions of the emerging theory of medical reasoning. Three dissertations were guided by him under aegis of this research program; these are reported in Chapters 7 through 10. He is senior author of Chapters 1 and 2; a slightly different version of Chapter 2 appeared in the 1975 *Review of Research in Education* (vol. 3).

In addition to performing the research for her own dissertation (Chapter 9), Sarah Sprafka was deeply involved in developing several versions of the scoring system for the high-fidelity simulations. She headed the team that scored protocols for the analyses in Chapter 4 and was a member of the group that analyzed the patient-management problems of Chapter 5. More recently, she has worked persistently and effectively at Michigan State University to help evolve practical means of instruction and evaluation based on the ideas discussed in this book.

Hilliard Jason conceived the idea for the project and was the principal investigator in its early years. The research program and OMERAD as a whole owe much to his creative leadership.

Norman Kagan developed the concepts and methods of simulated patients and videotape-stimulated recall that are central to our research methods. His insights about early hypothesis generation contributed significantly to the theoretical framework of the research program. In addition to working with several participating physicians as an uncommonly skilled interrogator, he trained and recruited other qualified interrogators: Anne Baucom, Mark Hector, Mary Heiserman, June Jacobson, Roger Landvoy, William Martin, Gary Price, Robert Van Noord, and Jeff Yager.

Like Sarah Sprafka, Linda Allal and Michael Gordon began their association with the project as graduate students and became valued and respected colleagues. Allal's doctoral dissertation forms the basis of Chapters 7 and 8. In addition, she set up and executed most of the statistical analyses reported in Chapters 4 and 6, developed the data analysis for Chapter 5, and participated in the research reported in Chapter 6.

Michael Gordon's doctoral dissertation is reported in Chapter 10, but his contributions go far beyond that work. He also served as consultant on problems arising with several subprojects covered in different chapters and shared responsibility for the scoring manual developed for the fixed-order problems (Chapter 6). Above all, he remained alert to the search for heuristics for medical problem solving, even when the particulars of each problem analyzed seemed to obscure the general. The portion of Chapter 11 dealing with medical heuristics owes much to his outlook, although he did not compile the list of heuristics proposed there.

Michael Loupe helped to design and pilot test the three high-fidelity simulations (Chapters 3 and 4) and to gather the first data in that series. He was actively involved in selecting instruments to study individual differences and in analyzing pilot data for formulation of the preliminary theory of medical inquiry.

Ronald Jordan directed the group that studied the fixed-order problems (Chapter 6), although the statistical analysis was done after he had left Michigan State University. He also provided substantial help as an interrogator and staffer during the hectic days when physicians were in the laboratory and simulations were staged.

Many physicians assisted in our work. Particular thanks are extended to Howard Barrows of McMaster University, who provided the scenario and training of an actress as patient for one of the simulations in Chapter 4. Brian Hennen and Hugh Scott helped greatly in the design of the other two high-fidelity simulations. Gilles Cormier was closely involved in scoring these protocols and in synthesizing other problems. Valuable aid in designing materials and consultation on scoring or on other questions was also provided by Alan Barnes, Alex Bryans, Bruce Challis, Marvin Clark, Michael Doyle, Dan English, Donald Gragg, David Greenbaum, Gerald Holzman, Carmi Margolis, Victor Neufeld, Michael Spooner, and Peter Ways.

We acknowledge the cooperation and interest of Christine McGuire, of the Center for Educational Development at the University of Illinois College of Medicine, who provided four patient-management problems in a format modified to our specifications and helped to clarify the differences among scoring systems. Her discussions with us of the special cognitive and measurement properties of patient-management problems were most helpful and contributed greatly to our deeper understanding of the subjects' performance.

Medical students who assisted with various phases of the project were David Hoisington, Robert Marra, Jon Overholt, Michael Shier, David Van Dyke, and Paul Werner. Randall Isaacson and Michael Petkovich were part-time graduate assistants from the departments of educational psychology and psychology respectively.

The following colleagues offered specific help and useful suggestions: Robert G. Bridgham, James B. Erdmann, Jack L. Maatsch, John Schneider, and Howard S. Teitelbaum. Rose Zacks assisted in relating our findings to the literature on memory organization. Paul Hoffman and Paul Slovic of the Oregon Research Institute and Kenneth Hammond of the Institute of Behavioral Science, University of Colorado, made valuable comments and significantly influenced our thinking.

The actors who played the roles of patients deserve special gratitude: Juliana Boehnlein, Nancy Gustafson, Holly Holdman, Marguerite Matthews, Laurel Montague, Roger Powell, Marshall Shnider, and Diane Bosley Taylor.

The physicians who took time from busy practices or used vacation days to join us in the project laboratory merit special recognition. We are also indebted to the medical students who served as subjects in the experimental studies. These individuals must remain anonymous, but they know that theirs was an essential contribution.

The Medical Inquiry Project was supported in part by Grant No. R01-PE-00041 from the Bureau of Health Manpower of the Health Resources Administration, U.S. Department of Health, Education, and Welfare. The patience of its officials during the project's long incubation and maturation is sincerely appreciated. The bureau is, of course, in no way responsible for our conclusions and interpretations.

The program has also received sustained support and encouragement from two medical schools at Michigan State University. We are grateful to Andrew D. Hunt, Jr., M.D., former dean of the College of Human Medicine, and Myron S. Magen, D.O., dean of the College of Osteopathic Medicine, for their support of this project and of the unusual academic unit in which it was housed.

A variety of circumstances has delayed the book. The complexity of the material and the problems of analysis consistently exceeded our estimates, and the concurrent challenges of developing two new medical schools drew heavily on our collective energies. Eventually a sabbatical leave for the senior author provided the time needed for reflection and writing. Support for this leave was provided by Michigan State University and by the Robert Wood Johnson Foundation through a grant to the Center for the Analysis of Health Practices, Harvard School of Public Health. The financial assistance of the Johnson Foundation does not in any way imply that it necessarily supports our research conclusions. The center provided a much-appreciated, appropriate environment for completing the book.

The secretarial tasks related to this project have been particularly complex. The painstaking transcription of lengthy taped physician-patient encounters and the typing of repeated drafts of the manuscript were accomplished by Prudence Barrett, Jean Bauman, Judy Carley, Marlene Dodge, Thelma Hadden, Sharon Jeffrey, Shermaine Shier, Karen Sutliff, and Nancy Teeter. Betty Kapp, who typed more than a fair share and supervised the typing of others, steered a steady course through a sea of details with remarkable calm; we are grateful for her organizational skill. Assistance in checking references was provided by Donna Edison and Kristina Olson. Nova Green's editorial contribution was most helpful.

We appreciate the advice and unfailing support of William Bennett, M.D., of the Harvard University Press. The manuscript was substantially improved by Vivian Wheeler's careful reading and intelligent editing.

A.S.E.
L.S.S.
S.A.S.

Contents

1	Introduction	1
2	Research in Problem Solving, Judgment, and Decision Making	10
3	High-Fidelity Simulation: Research Methods	46
4	High-Fidelity Simulation: Results	64
5	Patient-Management Problems	122
6	Fixed-Order Problems	152
7	Generation of Initial Problem Formulations: Performance of Experienced Physicians	168
8	Generation of Initial Problem Formulations: Training of Medical Students	199
9	Effects of Hypothesis Generation and Thinking Aloud	228
10	Use of Heuristics in Diagnostic Problem Solving	252
11	Conclusion	273
	Appendixes	305
	References	311
	Index	323

Medical
Problem
Solving

1 / Introduction

This book reports the investigations and findings of the Medical Inquiry Project, a five-year program of research on medical problem solving that began in early 1969 and continued through late spring 1973. The studies employed a broad range of methods and orientations—naturalistic, descriptive, experimental, anecdotal, psychometric—to examine a complex, multifaceted target. The research was pursued in the service of three disciplines: medicine, psychology, and education. We sought to understand medical practice better and thereby to improve the instruction and performance of present and future practitioners. Two perennial problems in psychology, the description and explanation of human thought and judgment, and the blending of laboratory research with daily concerns to improve human welfare, are paradigmatically represented by medical reasoning and decision making. For education, the special needs of medical training—of inculcating or fostering a broad range of knowledge, perceptual and psychomotor skills, strategies, attitudes, and personal dispositions—stood as a major challenge.

Background

As is true of many research programs, this one was motivated by both practical and theoretical concerns. The 1960s were a period of significant and rapid curriculum reform at all levels of formal education, from preschool to professional school. While some educators were urging that four-year-olds could learn to read and six-year-olds could master set theory and topology, others were advocating that first-year medical students could be taught clinical skills and be given introductory clinical responsibilities, so that the training period could be shortened by at least a year. In the decade of the fifties, the most important changes in the medical curriculum had been in the conceptions of subject matter, as exemplified by the shift from a discipline-centered to an organ-system–centered conception at Case Western Reserve University Medical School. During the next decade, attention was directed toward the manner in which the student was expected to learn the subject matter, however it was defined. With increasing frequency medical educators were told that their objective was to produce problem solvers, inquirers, individuals skilled in gathering and interpreting information for the purpose of rendering judgments, making decisions, and taking action. As dissatisfaction with the lockstep curriculum and with a sharp distinction between basic or preclinical and clinical education grew, it was at times argued that mastery of specific content was less important than mastery of a process, particularly since the content was likely to be obsolete in a relatively short time (say five to ten years). Efforts to introduce more electives into medical education were linked to the theory of guided discovery learning. By emphasizing the importance of proper habits of inquiry, as contrasted with the content learned (again a means of justifying electives), the medical student could safely be allowed to take more responsibility for his learning (Cope and Zacharias, 1966; Knowles, 1968). Thus it came about that admonitions for restructuring the learning *process* often sharply contrasted this process with a conception of the preclinical phase of medical education as a stage of amassing vast sums of knowledge.

The emphasis upon the primacy of process over content in medical education was a major stimulus for the present research. It was, however, one thing to talk about the importance of teaching medical students to solve clinical problems and quite another to define specifically what was meant by the term *problem solving*. The call for operationally defined objectives, a pervasive theme in the literature of medical education during that same period, made it difficult to remain vague on the subject of problem solving. Was there a set of general problem-solving skills that cut across the variety of specific medical problems? Or did each medical problem call for a particular set of processes? If there were general problem-solving skills, were they unique to medicine or were they medical manifestations of problem-solving processes, strategies, and heuristics employed in all intellectual pursuits? If the latter, was it not likely that a group of highly selected college graduates would already have mastered the general forms of these processes and now need only medical content to make them operative in that domain as well? Whether universal, medicine specific, problem specific, or some combination, what are the problem-solving processes characteristic of experienced physicians which, once identified and clearly formulated, could form the basis for empirically based statements of objectives for medical education?

Examination of the research literature in medical thinking, such as it was then, led rapidly to the conclusion that our understanding of how experienced physicians solve medical problems was based on everything but systematic empirical studies. The literature included admonitory papers detailing how clinicians *ought* to do their work, fortified with anecdotes provided by distinguished physicians. Similarly, computer, Bayesian, or logical models of the diagnostic process (Warner et al., 1961; Jacquez, 1964; Lusted, 1968) prescribed how clinical reasoning should be done or showed how a computer could do it, but left open the question of how humans, with a vastly different information-processing capability, in fact perform this task. Finally, the few empirical studies of medical reasoning that existed could be objected to on grounds of questionable external validity. There were studies that utilized paper-and-pencil problems, Twenty Questions formats, sequential formats, and the like, but a convincing relation between performance under these special test conditions and more realistic circumstances was not demonstrated.

The paucity of empirical data on clinical reasoning in the field was the major motivation for our decision to conduct the largest single piece of this work under conditions that approximated as closely as possible the natural environment of medical practice. From studies of medical reasoning conducted in this manner we hoped to be able to understand the skills, strategies, competencies, or attributes that characterize the performance of skilled clinicians. We would then move on to additional studies and investigate approaches to improving or accelerating the manner in which medical students might learn to master those capabilities. Perhaps it would turn out that some capabilities were not teachable, that students either did or did not possess them prior to entry to medical school. If so, what had been originally conceived as research for medical instruction could end up as research for medical school admission and/or certification. In either case we felt strongly that further progress was predicated on conducting serious empirical research to gather data on which decisions concerning instruction, admission, evaluation, or certification could be more soundly based.

Another stimulus for these studies arose from the history and status of psychological investigations of cognitive processes. One of the legacies of psychology's longstanding quest for the methodological objectivity of the physical sciences was the practice of employing artificial tasks to study learning and cognition. Rats were studied in mazes, cats in problem boxes, and human beings with memory drums, concept-attainment boards, or rooms with two strings suspended from the ceiling. The rationale was the same: to devise conditions where uncontrolled encroachments from the organism's prior experience could not influence performance. Doubtless these cautions did ensure that the problem-solving behavior observed was more a function of the novel structure of the presented problem than of unique and unobservable prior experience of the individual problem solver. Unfortunately, the price paid for this insurance was often exorbitant, in our opinion. While these tasks were employed in the interest of increasing generalizability by reducing individual and task variability, a psychology of problem solving based solely on such studies was likely to be generalizable only to a population of problem situations that were so novel or unstructured that the individual problem solver's prior knowledge, experience, and strategies were essentially neutralized.

Medicine, however, constitutes a striking illustration of a general characteristic of most human problem solving: problems are approached by a critical interplay of capabilities developed in the past and the particular features of the problem being attacked. The universe of such real problems fell outside the population of situations to which the findings of traditional psychological studies could be easily generalized. We shall pay close attention to matters like search strategies and the structure of memory, and explore how a particular problem is approached by blending general strategies and previously acquired knowledge.

The recognition that a psychology of "novel problem solving" was seriously incomplete made the study of medical inquiry all the more engaging. Here was a universe of tasks that seemed reasonably well defined, amenable to careful systematic study, and nevertheless clearly dependent for their solutions on previously acquired knowledge and capabilities. Hence, in addition to the practical value attached to conducting such research from the perspective of medical education, the studies were extremely attractive as contributions to the psychology of human problem solving under more nearly natural conditions. In this respect our studies are part of a larger movement within psychology to reemphasize the role of the environment, although not as pure empty-organism behaviorism. The study of rationality is the study of how humans adapt their thinking to diverse environmental demands. To understand the problem-solving process, then, the environments in which the solving occurs must be sampled just as carefully as psychologists have long sampled the persons doing the solving (Brunswik, 1956).

To connect these diverse strands, the objectives of the Medical Inquiry Project were formulated:

(a) To identify the intellectual processes characteristic of expert clinical reasoning, and in so doing, to clarify the pervasiveness, specificity, and degree of content-independence of these processes, as well as the degree to which the processes were consistent attributes of individuals.

(b) To generate a psychological theory to explain these features.

(c) To relate this new theory to existing theories of thinking, human information processing, decision making, and problem solving.

(d) To develop instructional methods and materials that could assist medical students to acquire and refine problem-solving skills.

General Methodological Considerations

Two major decisions relative to research strategy were made in our early deliberations and guided our study of physician performance. The first concerned the selection of subjects for in-depth simulation studies. We decided to study not a random or representative sample of physicians, but a sample of criterial physicians—practitioners whose reputations for diagnostic excellence set them apart in the opinion of their peers—and to compare them with a group of "average" physicians. How were these groups to be identified? In a field such as clinical medicine few viable alternatives to peer ratings exist, despite the obvious inaccuracies and distortions associated with that method. It is pointless to count publications or citations, since clinical expertise is unlikely to be a function of research productivity. Similarly, were there a valid test of clinical skill with which to identify criterial diagnosticians, a major reason for conducting the present research would have been obviated. The details of the peer nomination process used and the level of participation of the sample are discussed in Chapter 3.

Our second major decision was to study the behavior of the participating physicians intensively, with a comparatively small number of problems analyzed in detail. The rationale is characteristic of process-tracing studies as a whole. Recognizing that no single research study can hope to answer all conceivably relevant questions, researchers within this paradigm (Clarkson, 1962; de Groot, 1965; Newell and Simon, 1972) have preferred to concentrate on in-depth analysis, as a trade off for breadth of domain and subject sampling. It was foreseen that there might be serious problems in generalizing from the sample of problems studied to the entire domain of medicine. We planned to correct this methodological weakness by analyzing the protocols obtained from the experienced physicians statistically as well as descriptively (see Chapters 4 and 5) and by testing hypotheses suggested by these quasi-naturalistic studies in more formally controlled research with medical students and physicians (Chapters 7 through 10).

The use of peer nominations to identify a select sample for analysis of a field of endeavor is not unique to this study. The practice is perhaps best exemplified in the program of research at the University of California's Institute for Personality Assessment and Research (IPAR) at Berkeley, where studies have been conducted of creative members of several professions—mathematicians, architects, authors, advertising executives. The participants were selected through a process of peer nomination that resembles the one employed in the present study. However, there is a major difference between the use to which the results of peer nomination were put in IPAR studies and in our investigation. The questions raised in IPAR research centered on the personal characteristics of creative practitioners of the professions under study. The major variables were in the domains of personality, attitudes, cognitive style, and life history. For our medical inquiry, such variables were of secondary interest. We were most interested in gathering meaningful work samples, observations of what criterial physicians actually do—their approaches, skills, strategies, and tactics. We were less interested in the personal qualities that predisposed someone to becoming an outstanding physician, although this is a question not without value, than we were in the actual cognitive activities engaged in by outstanding diagnosticians "doing their thing." This was of interest, as we have said, both as a contribution to the general psychology of problem solving, and for the improvement of medical education. In analyzing and modeling their *performance*, we hoped to lay an empirical basis for rational approaches to instruction and evaluation in medicine.

Overall Design of the Project

Studies of Physicians

Our program of research comprised a variety of studies. The core study was an in-depth descriptive analysis of the reasoning process of a group of twenty-four carefully selected, experienced internists performing on a range of medical and nonmedical problems. The methods of this study are described in Chapter 3, and the results are presented in Chapter 4. Chapter 5 analyzes physician performance on a specially prepared set of patient-management problems (PMPs) that were independently evaluated using our own scoring system as well as the system developed at the Center for Educational Development of the University of Illinois College of Medicine.

Chapter 6 reports the findings from yet another set of medical "paper problems" addressed by the entire sample of experienced physicians. These were of lower fidelity than the PMPs, with sequence and numbers of data being carefully controlled by the research team.

Experimental Studies

The next section of the book comprises a series of experimental studies conducted to examine further a number of the points suggested by the descriptive and comparative studies of physicians. The goal was to explore with greater precision and control several variables potentially important in medical problem solving. The studies focused on early hypothesis generation, on the roles of hypothesis generation and verbalization in problem solving, and on the use of heuristics as aids in clinical diagnosis.

Chapters 7 and 8 report the first of three experimental training studies designed to test some concepts of instruction that emerged from the earlier studies. The study is in two parts. In the first, a small group of experienced physicians (a different group from those participating in the descriptive simulation studies) are observed as they respond to a set of special films produced to simulate a "physician's-eye view" of the first five minutes of an encounter with a new patient. In the second part of the investigation, alternative training procedures that employ different combinations of instructional films and written materials are experimentally compared in teaching second-year medical students. The objective was to explore the degree to which students can be taught to generate diagnostic hypotheses based on early information with the mental processes employed by experienced physicians.

Chapter 9 presents the results of an experimental study that deals with the roles of hypothesis generation and verbalization in the conduct of medical inquiry. Second-year medical students were encouraged to think aloud and generate hypotheses, or else urged to refrain from either or both. The consequences of this procedure for their performance on a set of modified patient-management problems are reported.

Chapter 10 is an account of an experimental study in which medical students were taught to use a variety of heuristics (strategies) in conducting a medical workup. The experiment contrasted two ways of developing and cuing the use of heuristics, and explored their effects on diagnostic accuracy and the cost of a workup.

The End and the Beginning

As a conclusion, Chapter 11 presents a general discussion of substantive theoretical and methodological issues in medical problem solving and decision making, as seen now in the light of this program of research. A reformulated theory of medical problem solving is advanced. Alternative models of clinical decision making are discussed, of both a logical and a statistical nature, and a list of problem-solving heuristics is developed that combines problem-solving and decision analytic approaches. Several methodological issues are reviewed in the areas of simulation and evaluation of clinical competence. Finally, needed programs of future research are presented in some detail; their implications for medical instruction and evaluation are discussed.

The next chapter will review some of the large body of literature to which we have turned in the course of this research. Some of these writings helped to stimulate and direct this investigation in its earlier phases. Others significantly influenced our thinking in the course of the investigation, or were consulted as we completed our research and sought to understand more fully the implications of our findings. A few clarified obscurities (or obscured what had otherwise seemed clear) as time passed and our understanding changed.

It is significant and encouraging that the years since this investigation began have seen a healthy increase in the volume and quality of research in human thought and judgment generally, and in medical reasoning and decision making specifically. Since we cannot cite all the studies performed, we hope that those reviewed are suitably representative of the diverse fields of study with which our own investigations share interests and concerns.

2 / Research in Problem Solving, Judgment, and Decision Making

The cognitive activities of the physician do not fit conveniently into a single category of psychological research. Indeed, the range of processes employed in medical inquiry cut across several distinct categories of psychological investigation that tend to be pursued quite separately. Even proposing to discuss the problem-solving, judgment, and decision-making aspects of medicine within the same research program is a departure from psychological tradition, which has treated thinking and decision making as separate domains. In the psychological literature these terms typically refer to different research paradigms and models. A recent volume of the *Annual Review of Psychology*, for example, reviewed thinking and individual decision behavior in consecutive articles whose references overlapped only trivially (Bourne and Dominowski, 1972; Rapoport and Wallsten, 1972). This is not simply the result of meticulous editing, but comes about also because experimental cognitive psychology permits and even encourages the isolation of these processes from each other. In complex real task environments such as are encountered in medicine, the processes of problem solving, judgment, and decision making relate to one another very closely.

In this chapter we review representative studies and theoretical proposals on thinking, human judgment, and decision making. Since the terms *judgment, decision making,* and *problem solving* are used in so many ways, we now outline the scope of our treatment.

First, the focus will be mostly on the performance of individuals rather than of small groups or organizations. The research literature on small-group problem solving and decision making and on decision making in complex organizations or bureaucracies is outside our scope. Though it may be possible to extrapolate from individuals' judgments to the aggregation of judgments within groups, we hesitate to do so.

Second, we are concerned only with those forms of decision making that involve processing of information to make judgments. The manner in which the processed information is acquired in sequence will sometimes itself be the object of inquiry. In other studies the information is presented in a "package" and the judgments alone are the objects of interest, varying over different patterns or amounts of information or forms of presentation. Other types of research attempt to trace the processes employed by decision makers. This is done either to simulate those processes on a computer or to develop a richer conceptual understanding of the processes without using artificial intelligence.

Third, we shall review a basic distinction between "process-tracing" approaches, which attempt to describe the intellectual processes used by subjects as they render judgments and make decisions or solve problems, and the "black-box" investigations, which attempt to model the processing of the judge mathematically through studies of input-output relations. In the process-tracing tradition, human thinking and problem solving are typically viewed as a series of operations susceptible to either verbal characterization or restatement in a computer simulation program. This approach will be contrasted with the major lines of research in the black-box tradition that have contributed to the field of judgment, emphasizing studies of clinical inference, the lens-model approach to judgment and decision theory, and a recent series of inventive studies on the psychology of prediction.

Process Tracing

Studies in process tracing differ greatly in the extent to which they select simple or complex tasks, and in whether they choose to investigate a total task—what Davis (1973) has dubbed the *complete problem solver*—or to isolate a particular part or subtask for examination.

Total Task Investigations

Total task studies, which investigate the sequential character of information seeking leading up to judgments or decisions, use forms of simulation to represent the task environment. The forms to be discussed here are "high-fidelity" programmed patient simulation involving trained actors; moderate-fidelity formats such as in-baskets or their equivalents; variations on the tab-item format which, while of lower fidelity, maintain realistic control by the subject over the selection and characteristics of information to be employed; and Twenty Questions formats, which constrain the subject to ask questions answerable by yes or no, although not predesignating the universe of possible questions in the manner of the tab-item approach.

The problem solving of the physician has been an attractive object of psychological study both for its social relevance and for the paradigm of expert judgment it represents. We shall not attempt to review comprehensively the growing research literature on medical diagnosis. Much of this work is well described in Kendell (1975). A major breakthrough in these studies occurred when Barrows and Abrahamson (1964) developed techniques for training actors and actresses to serve as "programmed patients," whereby they simulate both the history and the sensory and motor deficits associated with many medical problems.

Barrows and Bennett (1972) conducted studies of diagnostic problem solving in neurology at the same time that we were conducting the research described in the coming chapters. They reported that the problem-solving methods of neurology residents were characterized by early hypothesis generation followed by systematic hypothesis testing. Similarly, Dudley's studies (1970, 1971) of surgical diagnosis reported the ubiquity of early generated hypotheses. These quite independent findings of the noninductive character of medical diagnostic inquiry were reported at nearly the same time as our own earliest findings (Chapter 3) and served to confirm our emerging characterizations of medical work.

Most of the research we shall review now is not medical in content, but attempts to address the same set of cognitive processes that underlie medical inquiry.

Clarkson (1962) combined a variety of process-tracing tactics to model the decision processes of a bank trust investment officer. His study illustrates the multiple settings and methods in which useful process-tracing data can be gathered. It also reflects the slow, painstaking, and frequently artful manner in which "thinking aloud" and other process data are collected and transformed into information-processing models. Clarkson began his study by attending meetings of bank officers in which investment decisions were reviewed and during which the trust officer was questioned on the rationale for certain selections. This experience provided him with a general framework for examining investment decisions. He then began working intensively with a single trust investment officer. First, he carefully examined historical records of several of the officer's accounts and built "behavioral models" of invariant decision processes across account models of what was *actually* done. Next, he collected thinking-aloud protocols of the same officer's deliberations and decisions while working on accounts that arose in the course of his current work. He proceeded to develop a "prior-state" model in which he described the investment officer's formulation of expectations, knowledge about and valuation of various stocks, general conceptions of good portfolio characteristics, and so on. He collected data by having the officer read journal articles and company financial reports and comment aloud on these while Clarkson collected his comments in the form of further protocols. Finally, he generated a computer simulation model of the full set of prior-state and decision processes (comparable in some ways to models of knowledge structure and task structure) used by the officer. This program constituted a "theory" of cognitive functioning for portfolio selection.

The theory is validated by comparing the outputs of the program with the actual decisions and decision processes subsequently observed in the person who is being modeled, when he uses a totally new set of data. Clarkson's model successfully matched the actual portfolios selected by the trust officer during a subsequent six-month period. Also, the protocols of the computer's "thinking" while working on those problems closely approximated the trust officer's actual deliberations. This latter comparison, a variation of Turing's test, is of particular interest to the information-processing theorist, since his goal is not merely to replicate the product of thought, but to understand and explain thought processes.

Moderate-Fidelity Tasks

In the quest for situations or tasks that can be used to represent the decision-making responsibilities of administrators, the in-basket technique has long been a favorite of business and industry. The in-basket that gives the method its name is the conduit through which a decision maker receives the messages to which his decisions constitute responses. The in-basket may contain letters from clients or customers, memoranda from superiors, periodic reports on economic or personnel matters in the firm, telephone messages requiring immediate action, and the like. Hemphill, Griffiths, and Frederiksen (1962) adapted the in-basket technique for school administrators, supplementing the in-basket contents with a variety of information sources that described in detail the fictitious school district within which the subject taking the in-basket had just become high school principal. The administrator's in-basket was used as a training device for educational administrators and as a research instrument for the study of the behavior of educational administrators as it related to individual differences in personal and professional characteristics.

Shulman (1965, and Shulman, Loupe, and Piper, 1968) modified the in-basket format to create a task environment that simulated aspects of a classroom's problems suitable for the study of teacher inquiry behavior under circumstances in which subjects could be observed functioning in a highly unstructured, problem-rich environment. Rather than focusing on teacher behavior as such, the variables of interest were problem sensitivity, use of diverse information sources, use of time (tasks had no time limit), quality of decisions, task organization and sequence of activities, and the like. The in-basket was thus transformed into a setting for the study of individual inquiry behavior under conditions that left the subject responsible for defining the problems to be attacked. Allender (1969) created an in-basket–like task environment to simulate the problems of the mayor of a small town in order to study the inquiry activities of fifth-grade youngsters. He too was concerned with understanding the general problem-solving characteristics of subjects, though his *I Am the Mayor* was used as both an instructional and a research setting.

In these in-basket settings human beings are replaced with paper or film representations of people so that the inquiry activities of subjects can be studied without the expense of a sound studio. The sacrifice in fidelity of simulation presumably is offset by the feasibility of conducting the research at all. The result is a task environment still an order of magnitude greater in validity than the typical problem-solving task situation, albeit under better control than a totally naturalistic situation. The aspect of task validity (external validity) exemplified by these and similar studies is fidelity to the existential demand characteristics of at least that portion of the real world from which the task has been selected. The aspect or criterion of external validity that these tasks may not fulfill is representation of an adequate sample of the total universe of tasks with which the subject of study (physician, teacher, principal, mayor, fifth-grader) must cope in his normal activities. It is rare that these two dimensions of external task validity—situational representativeness and universe representativeness—are satisfied in any one study, even though both are important.

Kleinmuntz (1968) studied diagnostic decision making among clinical psychologists who were interpreting psychological test profiles and among clinical neurologists working with simulated data drawn from that specialty. In the study of psychological test profile interpretation, the Minnesota Multiphasic Personality Inventory (MMPI) was used. An expert was tape-recorded while thinking aloud as he sorted 126 test profiles into a fourteen-step forced normal distribution. Information was thus obtained about the heuristic principles used to assess MMPI data for degree of adjustment versus maladjustment. These heuristics were organized into a set of sequential decision rules from which flow charts were prepared. A computer program was written that could interpret MMPI profiles using rules. It reproduced the source clinician's judgments on the original sample and interpreted MMPI profiles from other samples about as well as expert clinicians. By using the heuristics and judgment of the best interpreter available and assuming that there are qualitative similarities among "good" interpreters, the study offers an explanation of how MMPI interpreters analyze profiles. There are problems with research of this kind, and psychologists were not long in finding them. Neisser (1968) restated a classical argument against introspectionistic research: the very process of thinking aloud alters the content and process of thought.

To study the reasoning of clinical neurologists, Kleinmuntz (1968) played Twenty Questions with them. Each game started with the interrogator's presenting only a few symptoms or biographical features. The sequences of questions used to seek the additional information needed to diagnose a patient were analyzed and found to consist in binary tree structures. The length of the decision chain varied as a function of the expertise and experience of the subject. Kleinmuntz found that more experienced diagnosticians asked fewer questions and focused on those most likely to maximize information yielded. They pursued a systematic general-to-specific search strategy. Wortman (1972) succeeded in writing a computer program that reproduced fairly well the reasoning steps taken by a single neurologist in a series of sixteen neurological problems. Hayes (1968), in a critique of Kleinmuntz's work, pointed out that any sequence of questions can be represented as proceeding from general to specific. It is also possible that the binary tree structure is, at least in part, a creation of the Twenty Questions format, with its requirement that all questions be answered either yes or no. Nevertheless, this research does open up the possibility of exploring the ways in which problem solvers who are experienced in a particular domain represent the task before them (organize the task in short-term memory) and relate it to their experience and know-how (relate the task to long-term memory).

One of the earliest studies to use process-tracing methods was de Groot's (1965) investigation of the thought processes of chess players. Much of the information for this research was collected before World War II. De Groot presented chess players of different ability levels with a midgame board position and asked them to think aloud as they pondered their next move. He collected verbal protocols of their subsequent deliberations as they weighed alternative moves and the likely consequences. His characterization of chess players' thinking has been extremely influential among information-processing psychologists. It has led to a variety of other investigations, from computer simulations of chess playing to studies of the perceptual skills and coding strategies of chess masters. De Groot sees himself as part of a long chain of tradition from the "thought psychologists" of the Würzburg group—Ach, Kulpe, Selz—to the Newell and Simon work at Carnegie-Mellon University, a line reaching, as it were, from Würzburg to Pittsburgh. Echoing de Groot's call for systematic description rather than strict hypothesis testing, Simon (1974) has advocated greater use of research strategies that utilize parameter estimation and less reliance on tests of hypotheses.

The work of de Groot, Kleinmuntz, and Clarkson has one striking similarity to the work of Piaget. All accept verbal reports as legitimate data and agree that knowledge of the process by which a problem is solved is at least as important to psychology as observing that it was solved. Because the problems studied by these investigators are more complex than Piaget's, heuristics and plans replace logical operations. Writing a computer program as a test of the sufficiency with which a particular sequence has been traced is a trademark of the contemporary information-processing approach developed by Newell and Simon. Other investigators have pursued what may be termed an ethnography of problem solving, in which detailed verbal and quantitative models are proposed as explanations of observed problem-solving processes.

In one discussion, de Groot (1966) gives a set of principles that characterize his work. They can serve as a credo for the process-tracing approach, ethnographic style:

> First, the research is directed toward systematic description of cognitive phenomena rather than to strict hypothesis testing. Second, we keep machine simulation in mind, but we hardly do it as yet. Third, the experimental settings are often more like real-life than the strictly controlled artificial conditions of the laboratory. Fourth, extensive use is made of introspective techniques of various kinds. Fifth, as a result, protocol coding and interpretation are of crucial importance (and consume a large part of our time). Sixth, prospective outcomes are expected to be primarily valuable to the extent we succeed in providing adequate, systematic process descriptions, possibly to be used as a basis for simulation (pp. 19–20).

Tab-Item Methods

A problem of both in-basket and high-fidelity programmed patient approaches is that the unit of analysis is frequently ambiguous. When has a subject sought information, and how much has he obtained? All tab-item methods share the important characteristic of predesignating the available items of information or choices of action available to the subject. By so defining the universe of possible information or alternative actions, problems of coding, analysis, and interpretation are greatly reduced. Units of analysis are treated as equivalent, and the paths taken by subjects can be described as sequences of moves through a finite set of alternatives. There is no need for subjects to think aloud or to introspect. Thus, while the task validity may be less compared with higher-fidelity simulation methods, there is an increase in objectivity and reliability. Similar considerations of "externalizing the operations of thought" motivated such efforts as the Rimoldi-John "problem-solving instrument" (John, 1957; Blatt and Stein, 1959) and the concept-attainment work of Bruner, Goodnow, and Austin (1956).

The earliest published tab-item study was conducted by Glaser, Damrin, and Gardner (1954). To study troubleshooting performance more objectively, they described a performance failure in a piece of electronic equipment, then listed all possible tests a troubleshooter might make in order to locate the source of difficulty. Next to each listed test was a paper tab covering the information gained as a result of the test. In order to perform a test, the subject would lift off the covering tab, then leave a record of the step he had taken.

Rimoldi (1955, 1963, and Rimoldi, Devane, and Haley, 1961) developed a large number of sequential problem-solving tests that used tab-item methods, and he experimented with a variety of scoring procedures. These procedures compared the order in which subjects gathered information with some optimal sequence, either as defined logically or as defined empirically by the performance of a criterion group. He devised pattern analysis procedures to characterize search sequences as well as a "utility index" that represented the degree to which information was sought in the optimal sequence for reducing uncertainty. One of Rimoldi's research instruments was directed at the study of medical problem solving by medical students and physicians. His test of diagnostic skills (Rimoldi, 1961) provided the model for some of the most widely used methods for assessing performance in medicine.

The tab-item approach to the study and evaluation of medical problem solving was further extended through a series of patient-management problems developed at the University of Illinois College of Medicine (McCarthy and Gonnella, 1967; McGuire and Babbott, 1967; McGuire and Solomon, 1971). Each problem begins with an introduction that contains some information about the patient, including the chief complaint. The task of the problem solver is to gather more information for diagnosis and management. The examinee is given a list of further available information. Figures including slides and X-rays are used to provide nonverbal answers to certain types of questions. The PMP format offers a number of alternative routes to a problem. A record is kept of the order in which sections of the problem are done and of all the questions ordered within a particular section. Cuing is reduced by offering a large number of options. The format facilitates observation of sequential decision making based on feedback from the answer sheet. The items are weighted by their value in diagnosis and management. Strongly positive weights are given to those items that helped the subject diagnose and manage the patient. Positive weights are also given to items that should be included in a thorough workup and conscientious management plan. Negative weights are assigned to items that are contraindicated, and zero weights are assigned to items that are noncontributory or are simply distractors. Subjects are evaluated for overall competence in working up and managing a patient, with the scores calculated for efficiency, proficiency, errors of omission, and errors of commission. The examinee also receives an overall score for attack strategy; he is rewarded for an appropriate sequence of actions and penalized for doing certain sections out of order.

These tests provide a more sophisticated evaluation of the medical student or physician's ability to collect and utilize medical information sequentially than do conventional multiple-choice examinations. The reliability of tests of this kind, however, presents difficulties. Reliability coefficients across problems are generally low—in the .20's and .30's—which indicates that true alternate forms have not been devised and that there is a large component of problem specificity in each of the tasks. As for predictive validity, there is evidence that PMPs provide an indication of inadequate clinical performance, but they do not suggest what a physician will actually do in practice. A physician who cannot manage a patient adequately on a PMP is unlikely to do so in actual practice, but those physicians who do manage a patient adequately on a PMP may not do so in actual practice (Goran, Williamson, and Gonnella, 1973). The instrument thus provides an estimate of an upper level of capability of performance but does not indicate what performance in a field setting will be.

General Remarks on Process-Tracing Studies

Research in the process-tracing tradition has been largely atheoretical, with the notable exception of the substantial contribution of Newell and Simon and their colleagues and students (Newell, Shaw, and Simon, 1958; Newell and Simon, 1972; Wortman, 1972). If there is a psychological theory of thinking or problem solving implicit in most process-tracing investigations (total task investigations, in-basket, and tab-item studies, as well as Kleinmuntz's research), it has been so embedded as to be invisible to all but the most careful and thoughtful reader. The major concern of workers within the research tradition we have just summarized has not been to develop psychological theory. Rather, their aim has been to observe the process of thinking and judgment within settings that resemble the actual task environment as closely as possible. The limits on the fidelity of the simulation were usually set by budgetary constraints and the need for some type of experimental control. For obvious reasons, it was desirable to observe a number of individuals solving the same problem or trouble-shooting the same defective apparatus. The actual task environment rarely provided the needed duplication of problems, and since neither the investigator's patience nor his budget permitted waiting until nature presented the desired repetitions, experimental task environments were created. The methodological justification for the experimental setting thus hinged on practicality rather than on psychological theory.

The research efforts of Newell and Simon may have been influenced by such considerations. It is certainly true that the task environments of symbolic logic, cryptarithmetic, and chess are conveniently reproduced within the psychological laboratory. Interest in developing a psychological theory of problem solving, however, has led Newell and Simon to a rationale for their experiments quite apart from expediency. This rationale characterizes all contemporary process-tracing or information-processing research on judgment and thinking.

The information-processing approach attempts to account for two bodies of fact. First, humans can and do learn to solve a variety of complicated problems. Some of these are so complex that if all potential steps toward a solution were explored, the time needed would be far greater than is ever observed and would in some cases exceed a lifetime. Evidently some planning is required, and labor-saving strategies must be developed. On the other hand, the planning and strategy must be consistent with those characteristics of the human mind that set limits on capability for processing information. As an example of a relevant limit, it appears that human long-term memory (LTM) is essentially infinite, but that short-term memory (STM) has a capacity of only a few symbols. The time required to transfer an item from STM to LTM is on the order of seconds or tens of seconds (Norman, 1969; Kumar, 1971; Simon, 1974). The behavior that is adaptive to these two constraints can be accounted for by a theory of thinking with four fundamental propositions (Newell and Simon, 1972, pp. 788–789):

> 1. A few, and only a few, gross characteristics of the human information processing system (IPS) are invariant over task and problem solver.
> 2. These characteristics are sufficient to determine that a task environment is represented (in the IPS) as a problem space, and that problem solving takes place in a problem space.

3. The structure of the task environment determines the possible structures of the problem space.
4. The structure of the problem space determines the possible programs that can be used for problem solving.

Methodologically, information-processing research generally relies on introspective reports to determine the thought processes, heuristics, symbolic manipulations, or decision rules needed to solve a particular problem. These are formalized by the investigator into a computer program or other model that should perform the task much as the human did, if the detailed specifications are adequate. A major feature of many of the situations studied with this approach, and indeed of many of the puzzles and problems used to study "problem solving," is that the starting situation and a desired end point are both given. The problem solver's task is to find a set of legal moves that will transform the opening position into the desired termination. Problems in trigonometric identities, logic, or chess are good examples. A general heuristic for solving these problems is to evaluate the difference between the present situation and the goal and to reduce it one step at a time. Newell and Simon call this procedure means-end analysis. Other problems, such as those studied by medical simulators, do not immediately appear to fit this general format, since the task in a diagnostic problem is to identify what the goal will be as well as to provide a sufficient proof for it. There is an underlying similarity of approach, however. As we shall repeatedly see in the chapters that follow, medical problem solving proceeds by selecting a number of diagnostic hypotheses as possible goals, and then testing to see whether one or more of the hypotheses selected can be justified. In general, the open problem apparently without goals is transformed into a problem with a set of hypothetical solutions, and the discrepancy between the present state and a number of possible goals is repeatedly evaluated (Elstein et al., 1972). This procedure was anticipated by Bartlett (1958) in his discussion of thinking in open systems.

Newell and Simon's theory emphasizes that rational human problem solving is characterized by adaptation to the problem to be solved. Since it is adaptive, the behavior of a person solving a problem tells us more about the structure of the task than about the personality dynamics of the problem solver. Different problems—chess, cryptarithmetic, anagrams, syllogisms—have different structures and demands, and people *can* learn to solve all of them. A theory of problem solving must be, first, a description of how different kinds of problems are solved, and second, a taxonomic or logical analysis of the interrelations among problem types. Psychologists have long investigated individual differences in abilities (Guilford, 1967) or experimentally induced variables like functional fixedness (Duncker, 1945) or set (Maier, 1930) as determinants of performance. The information-processing approach argues that these traditions have treated problems essentially as interchangeable and suggests instead that we consider the task itself as a major determinant of human behavior. The valuable contribution made to an information-processing theory by the simulation, in-basket, tab-item, and process-tracing studies reviewed is the data they provide on how different types of problems are solved. Newell and Simon would, we think, applaud the effort to study problem solving or judgment in a broad spectrum of environments. However, they would justify this approach on the grounds that problem-solving strategies are largely determined by the structure of the task environment, not because it is more expedient to study problem solving in such environments.

Judgment

What is judgment? Newell (1968) has attempted to provide some guidelines that characterize the research on human judgment. The present section bears the clear imprint of his analysis. Newell cites Johnson (1955), who distinguished between three functions of thought processes: *preparation, production,* and *judgment.* To quote from Johnson,

> The third process, judgment, may be identified as the evaluation or categorizing of an object of thought. This is logically differentiated from productive thought in that typically nothing is produced. The material is merely judged; i.e., put into one category or another. Many of the subjective analyses of thinking have included a concluding phase of hypothesis testing or verification during which the thoughts previously produced are judged. In experimental psychology, judgment is a well developed topic, studied chiefly under the headings of psychophysics, aesthetics, attitudes and rating of personnel (p. 51).

Newell has abstracted the "definitional strands" that appear to characterize the act of judging as a cognitive process studied by psychologists: (a) The main inputs to the process are given and available; obtaining, discovering, or formulating them is not part of judgment. (b) The domain of output is simple and well defined prior to the judgment. The judgment itself is one of a set of admissible responses; where classes or categories are given, it is usually called a selection, estimation, or classification. (c) The process is not simple transduction of information; judgment goes beyond the information given and adds information to the output. (d) Judgment is not simply a calculation or the application of a given rule. (e) The process of judgment concludes or occurs at the end of a more extended process. (f) The process is immediate, not extended through time with subprocesses, in which case we would refer to *preparation* for judgment. (g) The process is distinguished from searching, discovering, or creating, as well as from musing, browsing, or idly observing. (Selected or paraphrased from Newell, 1968, pp. 5–6.)

Newell then proceeds to analyze the major questions investigators ask about judgment and why those questions are important to them. First, what are the major scientific questions asked about judgment? (a) Upon what information is the judgment based? (b) What is the judgmental law? That is, what is the rule that explains how the information which serves as input is transformed into the output, a judgment? (c) What is the psychological process or processes that make possible the lawfully operating judgment? This can be a verbally stated theoretical model describing stages of judgment, or it can be as elaborate as a total computer simulation program. (d) What are the other conditions that influence the judgment and how do they work? These are conditions external to the input itself, such as instructions and personality variables.

Second, why do people ask these questions? Because they have other underlying questions in mind such as the following: Why doesn't a human make optimal judgments? Can a machine or an algorithm make judgments as *valid* as those of humans? How do humans manage to achieve so simply what appears so complex?

Finally, Newell distinguishes among several basic formulations with which investigators attempt to represent the process of judgment as they work:

(a) *Models with maximum formal generality.* Here the formal model comes first and is chosen for its universal characteristics. The approach is typically abstract, formal, and general. The focus is on the discovery and refinement of the judgmental law; the work of Edwards (1968) and Goldberg (1970) are examples. Both investigators aver that human judgments in a variety of situations are less than optimal, and each proposes a general method to improve judgments or decisions. Both advocate a mechanical or statistical rule for combining inputs into a decision more consistently and accurately than people do, and each has a general form for the recommended rule. Edwards prefers Bayes' theorem, whereas Goldberg opts for regression equations. Both maintain that for any particular judgmental problem, the substance to be clothed in the recommended quantitative garment should be derived from an appropriate analysis of a series of judgments or estimates obtained from judges.

Note that the generality of their proposals rests on the proposition that either the Bayesian or regression approaches can, in principle, model any judgmental or decision task, provided that the variables employed in the decision are scaled in the form needed by the model. The task of research then becomes to disclose the variables needed in a particular problem and to obtain suitable estimates of the scale weights, either regression coefficients or probabilities, to be assigned to each variable. Users of the regression model typically study the one who judges as a static policyholder and employ the model to discover the stable underlying weighting scheme that best represents the judge's processing of information. Users of the Bayesian model are most interested in *changes* in judges' beliefs as a function of new information. The regression model treats the available information as given; the Bayesian model sees information aggregating either until it has been exhausted, or until the judge has deemed it no longer necessary for a decision.

(b) *Models of the task environment.* These approaches begin with highly specific models of particular task environments: chess, faces, personality types, and so forth. The models are not general, and the judgmental law is secondary to the attempt to represent explicitly the major distinctive features of the unique task environments of interest.

(c) *Models of the information processes.* The purpose of a process model is to explain, by the cognitive processes involved, the relation between the information used in a judgment and the law or principles used to form a judgment based thereon. The modeling task is more difficult when the characteristics of the task environment to which the subjects respond are less understood. As an illustration, Newell contrasts Kleinmuntz's studies of MMPI interpretation (clean task environment) and neurology (messy task environment). When the processes are expressed in the form of computer simulation programs, the program comes first; and only out of it may emerge a judgmental law.

Modeling the Judgment Process

Dawes and Corrigan (1974) have cited Benjamin Franklin's letter to his friend Priestly wherein Franklin described his method for making systematic use of available information before rendering a practical judgment. He would list all the factors supporting or militating against a particular decision, would assign greater or lesser weights to individual factors according to their perceived importance, and then sum the values in the pro and con columns to make his judgment. He dubbed this approach "moral or prudential algebra." It seems that men of practical wisdom have long recognized that pragmatic judgments can be made better through intuitive application of a systematic approach to weighing evidence. In fact, our Western epitomization of fair judgment is the representation of Justice standing blindfolded to prevent the inadvertent effects of extraneous irrelevant influences, holding aloft a balance scale that registers objectively the weight of evidence on both sides of a question. This image of justice, which dates back to Greek sources, is itself a version of Franklin's prudential algebra. Both are intuitive applications of a simple additive model as a method for making judgments.

It is often not perfectly clear, however, what are the variables the sum of whose weights leads to the judgment. We can see that judgments are made, but we have no method for directly estimating the weights. This is frequently the case because Justice's blindfold does not permit her to see even those sources that are meant to influence the judgment. That is, like the shortstop unerringly moving in for a slow ground ball, or the middle linebacker swiftly changing direction to cut off a reverse play, the judgment is made without conscious knowledge of which variables have been employed and how they have been weighted and aggregated. Research later described will demonstrate that when judges are asked to supply such information, they typically believe that they make use of more variables than they actually do. They also erroneously claim to give serious weight to what appear to be minor variables. Furthermore, the complexity of the combination rule used in making judgments tends to be overestimated.

It was this sort of problem that in 1923 motivated an Iowa agricultural researcher to construct what was apparently the first statistical model of the ways in which judges weighted and aggregated variables in making an evaluation classification. Henry A. Wallace, later secretary of agriculture and vice-president under Franklin D. Roosevelt, asked, "What is in the corn judge's mind?", presenting experienced corn judges with ears that varied systematically across the parameters of corn quality, such as kernel size and color (Wallace, 1923). After they had made their judgments, Wallace modeled their underlying policies by calculating path coefficients representing the relative weights assigned to each characteristic by each judge. Wallace interpreted the relative weights as representing the actual ways in which the judges processed the information to make their judgments. As has been the case in countless similar studies, the variance in judges' classifications could be accounted for by a relatively small subset of the total number of possible characteristics ostensibly taken into account. Wallace's study, published in an agronomy research journal, went unnoticed by psychologists or educators. Thirty-seven years later, Hoffman (1960) suggested using multiple regression equations to model the policies of clinical psychologists making clinical judgments. He was careful to emphasize that the statistical model was a "paramorphic representation" of the clinician's policy, not an isomorphic one. That is, the multiple regression equation performs *like* the judge, but cannot be interpreted as a veridical model *of* the judge's own information-processing strategies.

Investigators using the paradigm, however, have often fallen into the trap of treating it as if it were in fact describing how a judge used a set of cues, despite the admonition (Hoffman, Slovic, and Rorer, 1968) that the model could not be viewed as explanatory unless an orthogonal set of cues were selected for analysis. In the same connection, these writers point out that while regression techniques may improve accuracy of judgment, it is not necessarily the case that the judge was using a particular item at all, much less in the way stipulated by the model.

The concluding paragraphs of Slovic and Lichtenstein's (1971) comprehensive monograph recognized this issue. They urged a rapprochement between research in cognition and information processing, which indicates that humans do not process information by using a stripped-down version of the Bayesian or regression model, and research on decision making that employs these models. The cognitive approach may be best at helping us to understand how people reason, judge, and make decisions, given the limitations on their capacities. Another type of model (Bayesian or regression) may be more useful for improving judgments and decisions while not engaging people in programs to modify their judgment procedures. This is the direction implied by Goldberg's (1970) work on diagnostic judgment in clinical psychology and Dawes' (1971) study of college admissions procedures.

When Hoffman wrote his now-classic paper in 1960, psychologists were vigorously engaged in a controversy concerning the relative merits of clinical versus actuarial prediction in clinical work. The history of this debate is well told by Gough (1962). Meehl (1954) had earlier summarized the controversy and had declared the actuarial position the clear winner under the rules of the game. These rules clarified the basic difference between the two positions as residing in the manner in which information is *combined* to predict patient outcome or diagnose client condition. Thus, a clinical judgment can be based upon both "objective" data—MMPI scores, Kuder profiles, a group intelligence test—and "subjective" data—impressions following an interview, projective test results. The method is defined not by the data used, but by whether or not they are evaluated impressionistically by a clinician. The same input data, if amenable to quantitative or scalar representation, could be treated actuarially if combined by statistical means, using an (empirically derived) judgmental law for weighting and combining the information. Meehl concluded that given the same quantitative and/or impressionistic (but scalable) data as input, actuarial methods of combining the data to render a judgment are consistently as good or better than clinical methods.

In a cogent reply, Holt (1958) argued that these studies were fundamentally unfair to clinicians, because the terms of the contest were set so that the actuarial approach was placed in a more favorable light. In particular, he stressed that the proactuarial group had focused excessively on the problem of combining a set of data into a decision, a task that might well be accomplished in a mechanical way. However, they had slighted the importance of the tasks of selecting and gathering relevant data, especially qualitative data, and of working them into a form suitable for an actuarial rule. These tasks, claimed Holt, were fundamental aspects of clinical activity and could not be dismissed as trivial or irrelevant.

Later discussions by Sawyer (1966), Goldberg (1968, 1970), and

Einhorn (1972), among others, explored optimal blends of clinical and actuarial processing. These typically involved using clinical methods to gather preliminary information or to make subtle observations, and used actuarial methods to combine the data for final decisions. Hence Einhorn's apt phrase, "expert measurement and mechanical combination."

By the 1960s it was the *form* of that mechanical combination that had become the subject of interest. Hoffman's paramorphic representation of human judgment was, like Ben Franklin's, a linear model. Study after study was henceforth to demonstrate that despite clinical intuitions ascribing highly complex, configural strategies to expert judges, their judgmental policies could be well represented, albeit paramorphically, by linear models. The addition of configural terms to the model (exponential components, for instance) generally failed to improve the accuracy of the model as assessed by the proportion of variance in human judges' performance accounted for by the statistical representation (Goldberg, 1971). Why did simple linear models perform so well as representations of a clinical process that few of even the most skeptical argued was in fact linear in the minds of the judges? This question and several others growing out of statistical methods of modeling the judge have occupied many investigators.

Following Hoffman's paper, a series of studies issued primarily from the Oregon Research Institute. The method of modeling a judge from multiple regression equations or analysis of variance came to be known as "policy capturing." Hoffman and his colleagues demonstrated how policy capturing could be applied to a wider range of situations than those involving clinical psychologists. Radiologists (Slovic, Rorer, and Hoffman, 1971), stockbrokers (Slovic, 1969), admissions committees (Dawes, 1971), draft boards (Gregory and Dawes, 1972), even girl watchers (Wiggins and Wiggins, 1969), could and did have their policies captured. Moreover, concluded these investigators, the resulting model not only approximated the future judgments of the human decision maker upon whose performance it was based, it frequently surpassed the accuracy of that very judge from whom it was derived! Apparently, unlike the human being who is distractible, unreliable, susceptible to inevitable "slips of the blindfold," the statistical representation, based on a long series of individual judgments that irons out or corrects for these occasional sources of error, serves as an idealization of the judge's policy under optimal conditions. Once it has been captured, the policy continues chugging along, immune to the countless distractions that may hinder its human ancestor. This use of statistical methods to improve judgment was dubbed *bootstrapping* (Goldberg, 1970).

A fine example of bootstrapping is Dawes' (1971) study of graduate admissions in a psychology department. He demonstrated that a multiple regression model based on the admissions committee's weighting of three variables—scores on the Graduate Record Examination, undergraduate grade-point average, and a scaling of "quality of undergraduate institution"—did a better job of predicting applicant success in the program than did the admissions committee members themselves. The equation that achieved this feat was a simple linear model that assigned weights to the predictors in accordance with the contribution of each to the prediction of the judgments.

The remarkable success of policy capturing and bootstrapping using the linear model contributed ironically to the realization that it was both more and less than it had seemed. Dawes and Corrigan (1974) described a series of studies designed to test the limits of the linear model's robustness. The underlying hypothesis had always been that models of judges' policies worked as well as they did because they managed to approximate the ways judges cognitively processed information. Hammond and several of his coworkers (see, for example, Hammond and Summers, 1972) treated feedback to judges on their own policies as a mirror of the mind. But Dawes, Rorer, and their colleagues remained skeptical about their own investigations. It had long been clear that the precise beta weights computed in any particular linear model were intrinsically unstable. To the extent that predictors were intercorrelated, which they usually were, weights assigned to individual independent variables could vary greatly. Special techniques, such as ridge regression, were studied as possible methods of increasing the reliability of betas under such circumstances. For if the beta weights, which in some way represented the cognitive operations of judges, should turn out to be evanescent statistical artifacts, what sense did policy capturing make?

One way of testing the degree to which the linear model can survive "errors" in beta values is to replace the values actually calculated for a given data set with randomly generated weights of the same sign. When this was done, the resulting linear model still did as well or better than the original. Furthermore, when these random weights were replaced by unit weights, that is, giving each predictor variable in the equation equal weight, the resulting linear model worked best of all! Dawes and Corrigan concluded that the simple additive model of Franklin's prudential algebra, devoid of multivariate refinements, probably represents how most clinical decision makers really operate. One need not even go through the laborious process of differential weighting. Just identify the "big variables" and add. Moreover, this very approach had been anticipated by Thorndike (1918).

At present, the situation appears to be as follows. Actuarial models derived from expert clinicians, often working with data inputs that could only be supplied via clinical impressions, are more effective in making decisions than are the clinicians themselves. In fact, a powerful linear model can be constructed if one can identify the relevant cues, measure them adequately, detect the sign (+ or −) appropriate to the cue, and ascertain that the function form for the cue-criterion relation is suitably monotonic. In that case, the resulting model will be a simple additive representation with unit weights.

Man as Decision Maker

Policy-capturing research has focused on deriving statistical models from human judges. Other investigations have compared human performance in decision making with an optimal mathematical model. Bayes' theorem is a precise mathematical formula for calculating the degree of change that should take place in a belief to reflect accurately the impact of new information. Psychologists were introduced to the Bayesian approach to decision making through the energetic work of Edwards and his collaborators (Edwards, 1954, 1961; Edwards, Lindman, and Phillips, 1965; Edwards and Tversky, 1967). Derivations of a number of forms of Bayes' theorem are found in several texts on statistical inference (for instance, Chernoff and Moses, 1959; Hays and Winkler, 1970) and in Slovic and Lichtenstein (1971). A technology is developing that will soon make it as simple to work out a Bayesian analysis of a decision problem as to do a one-way analysis of variance at a desk calculator. Problems remain, however, with generating the matrices of conditional probabilities needed as an input to decision analysis.

The Bayesian model can be applied to any situation where observation of the presence or absence of a certain event or item of information (the datum) should cause a revision of opinion on the probability of another event (the hypothesis) that is associated with the datum and also with other data. Bayes' theorem can also be used to measure the impact of several data, provided they are conditionally independent events. Even if they are not, it is sometimes possible to cluster events into subsets that are conditionally independent. A variety of experiments then becomes possible, concerned with how well people can estimate the probability of events compared to objective data, how sensitive people are to data of varying diagnostic power, and the degree to which people revise their opinions when confronted with sequences of data or complex choices. Reviews of the psychological literature on this topic are found in Slovic and Lichtenstein (1971) and Rapoport and Wallsten (1972).

According to Bayes' theorem, accurate decision making depends on the prior probabilities of the hypotheses and the data, and on their probability of joint occurrence. The strength of an association or the weight to be assigned to a cue is indicated with probabilities or odds rather than with correlation coefficients or regression weights.

Several parameters must be known or estimated to analyze a problem in Bayesian terms. In the simplest case there must be a prior probability associated with the belief or hypothesis, which reflects either an objective accounting of the base rate for the occurrence in question or a subjective estimate of likelihood derived from impressions of base rates. A fascinating area of research examines the accuracy of subjective estimates for prior probability when objective base rate information is available but is typically unknown. A second parameter to be considered is the *diagnosticity* of the new data, a combination of reliability and relevance that dictates how much impact on the prior hypothesis the new datum ought to have. Given this information, Bayes' theorem calculates how the information should be aggregated to result in a new posterior belief—that is, how much the prior belief should change in light of the new evidence. A decision maker is said to be performing suboptimally when his posterior confidence in a hypothesis departs from the posterior probability as calculated by Bayes' theorem.

When the data are of poor quality and low validity, they should contribute little to altering our judgments. In this situation, the judge should stick to the base rate as the best predictor of an event. However, at least in clinical psychology, there is some evidence that with increasing amounts of data, accuracy levels off while confidence continues to grow (Oskamp, 1965). This result was replicated in a study of expert horse-race handicappers (Slovic, personal communication). Kahneman and Tversky (1973) have shown clearly that unreliability is often ignored, poor data being treated as if they had the same diagnostic power as adequate data. Some recent work in the psychology of decision making has been concerned with drawing inferences from unreliable reports (Snapper and Fryback, 1971; Schum and Kelly, 1973), a matter that probably should concern educators and physicians as much as it concerns military intelligence analysts.

The first Bayesian studies of man as an intuitive statistician disclosed repeatedly that human decision makers are notoriously conservative. Given new data, they change their beliefs far less than they should; hence they are prone to seek much more information than is necessary for making a decision at a desired level of confidence. Vigorous debate centered on whether conservatism was a function of misaggregation of the evidence (not following Bayes' rule), or of misreading the diagnosticity but subsequently aggregating correctly, or was an artifact of psychological experiments involving bookbags and poker chips (Edwards, 1968). The entire December 1973 issue of *Organizational Behavior and Human Performance* was devoted to the topic of multistage or cascaded inference. Subjects frequently revise their opinions excessively when drawing inferences in stages or sequences. Research is now aimed at understanding why this occurs (for example, Gettys, Kelly, and Peterson, 1973). Conservatism may not be a universal, invariant characteristic of human information processing; it may instead be the outcome of human functioning in particular task environments.

In either case, the remedy recommended by Bayesians for suboptimal opinion revision has generally been Edwards' Probabilistic Information Processing system (PIP), in which people estimate the probabilities of data given certain hypotheses, and machines use Bayes' theorem to aggregate these estimates across data and hypotheses into estimates of the probabilities of hypotheses given certain observed data. The soundness of this recommendation rests upon the degree to which people can accurately estimate the probabilities of observing data under different conditions. For some purposes these estimates seem to be quite accurate (Gustafson et al., 1971). However, recent research has suggested that subjective probabilities are biased when not estimated by direct reference to frequency. Availability, or the ease with which instances can be recalled (Tversky and Kahneman, 1973), and representativeness, the similarity between two events (Kahneman and Tversky, 1972), are two rules of thumb regularly employed instead of frequency to estimate probability. Like other such rules of thumb, they sometimes lead to reasonably correct estimates but at other times are grossly in error.

In a particularly inventive set of studies on intuitive statistical thinking, Kahneman and Tversky have further demonstrated that, whether or not they have received formal instruction in probability and statistics, human judges consistently err in using information on base rates and data diagnosticity to make decisions. For example, believing in the "law of small numbers," they place inappropriate faith in early trends that appear in the data and hence in conclusions that derive from exceedingly small samples (Tversky and Kahneman, 1971). Moreover, even when given (or presumed to have knowledge of) base rates for a particular phenomenon, subjects will consistently disregard this knowledge in favor of stereotypes of the representativeness of particular characteristics. (The failure to recognize those situations when the best prediction is based solely on base rates also played a role in early debates regarding clinical versus actuarial prediction—see Gough, 1962.) Judges also tend to make predictions as if all information were perfectly reliable. Finally, they tend to ignore such well-understood phenomena as statistical regression, preferring always to consider individual events as directly caused rather than as products of chance fluctuations (Kahneman and Tversky, 1973).

The following example is a particularly impressive instance of this last tendency. Flight instructors in the Israeli Air Force had adopted the policy of providing positive reinforcement for student pilots after each session. After some time they informed the Air Force psychologists that the policy was not uniformly effective. In fact, it appeared that positive reinforcement following extremely fine performance led to decrements in succeeding sessions, rather than improvements. This misunderstanding of the normal phenomenon of regression eluded an entire class of graduate students in psychology who were presented with this anecdote and then asked how they would explain the decrement in performance following reinforcement. They came up with a host of elaborate psychological rationales—everything *except* simple regression after extreme performance, easily the most likely hypothesis.

Much of our functioning on a day-to-day basis, whether as teachers, physicians, or parents, involves predictions of future events based on data of variable quality or on interpretations of the efficacy of past actions or decisions based on records of past events. Hence, a thorough understanding of how humans aggregate information and expectancies in judgment becomes important. Studies of how typical error patterns can be reduced are critical. There is a pervasive tendency to interpret behavior as strictly determined, although the variety of determinism that is preferred ranges from classical behaviorism to psychoanalysis. This perspective has been invaluable in creating scientific as well as common-sense explanations of human behavior. Yet it must be tempered by insights regarding a probabilistic world where causality is attenuated by the fact that co-occurring events are correlated at substantially less than 1.00, where sources of information are less than perfectly dependable, and where the illusion of validity can lead to judgments of lifelong consequence for oneself and for other human beings.

Bayesian reasoning and equations teach us that we should attend to instances when an event does not confirm our expectations as well as to instances when it does. Here we find a convergence between studies that derive from the Bayesian paradigm and studies of human estimation of the strength of a correlation. Most clinical case studies derive their implied validity from the supposition that the selected cases are representative of a general trend that the clinician has detected in the population. They are used to illustrate the intuited correlation among observed events or characteristics. Yet Smedslund (1963) has demonstrated that when nurses were presented with a series of cases in which a particular symptom was associated with a particular diagnosis precisely as often as it was not, hence where the correlation between presence of the symptom and the diagnosis was zero, the subjects concluded that the symptom and the diagnosis were positively correlated! Naturally, since 50 percent of the cases reviewed were consistent with the belief that the symptom and the diagnosis were perfectly correlated, they could cite numerous cases as supporting evidence. The same result has been reported by Chapman and Chapman (1967, 1969) with somewhat different methods. These are only some of the problems of using case materials as evidence for the correlation between variables.

The tendency of intuitive statisticians to overemphasize positive information, information that supports a belief or reflects a positive co-occurrence of two variables, is also consistent with findings from research in concept attainment. Failure to give adequate weight to negative instances of a concept has been noted by Bruner, Goodnow, and Austin (1956), Bourne (1966), and, most convincingly, by Wason (1968). Recognition of these human tendencies to self-deception in the processing of information are not new discoveries. Contemporary psychologists have merely provided experimental confirmation of observations made several centuries ago by Francis Bacon in a discussion of the "idols of the mind."

> The human understanding when it has adopted an opinion, either as being the received opinion or as being aggreeable to itself, draws all things else to support and agree with it. And though there be a greater number and weight of instances to be found on the other side, yet these it either neglects and despises, or else by some distinction sets aside, and rejects; in order that by this great and pernicious predetermination the authority of its former conclusions may remain inviolate. And therefore it was a good answer that was made by the man who was shown hanging in a temple a picture of those who had paid their vows as having escaped shipwreck. They would have him say whether he did not now acknowledge the power of the gods—"Aye," asked he again, "but where are they painted that were drowned after their vows?" . . .
>
> It is the peculiar and perpetual error of the human intellect to be more moved and excited by affirmatives than by negatives; whereas it ought properly to hold itself indifferently disposed toward both alike. Indeed in the establishment of any true axiom, the negative instance is the more forcible (Bacon, in Curtis and Greenslet, 1962).

Bacon's solution to these dilemmas was the recommendation that science proceed by a mechanical form of hypothesis-free induction and aggregate observations without prejudice until a generalization is clearly warranted. Both contemporary philosophy of science (for instance, Popper, 1959; Medawar, 1969; Kuhn, 1970) and cognitive psychology, however, have demonstrated the impossibility of Bacon's dream of a science free of the burdens of prior beliefs or hypotheses. Man does hypothesize; apparently he must. The solution to the Baconian problem lies not in the invention of science machines that ignore prior beliefs, but in the recognition of the adaptive value of hypotheses for selecting and managing information, and the development of optimal man-machine systems for achieving "expert measurement and mechanical combination" (Einhorn, 1972). For many reasons we cannot function without hypotheses and judgments, but we must learn to avoid the pitfalls involved in using them.

The Lens Model

Egon Brunswik's probabilistic functionalism (1955, 1956) was a response to American behaviorism. His most noteworthy theoretical contribution was the lens model, and in the hands of Kenneth Hammond and his students and colleagues the model has been extended and applied to a wide range of situations.

The terminology associated with the lens model befits its Brunswikian heritage, and the number of correlation coefficients involved in working out an example completely can be formidable, especially for teachers and administrators who are practitioners of their arts first and numerically proficient researchers second. Certainly we have found this to be the case as we have attempted to understand the relevance of the lens model for studying medical judgment and the process of medical education and then to transmit our comprehension to the medical educators and practitioners with whom we work. Yet as we have become more comfortable with the model and have understood better its relevance to these tasks, it has become clear to us that many aspects of medical training and practice can be illuminated by it.

Brunswik insisted that the object of psychological study must be the relation between the person and an environment that is in principle uncertain or probabilistic. A crucial issue is how people come to interpret the cues available to them. This concern with "definition of the situation" puts the Brunswikian perspective philosophically close to the symbolic interactionist school of sociology and social psychology (Mead, 1934; Goffman, 1959). But Hammond and his collaborators have pursued this concern largely as experimental psychologists, and they and the symbolic interactionists cite one another rarely. Although their language is not that of medicine or education, Brunswik and Hammond both argue for the study of judgment in real situations. They prefer representative experimental designs to systematic orthogonal designs of probably reduced task validity. This point of view is shared by teachers and clinicians alike, who ask for research that deals with real-life problems and situations. Furthermore, programs for training both physicians and teachers are concerned with assessing the degree to which a student comes to view and evaluate the environment in the way that experienced practitioners do. This concern can be translated into an information-processing model strikingly similar to the lens model.

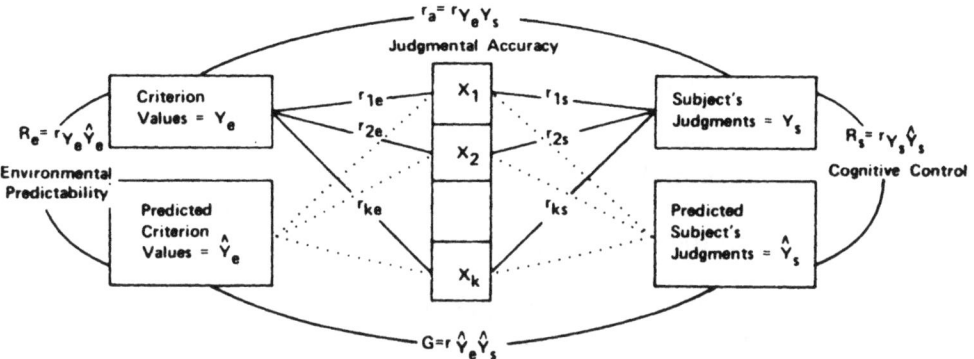

Figure 2.1 The Brunswikian lens model of the relation between a perceiver and the objects of perception.

The lens model (Figure 2.1) represents the relation between a perceiver (or judge) and the objects of perception (or judgment), as mediated by cues whose relation to both the perceiver and the object is probabilistic. Thus we never see an object per se, only via a set of cues—some associated with the object from one perspective, others from a different perspective. (Brunswik's formulation is thus a psychological version of Kant's distinction between the *Ding an sich* and the *Ding für sich*—the thing-in-itself, the noumenon that is fundamentally unknowable, and the thing-as-perceived, the phenomenon that we can know.) To understand the cognizance of anything, whether in an act of perception, judgment, or learning, is to comprehend the ways in which the knower comes to relate the observable cues to one another and to the object of perceptual or judgmental interest.

The lens model uses correlations to express and to assess the relation between observable multiple cues and the non–directly observable criterion states that produce them. In Figure 2.1 the cues or stimuli $X_1, X_2, \ldots, X_k$, arrayed in the central vertical axis of the lens, are information sources defining each stimulus object. Criterion states are on the left-hand side in the environment and judgments or inferences are on the right, products of the cognitive or judgmental process. The objects to be judged and the cues used in judgment form the task system or environment. The cues and the judgments made from them form the cognitive system (Brehmer, 1974). Each cue (X_k) is individually correlated with the criterion value (Y_e) and with the judgment of the criterion (Y_s). The correlation between any particular cue and the criterion is sometimes called the ecological validity of that cue; the correlation of a subject's judgment with a given cue is also known as the subject's utilization coefficient for that cue. Because the model assumes representative design and because cues are often correlated in reality, the possibility of intercorrelation among cues across criterion objects[1] is indicated in Figure 2.1.

The four central terms in the model are related in a formula that has come to be known as the lens-model equation: $r_a = GR_eR_s$. The form of the equation given here applies strictly to linear systems only, but since most studies of clinical judgment have shown that linear models are perfectly adequate representations and only a small fraction of additional variance is accounted for by adding nonlinear terms, it is sufficient for most purposes (Goldberg, 1970; Dawes and Corrigan, 1974).

The lens-model equation states that judgmental accuracy is limited first by the degree to which the task is predictable, R_e. Beyond that, accuracy is determined by knowledge of the properties of the task, G, and by cognitive control over the utilization of that knowledge, R_s. Moreover, knowledge and cognitive control are statistically independent. Thus, to improve judgments or decisions, one may either increase knowledge of the task or increase the consistency with which existing knowledge is utilized (Hammond and Summers, 1972).

The paradigmatic task for lens-model research is multiple-cue probability learning (MCPL). Subjects must learn to make judgments based on the values of multiple cues that bear a probabilistic relationship to a criterion. For example, a medical student may be learning to diagnose the severity of a particular liver disease by means of data from three laboratory tests. He is presented with a long series of laboratory test results, each of which comprises combinations of the three test values, and in each case he is asked to judge the severity of disease. Three basic forms of feedback are possible. *Outcome feedback* is the familiar form of knowledge of results so popular in concept-learning research, where the subject is informed after each trial of the correctness of his judgment. *Lens-model* (or *process*) feedback involves with-

---

[1] In practice, however, cue intercorrelations do not enter significantly into the variables highlighted by the model. And, indeed, one weakness of the model is the problem of the stability of regression weights assigned to correlated cues, a point we have touched on earlier. This is a critical question for the lens model, since it is anti-introspectionist and since Hammond, like Hoffman, claims that a judge's verbal report cannot be used as a reliable indicator of what he is actually doing.

holding knowledge of results until sufficient judgments have accumulated to make possible a reliable modeling of the judge's own underlying policy and form-function curve. Subjects are presented with graphic displays of their own model as compared with the ideal model. This is especially critical for learning probabilistic and nonlinear relations. In *feedforward* (Bjorkman, 1972), the learner is shown the properties of the task prior to making judgments.

Studies conducted by Hammond (1971) and others have demonstrated that simple outcome feedback is practically worthless for improving judgments, since it does not aid learning the ecology of relations among cues and criteria. On the other hand, lens-model feedback and feedforward are powerful and dramatic aids to learning. Rappoport and Summers (1973) say:

> The potential benefits of applying computer graphic displays in practical situations can in many ways stagger the imagination. But it should be emphasized most emphatically that although the technique has remarkable facilitating effects upon judgment and related phenomena, the effects are *not* accomplished by programming persons to think according to predetermined patterns. The computer is used to give persons information about how they themselves are thinking. To put it simply and candidly, this is a type of process information that has never been available in the history of mankind. Just as technical developments in the field of electrophysiology now permit men to gain process information (biofeedback) about the workings of the central nervous system, the development of computer graphic technology provides a similar caliber of information about higher mental processes associated with judgment (p. 11).

Note that these remarks apply more to process feedback than to feedforward, since the latter attempts to guide the judge more explicitly about the properties of the judgmental task.

What has excited lens-model researchers even more than the implications for research on single-subject MCPL tasks is the applicability of the paradigm to the resolution of conflicts between individuals or groups. A fine example can be taken from labor negotiations. Imagine negotiators from labor and management who are seriously deadlocked in their bargaining. One reasonable supposition is that the precise basis of their stalemate may not be evident to the participants, since each side may not have a clear picture of what the other side values, or how they assign relative weights to the items being negotiated. Lens-model researchers, in an attempt to clarify the basis of the dispute, now present a series of possible contracts to both sides separately, asking them to consider the terms of each proposed settlement and to judge its acceptability. The parameters systematically varied in the proposals may be wages, fringe benefits, working conditions, and policies on the rehiring of striking workers. Negotiators are asked to judge each contract as they would themselves—and as they believe their adversaries would. Then a series of regression equations can be calculated for each side, representing their own weighting of the variables in the contracts, as well as their perceptions of the weights of those with whom they are in conflict.

In a study actually conducted in this manner, Balke, Hammond, and Meyer (1973) discovered that management negotiators consistently assumed that labor's major concern was increased wages, while in fact the issue of rehiring strikers carried far more weight for labor than did wages. Had this basic misperception of the nature of the conflict been clarified earlier, subsequent negotiations could have proceeded more smoothly. Similar studies have been conducted in such areas as police-community relations and international affairs.

The concept of lens-model feedback is also important in a situation where a teacher is attempting to teach students how to make better diagnoses, judgments, or decisions. These circumstances arise in nearly all forms of professional training. Hammond (1971) argued that the teacher is frequently unaware of the real system he uses to make his expert judgments. He may even believe that he operates in a very different fashion from the way in which he actually does operate. Imagine the frustration of students who must learn to ignore what he *says* they should do, and instead must themselves infer the model of his judgments. Alas, claims Hammond, this is far more frequent in the teaching of clinical judgment than has been admitted or recognized.

Comparison of Approaches

As the organization of this chapter implies, psychological research on problem solving, thinking, judgment, and decision making departs from our common-sense notions of these phenomena by treating them largely as separate, relatively nonoverlapping areas. There are encouraging signs of convergence in these research traditions and movement toward common conceptualizations. A unified theory of problem solving and judgment, however, is not yet available. Let us compare the information-processing, Bayesian, and regression (including lens-model) approaches to judgment and thinking and note major points of convergence and divergence. This summary will be phrased as a set of answers to common questions.

(a) What is the aim of the theory or approach? Information-processing theory purports to be a theory that illuminates the processes by which humans reach judgments and solve problems. The adequacy of the account may be tested by writing a computer program based on analysis of verbal protocols produced as the problem is solved and observing if the steps taken and conclusions reached by a human thinker are reproduced. Because it is based on analysis of these protocols, the term *process tracing* has also been applied. Hence the information-processing approach is avowedly isomorphic in intention. It aims to provide an *explanation* of human thought by use of more elementary processes, operations, or capabilities. The aim of the other approaches is less clear. Green (1968) has argued cogently that both the Bayesian and regression models of judgment are fundamentally descriptive models that have a high probability of fitting a variety of data. Simply because a regression equation can be found that will relate a series of judgments to a set of predictor variables is no guarantee that the judgments were in fact generated by this equation. On the other hand, the effectiveness of lens-model feedback as an educational technique seems to imply that humans are using a system of weighted cues and function forms to combine variables, although admittedly it does not prove that they do. Investigators using the Bayesian model to study decision making have generally treated it as prescriptive as well as descriptive or explanatory. They have argued that some version or other of Bayes' theorem is a better way of revising opinions or estimating probabilities than the methods customarily used. The phenomenon of conservatism was important largely as evidence of the inefficiency of human information processing. Much effort has been devoted to explaining the principles that account for nonoptimal human performance.

The term *policy capturing* obscures the extent to which the regression model is descriptive rather than explanatory. It seems to imply that the judge's actual method of weighting cues has been captured, a view preferred by most investigators to the less ambitious one that the policy is a means of duplicating the judge's output. Indeed, it is often exceedingly attractive to neglect this distinction. Take studies that purport to show that judges use fewer cues than they believe they do, or that they cannot accurately estimate the weights assigned to cues, or that they believe the combination rule is complex while the regression equation is a series of simple linear terms. The authors of these studies want us to believe that something about human judgment has been explained, not merely represented. These researchers argue, in effect, that they are searching for principles to explain human behavior in a particular area, that some of this explanation is to be found in the inability of humans to apply consistently a rational decision rule or policy, and that it is an error to view this endeavor as purely or even chiefly descriptive, when the aim is to explain decision making and judgment. Thus the excellent review by Slovic and Lichtenstein (1971) collapses the distinction between paramorphic and isomorphic representations when it states that the linear model "is capable of highlighting individual differences and misuse of information as well as making explicit the causes of underlying disagreements among judges" (p. 679).

(b) What is the position of the theory on the legitimacy of introspective data in the psychology of thinking and judgment? Bayesian and regression approaches concur in their distrust of verbal testimony. As we have seen, one of the favorite tactics of policy-capturing research is to show that cue weights or combination rules determined by regression analysis are markedly different from those obtained from judges' verbal reports. This research tradition holds that judges' introspections about their judgments are not a source of legitimate data because in general judges have accurate knowledge of neither the variables they use nor the weights they assign. The finding that judges profit from process feedback implies, however, that the lens-model or regression representation is somehow isomorphic with the mental processes used, and that telling judges what they are doing improves their judgment. That is, while a judge may not know what he is doing, he can be brought to know.

The information-processing theorists, on the other hand, rely heavily on verbal reports to obtain data about the operations performed to solve a problem. Unlike classic introspectionism, the modern version does not require the informant to undergo elaborate training to be able to report accurately the contents of consciousness. Nevertheless, some training of subjects is probably wise, since thinking aloud while performing a cognitive task is not a frequently practiced skill. It may be significant that the process-tracing investigator primarily asks subjects to introspect regarding the *processes* or algorithms they employ, rather than the specific cues and weights. It is therefore conceivable that the two approaches are more complementary than contradictory, each supplying a kind of data unavailable in reliable form from the other. We foresee a growing methodological literature on introspective data gathering with the increased acceptance of process-tracing approaches. Currently, the methods involve at least as much art as science, with few well-calibrated procedures available for use. As attested by the recent renewal of debate in the psychological literature (Hebb, 1974; Radford, 1974), research on mental processes is no longer treated as a skeleton in psychology's closet.

(c) What is the position of the theory on the relative importance of understanding and prediction as aims of scientific inquiry? Whatever their weaknesses as explanations of human performance, the regression and Bayesian models have one powerful advantage over information-processing approaches. They provide methods for reducing human error and for increasing the control and consistency with which complex, multidimensional data are managed. The major claim for scientific status made by these theories relies on their capacity to improve on or predict judgments and decisions. Information-processing researchers, on the other hand, have been chiefly concerned with understanding how humans solve problems and only secondarily interested in building a computer program that can beat a human at chess or other similar projects more closely identified with the domain of artificial intelligence. For information-processing researchers, understanding and explanation take precedence over prediction and control as the scientific contribution of the theory. Like Toulmin (1961), we believe that the contribution to explanation, rather than the contribution to prediction, will ultimately determine the scientific community's verdict on the significance of a particular line of work. But for the important task of developing practical means for assisting decision making in complex situations, we find Bayesian and regression approaches more relevant.

(d) What is the role of mathematical modeling in the theory? Bayesian and regression approaches are clearly mathematical models of how people behave or ought to behave. The information-processing approach is practically nonmathematical, or at most uses a simple variety of mathematics. Newell and Simon (1972) explicitly point out that their theory of human problem solving is intentionally nonexperimental and nonstatistical. Nonmathematical representations of hierarchical associative networks presumed to be used in problem solving are found in Wortman and Kleinmuntz (1972) and Schwartz and Simon (1972).

(e) How is the theory integrated with other topics in psychology? Slovic and Lichtenstein (1971) pointed out that Bayesian and regression approaches had become quite specialized and self-contained modes of research, and that little effort had been made to articulate points of contact with other areas of psychology. They recommended that this task be undertaken. Some work has been done, and we shall turn to it when we examine points of convergence among theories. The information-processing theory of problem solving has tried more systematically to link up with psychological research on memory, cognition, language, and logic. Individual differences have been studied by policy-capturing research and largely ignored by the other approaches, which have treated them as errors of measurement in the spirit of classical experimental psychology. Within policy-capturing research, interest has focused chiefly on the demonstration of differences between judges rather than on the personality correlates of these differences.

Having enumerated these points of contrast, where are the encouraging signs of convergence among approaches which, at the start of this section, we claimed could be observed? They are to be found chiefly in shifts of position regarding the role of quantification and in the emergence of deliberate efforts to integrate with other areas of psychology.

The Bayesian and regression approaches seem to be shifting toward the degree and type of quantification employed by the information-processing approach. Research in the decision-making tradition early established that humans do not combine probabilities well and that it was more appropriate to ask them to provide subjective estimates of probability, which could subsequently be combined according to a decision rule. Martin and Gettys (1969) and the incisive series of papers by Kahneman and Tversky (1972, 1973; Tversky and Kahneman, 1971, 1973, 1974) have shown that humans often make substantial errors in estimating probabilities on a continuous scale, while they may do better with categorical classification of likelihoods. Even more critical for the state of theory, the studies of Tversky and Kahneman link subjective probability to the topics of perception and memory, since investigating the heuristics of availability and representativeness so characteristically employed when human judges estimate frequency is really a way of assessing what has been perceived and remembered. Brehmer (1974) introduced the concepts of hypothesis and hypothesis generation into a lens-model study of judgment and thereby shifted this approach closer to cognitive theory. Similarly, Dawes and Corrigan (1974) reworked the linear regression model of judgment, eliminated regression coefficients, and showed that regression equations are a special case of a simpler, more general system for weighting and combining variables that humans could and probably do utilize. Thus mathematical, prescriptive decision theories appear to be moving toward greater simplicity as they focus on the task of information-processing theory: to provide an account of how people *actually* think and reach decisions, not how they *ought* to.

At the same time, information-processing theorists are beginning to consider some of the problems addressed in decision-making research. We have already noted that many of the problems studied by information-processing theorists were those in which a goal was set and the task of the problem solver was to construct a set of logical or legal steps from the starting point toward that goal. Many problems, however, require a stage of hypothesis generation in which a goal or set of goals is constructed by the problem solver. Then the problem solver elaborates a set of moves toward the goal or goals. To solve problems of this type, hypotheses must be retrieved from memory, and the principles governing this retrieval may be those that govern estimates of subjective probability. That is, hypotheses may be retrieved on the basis of availability, representativeness, or perceived usefulness or worth.

We have reviewed in this chapter several quite different approaches to the study of human thinking and problem solving. Not all of these are equally reflected in the research program to be described in the chapters that follow. We shall discuss in detail the methods we employed in the study of medical diagnostic thinking by a group of experienced internists. Our efforts were clearly in the process-tracing tradition, directed at development of an information-processing model. Our awareness of the judgment and decision models came later in the research program; they are reflected mainly in variations in scoring systems for high-fidelity simulations or in conceptual reinterpretations of data collected by means of process-tracing methods.

3 / High-Fidelity Simulation: Research Methods

Chapters 3 to 6 report the results of studies of the problem solving and reasoning of a panel of experienced physicians. Several formats were employed in these studies, and the most complex is the subject of this chapter and the next.

Once a physician arrived at the Medical Inquiry Project laboratory, the bulk of his/her time was devoted to working up and discussing with the project staff three simulated medical problems intended to represent some of the complexities often encountered in clinical practice. These three simulations were intriguing to physicians and research psychologists alike, because high face validity was achieved by training actors to play the roles of patients. The use of actors in this way was intended to present physicians with as faithful a representation of clinical reality as could be devised within the constraints of our ingenuity and financial resources. The term *high-fidelity simulations* will be used to refer to these particular simulations and to distinguish them from other, "lower-fidelity" simulations analyzed in Chapters 5 and 6.

This chapter describes the experimental setting and the variables developed for scoring and analyzing the protocols obtained. The results of the analyses will be presented in Chapter 4.

Research Method

Selection of Physicians

All the participants were boarded or board eligible in internal medicine.[1] They were identified by peer nominations, the peers

---

[1] This means that each physician had completed a certified residency training program in internal medicine and had either passed an examination administered by the American Board of Internal Medicine or was eligible to stand for this examination.

Table 3.1 Numbers of physicians participating in Medical Inquiry Project, by practice setting and criterial status.

	Practice setting		
Status	Salaried group practice	Private practice	Academic medicine
Criterial	7	6	4
Noncriterial	2	3	2

being the other physicians on the staff of the Department of Medicine in the hospital where each had his/her inpatient practice. Three practice settings were sampled: salaried group practice, private practice, and academic medicine. Ballots were sent to all members of the medical staff of four hospitals in three Michigan cities, asking for nomination of four physicians judged to be the best diagnosticians known to the respondent. Those physicians receiving at least five votes were designated as "criterial," while those who received one or none were identified as "noncriterial." Approximately forty-five physicians were contacted and asked to participate in the study. Each was told that he/she had been recommended by peer nominations, the only deception in the entire project. Twenty-four agreed to participate. The distribution is shown in Table 3.1.

Each physician on this panel of voluntary participants spent approximately two days in the project laboratory at Michigan State University. The bulk of the time was spent with the three problems described and analyzed in Chapter 4. Several hours were also devoted to the medical problems analyzed in Chapters 5 and 6 and to personality scales and logical problems.

Procedure

A room was designed to resemble a physician's office; two television cameras were mounted near the ceiling so that the entire interaction between the doctor and the simulated patient could be videotaped. The scenarios used to prepare the actors and to develop the physical examination and laboratory findings were based upon actual clinical records. The cases were intended to be problems that a general internist practicing in a community hospital of moderate size could be reasonably expected to see, at least for an initial encounter. As in real-world medicine, each physician could decide how many data to collect and had the options of calling a consultant or referring the patient whenever he chose.

The subject matter was hematology in simulation 1, gastroenterology in simulation 2, and neurology in simulation 3.

Actors from the Department of Theater at Michigan State University were carefully trained to simulate the patients. Each was provided with a detailed synopsis of the problem and had available far more data about the patient's medical and personal history than were ordinarily requested during the course of the workup. The actor was coached in all details needed for a convincing performance, but was given no fixed script beyond the opening statement of the chief complaint, so that the interaction of the actor and the physician could be natural. In two cases the actor-patient was interviewed for a history of the present illness and a review of systems. When the physician was ready to begin the physical examination, the actor left the room and an assistant entered who served as a "data bank." The physician was told that the data bank contained all possible information from the physical examination, available upon questioning. The data bank could offer only physical findings, not interpretations. For example, if the physician asked for blood pressure, a reading was provided without comment as to its significance. In the third case an actress was trained to simulate both history and physical findings of an illness involving sensory and motor losses, so that the physician could conduct both an interview and a physical examination. A data bank for laboratory tests was provided in all three cases.

Instructions to the physician stressed that he was free to elicit whatever data were felt to be necessary and in whatever order was appropriate. Laboratory tests could be ordered at any time, the requested reports being provided on the standard forms used by the University Health Center. The physician was asked to work in his customary manner and to do whatever he felt was appropriate for the case at hand. Each physician was advised that he was the first to see the patient regarding the present complaint, that there were no time pressures, and that the extent of the workup was entirely discretionary.

Whenever possible, and particularly when natural breaks occurred in the workup of the patient (usually between the history and the physical examination, and at the conclusion of the examination prior to ordering laboratory tests), the physician was asked to think aloud and to provide an ongoing account of his reasoning. This was not difficult for most participants, since it was a minor variation of their conduct on ward rounds or when reviewing cases with students. Some preferred to confine their comments to the natural breaks previously mentioned; others felt comfortable in pausing to review at much more frequent intervals. The physicians knew that the patients were actors and were assured that interruptions for the purpose of review and thinking aloud would not disturb the actors. The actors had been alerted to the fact that reviews would occur; part of their training was devoted to acquainting them with this procedure and to maintaining the proper atmosphere during the pauses. Three episodic, retrospective reviews were an essential feature of the research method, since it was early realized that the physician's strategy would not be accurately inferred only from the record of his interaction with the patient. While we were pilot testing the simulations and the thinking-aloud method, it became clear that physicians covertly generated and evaluated preliminary diagnostic formulations long before they would be willing to share these with a patient.

Most physicians reported that the simulations were convincing and provided a satisfactory approximation of the atmosphere of a real case. Some pointed out that certain departures from their usual procedures were necessary because of the simulation technique, most notably that two of the cases required a definite separation between history taking and physical examination. These clinicians observed that this separation would not be maintained in their usual method of assessment, since they were accustomed to conducting the review of systems while performing the physical examination and could easily recycle to obtain additional history if the physical findings were suggestive. It was possible to do this in the simulation by bringing the actor-patient into the room with the data-bank assistant, but this procedure was not as natural as examining a real patient. A few physicians noted that they would have detected jaundice upon examination of the eyeballs of one patient whose laboratory reports showed an elevated bilirubin (the actor was not so afflicted), but this deficiency was not critical to the case.

Other comments related to the primary care setting and lack of time constraints. Several clinicians noted that a real practice either provided time for lengthy workups or else for "brief-encounter" primary care, but that the two were usually incompatible. They were therefore aware of a certain staged quality in the simulations.

On the whole, however, the sample felt that these were minor differences that exerted little if any effect on their usual methods of gathering data. Since we do not have data from the physicians' practices, this testimonial cannot be verified or refuted. Other studies (Goran, Williamson, and Gonnella, 1973) have suggested that physicians tend to be more thorough in collecting data in simulated settings than in actual practice.

After the full workup had been completed, the "stimulated-recall" section of the experiment began (Kagan, 1973, 1975). The videotape of the physician's workup was replayed for him. He was given a stop/start switch with which to control the playback. A specially trained research assistant served as recall interrogator (Kagan et al., 1967), a person trained in encouraging the physician to use the videotape as a vehicle to stimulate his memory and relate what he was thinking throughout the session being reviewed. The stimulated recall was another attempt to move beyond the observable behavior into the thoughts, feelings, associations, and strategies going through the mind of the physician at the moment when the events being reviewed were occurring. Review of an entire diagnostic workup is a lengthy and demanding process. Generally, it was found that the scrutiny of the first thirty minutes of the encounter provided sufficient information about the thinking of the physician during the patient contact to clarify how data obtained were being utilized. Review of the first half-hour of the workup ordinarily required one to one and a half hours. The stimulated recall was itself recorded on audiotape and transcribed for subsequent analysis.

Three kinds of data thus were available to supplement the analysis of the workup itself. First, there was material from concurrent thinking aloud, usually brief statements of what the clinician had learned or was about to do and why. Second, there were longer episodic reviews usually conducted at natural breaks in the action. The third source consisted in material obtained from reviewing the videotape of the workup with an interrogator in videotape-stimulated recall. Where discrepancies were found among these three sources, they were weighted highest to lowest in the order given.

The Scoring System

Principles

Four principles directed the formulation of the present scoring system:

(a) *Objectivity and reliability.* Given formal statements of the rule for each scoring category, independent judges ought to reach at least 85 percent agreement on the specific categories to which any particular unit of behavior is assigned.

(b) *Task relevance.* The method must reflect the critical and relevant characteristics of the particular mode of cognitive functioning under study. The scoring system should draw attention to the more relevant aspects of functioning and pay less heed to irrelevant aspects.

(c) *Theoretical relevance.* The scoring system should measure aspects of the activity under study that can be related to parallel variables in other theories of problem solving and/or studies of similar processes in other content domains. That is, the scoring system should describe physician performance in medically relevant terms, and should also afford a way of describing the cognitive functioning of the subject that is meaningful in the light of broader theories of cognitive functioning and problem solving.

(d) *Discriminant validity.* The specific scores or assessments generated by the scoring procedure should distinguish effectively between clearly different levels of competence in medical functioning.

Units of Analysis

A major rationale for utilizing high-fidelity simulation was that the fundamental units of analysis appropriate for the study of medical reasoning were unknown to us. Other scoring systems (such as Rimoldi, 1961; McGuire and Babbott, 1967) had made some assumptions about the fundamental units, but the measures developed did not articulate clearly with current trends in cognitive psychology. Our strategy was to develop the fundamental units of analysis from observations of physicians' performance in the setting of high-fidelity simulation, utilizing the episodic-review and stimulated-recall techniques to identify the fundamental elements in terms of which the solution of medical problems was organized. In the analysis of simulation data, much time was devoted to refining and sharpening the concepts by developing more operational definitions with satisfactory interrater reliability. The three fundamental units of protocol analysis identified in this manner are information search units, cues, and hypotheses. The latter two terms are related to similar concepts in other theories of judgment and problem solving and serve as links to those theories; the information search units describe subject performance in traditional medical categories. The analytic concepts thus relate the performance of any particular physician to both familiar medical categories and to contemporary thinking in cognitive psychology.

Information search units index the data-gathering behavior of the physician. To solve diagnostic problems, physicians collect data. This search for information encompasses general interrogation regarding personal habits and life-style of the patient, maneuvers in the physical examination such as measuring the pulse or examining the eyes, and specific requests for laboratory tests. Questions may be leading or nonleading. Cues are the data or findings obtained via the physician's inquiry. They may be volunteered by a patient, nonverbally displayed by a patient, or elicited by search activated by the inquiring physician. Hypotheses are the physician's formulations of possible solutions of the problem. They are concepts of medical significance used to cluster cues and are in turn verified or disproved by the evidence.

INFORMATION SEARCH UNITS. An information search unit is defined as any statement or act of the physician that either seeks information from the patient, instructs the patient concerning a procedure in the examination, or establishes rapport between the physician and the patient. Eight content categories were developed into which any information search unit could be assigned: history of present illness, personal and social history, previous medical history, family history, physical examination, laboratory, instructions, and rapport. The first six are minor modifications of a widely used outline for examining patients (Harvey et al., 1972). History of present illness was subdivided into effects on the patient, time variables, patient's view of precipitant or symptoms, modifying factors, contacts, and other.

Scoring of protocols according to these categories was done by physicians and senior medical students. To assess reliability, several protocols were scored by two judges independently. Agreement on the identification of information search units was 91 percent; on the assignment of information search units to content categories, it was 86 percent.

Nearly a year was spent trying to develop a scoring scheme and a set of rules that could reliably and consistently categorize questions as either hypothesis directed or routine. The rules and procedures developed were uniformly unsuccessful. Discriminations made for one case by two judges could not be used as a set of rules that would distinguish in another case. We are unable to offer a set of rules that will reliably discriminate between information search units belonging to routine searches for information and those that are hypothesis directed. Intuitively, the distinction makes sense to us, and to physicians who have discussed the problem with us, but specific information search units still cannot be placed reliably in one or the other category. We were similarly unsuccessful in developing rules for reliably categorizing questions on the history as open or closed, nonleading or leading; with regret we abandoned this line of analysis.

CUES. A list of potential cues for each case was compiled based on the synopsis used in training the actor, the pertinent physical findings, and experience in pilot testing. It included all laboratory tests ordered in the real case that was the basis of the simulation scenario, plus additional tests ordered in pilot testing. Physical findings in the potential cue list included all positive findings and all pertinent negatives. The cue list also included the chief complaint and routine basic data presented to the physician at the start of the problem. Once each cue was numbered, it was a relatively simple matter to record the sequence of cue acquisition on a summary sheet compiled by careful reading of the transcription of the workup. Any cues not on this list but identified by participants were designated by letter rather than number. These were idiosyncratic and no consistent pattern was observed.

HYPOTHESES. A hypothesis may be generated alone or in the company of competitors. It may be a fairly specific diagnostic label (infectious mononucleosis, for instance), or a complex multilevel formulation (such as acute infection, probably viral in origin, possibly infectious mononucleosis). It not only has a moment of birth but also an ultimate fate. It may be entertained and then rejected; it may never be explicitly rejected, but simply allowed to fade away as better alternatives move into place; it may be confirmed, in which case it moves from the status of hypothesis to that of tentative or final diagnosis. The purpose of asking specific questions to elicit cues is to manipulate the status of these hypotheses in order to reach a satisfactory diagnosis.

In the pilot stage of our work, criteria for identifying hypotheses were not defined by a set of explicit rules. Hypotheses were identified through analysis of the physician's thinking aloud and from his reflections during the stimulated recall. At the time we thought that a physician was entertaining a particular hypothesis because he told us so or because it seemed apparent that he was. The seriousness of the hypothesis was judged subjectively by members of the research team. As the scoring system developed, it became apparent that these informal rules led to unsatisfactory levels of interjudge reliability. Clearer rules for identifying hypotheses were gradually developed and were incorporated into a manual for scoring the cognitive aspects of diagnostic problem solving. This manual contains rules for coding a subject's use of information search units to obtain *cues,* for identifying hypotheses as well as points where they are *generated* and *terminated,* and for scoring the way a subject relates cues obtained to hypotheses generated. The final version of the manual is available from the senior author. Its rules are deliberately quite conservative. A hypothesis can be very general or very specific, but the rules led to exclusion of some very general hypotheses entertained early in the session because the physician quickly reformulated more specifically and did not again mention the initial general hypothesis.

Cue-Hypothesis Matrix

Subsequently the hypotheses most frequently entertained in each case were determined. These hypotheses and all cues were compiled into a matrix or grid having cues on one dimension and hypotheses on the other. The matrix was then given to an expert in each field represented by the cases, who was asked to weight each cue relevant to each hypothesis on a seven-point scale that ranged from -3, strongly negative, through 0, equivocal or noncontributory, to $+3$, strongly positive. A sample page of one matrix is provided in Figure 3.1. Each physician's interpretation of cues with respect to hypotheses was assessed by comparing the weights he explicitly assigned to the cues he interpreted with the weights entered in the cue-hypothesis matrix.

We recognize that a panel of raters might assign somewhat different weights in the cells of each matrix, although in one or two instances where it was possible to have the grid completed by two independent experts, their agreement was substantial. The method is presented as a demonstration of an approach to evaluating clinical process, not as a definitive statement of the cue weights for three specific medical problems.

To summarize the discussion to this point, it is possible to take the transcribed protocol of a doctor-patient interaction and divide a physician's activity into basic components called information search units, which can be assigned to medically relevant content categories. The cues acquired by the physician as a result

Figure 3.1 First page of the cue-hypothesis matrix for simulation 1. An asterisk signifies a critical finding, as defined in text.

FINDINGS / HYPOTHESES OFTEN ENTERTAINED

FINDINGS	INFEC	STREP	CNS	MONO	FLU	HEPAT	LEUK	LYM	ANEM	MEA	IPA	HA	CSA	ASA
GIVEN AT START OF PROBLEM:														
1. 19 year-old female												+1	+1	
2. Chief complaint: Fatigue, poor appetite														
*3. Temperature 102°F oral	+3	+1	+1	+1		+1		+1	+1	+1	+2			
4. Ambulatory, alert														+2
PRESENT ILLNESS:														
*5. Excessive sleeping	+1	+1	+2	+1	+1	+1	+1	+1	+1	+1				
6. Anorexia – 3 days	+1	+1	+1	+1	+1	+1	+1	+1						
*7. Severe throbbing frontal headache	+1	+1	+1	+2	+1	+1			+1	+1				
8. No visual disturbances			−1											
9. Generalized weakness	+1	+1	+1	+1	+1	+1			+1	+1				
*10. Mild chills and fever	+3	+1	+1	+1	+1	+1	+1	+2			+2			
*11. General achiness, 5 days' duration	+1	+1	+1	+1	+2	+1	+1	+1						
12. No cold or runny nose now	−1	−1			−1	−1								
*13. Probable exposure to influenza	+2		+1	+1	+2	−1	−2	−1			+2			

KEY — INFEC = Infection
STREP = Strep Infection
CNS = CNS Infection
MONO = Infectious Mono
FLU = Influenza

HEPAT = Infectious Hepatitis
LEUK = Leukemia
LYM = Lymphoma
ANEM = Anemia
MEA = Mixed etiology anemia

IPA = Inflam. Produced Anemia
HA = Hemolytic Anemia
CSA = Congenital Spherocytic Anemia
ASA = Autoimmune Spherocytic Anemia

Blank equals 0

of his inquiry can be identified. Through use of information from the physician's comments during the workup and from the stimulated recall, the hypotheses entertained during the workup as well as the way cues were applied to these hypotheses can be determined. A tally sheet or symbolic map of each subject's progress through each case can be developed. On each tally sheet the information search units are listed by number down the left-hand margin, and the hypotheses entertained by the subject are entered across the top. In the body of the tally sheet the following are noted: the point at which each hypothesis was generated, the points at which cues were acquired by the inquirer and at which they were applied to hypotheses, and the point at which each hypothesis was terminated. Cue numbers are the same as those used on the cue-hypotheis matrix. Letters are used to indicate an occasional cue mentioned by a physician but not included in the matrix. An example of a tally sheet is shown in Figure 3.2. By carefully examining the relations of the hypotheses and cues, we can compare the number of positive and negative cues that the doctor elicited for any considered hypotheses.

Scoring Variables

The scores developed in this study are essentially different combinations built on these three basic building blocks: information search units, cues (and critical findings), and hypotheses. We turn now to definitions of the variables derived from these fundamental concepts.

(a) *Total information search units.* This variable is a measure of the length of the workup and includes search units in the rapport and instructions categories. Workup length is measured in total information search units, rather than time, so that differences in thinking aloud time do not affect the assessment.

(b) *Point of generation of first hypothesis.* In pilot observations of medical problem solving (Elstein et al., 1972) early generation of relatively specific hypotheses was regularly noted. This variable was developed to determine more rigorously the frequency of this event and to specify more precisely what is meant by "early." The rules for determining when a hypothesis was generated were deliberately conservative, as we wished to establish conclusively that the first hypothesis was generated no later than the point specified and that it could conceivably have been earlier.

(c) *Number of hypotheses active one-quarter of the way through workup.*

Figure 3.2 Tally sheet for analysis of medical reasoning.

Case # **1**   Dr. **A**   Page **2** B of **3**

Coded by **SS**

ANALYSIS OF WORK-UP

ISU #	FINDINGS Elicited	Presented		Induction	4. maxim 2:	4. max 2:	5. yl 2:	HYPOTHESES			
5 A-H	18										
6 A-P	(11), 13										
7 A				G?							
8 A				G							
B	(27)(32), 42										
C											
D											
E	(35)(40)										
F	(37)										
G											
H											
I											
J											
9 A-H	28, 30, (31)										
	36										
10 A-H	38, (39)			31+	C						
I					a⁻						
J				33+	33+						
K	(34), 33										
L											
M											

a. 3 days' duration of all symptoms

(d) *Number of hypotheses active halfway through workup.* These two variables were developed to provide measures of the process of converging on a diagnostic solution and the number of working hypotheses in memory at a given moment, and thereby relate the analysis to cognitive theory. The variables represent the number of hypotheses being actively entertained at two particular points.

(e) *Total number of hypotheses generated.* This is a count of the number of hypotheses generated at any point in the workup without regard to specificity or duration of a hypothesis. Variables (c) to (e) provide some insight into the rate of turnover of hypotheses. Very short-lived hypotheses generated quite early in the workup and terminated quickly will appear in the count of total hypotheses, but not in the list of those active at the one-quarter mark. Longer-lived hypotheses will appear in the counts of both variables (c) and (d). Little variation among scores on variables (c) to (e) for a particular clinician shows that the same hypotheses were retained for a longer period of time.

(f) *Number of hypotheses retained.* Two of the simulations converged on a single solution. The third had two accurate outcomes. Despite the convergent nature of the cases, not all subjects reached a single (or dual) solution. Therefore, the hypotheses each physician was still considering at the conclusion of a workup were counted.

(g) *Number of cues acquired.*

(h) *Percentage of cues acquired.* The number of cues acquired by each subject in working up the problem is one measure of the thoroughness of data collection. Percentage of cues acquired is calculated by dividing the number of cues acquired (excluding cues not in the cue-hypothesis matrix) by the total number of cues listed on the matrix for that case, a constant for each case.

(i) *Number of critical findings acquired.*

(j) *Percentage of critical findings acquired.* These two variables are defined similarly to variables (g) and (h). Critical findings are cues assigned a weight of ±2 or ±3 relative to at least one hypothesis on the cue-hypothesis matrix. Variable (i) is a count of the number of critical findings acquired by any subject, irrespective of whether he was entertaining the hypothesis for which a cue was critical. The percentage of critical findings acquired is the number of critical findings acquired divided by the total number of critical findings listed in the cue-hypothesis matrix. Variables (i) and (j) constitute a measure of how many potentially *high-yield* data a subject collects. Comparing scores on variable (j) with those on variable (h) tells us to what extent the inquiry focused on high-yield data.

(k) *Efficiency.* It was noted earlier that it was not possible to determine whether an information search unit was being used to test a hypothesis. Enduring interest in the role of hypotheses in clinical problem solving led to development of the efficiency variable to try to assess hypothesis-related activity. Efficiency is the percentage of critical findings elicited by a clinician that are weighted ±2 or ±3 for at least one of the hypotheses being entertained. Efficiency focuses more on a physician's own hypothesis-evaluation activities than variable (j). Comparing this ratio to (j) for any one subject shows that his ability to gather potentially high-yield data relates to his opportunities to apply these data to his own hypotheses. Since subjects were not constrained to interpret every cue they obtained relative to every hypothesis they entertained, a direct measure of each subject's hypothesis testing was not possible. The alternative is this efficiency variable, which gives an upper limit of hypothesis-related activity for any subject.

(l) *Accuracy of interpretation.* This variable assesses the correspondence between a physician's interpretation of the data he obtained and the interpretation offered by the cue-hypothesis matrix. The cues applied to any hypothesis and the weights assigned were determined from the entire protocol of each workup, including recall. From these materials it became clear that subjects generally used a three-point weighting scale—positive, noncontributory, and negative. Therefore it seemed likely that the distinction between cues and critical findings was not made by the physicians in the study. For these reasons each participant's cue interpretation was compared to the cue-hypothesis matrix according to the scheme displayed in Table 3.2.

Table 3.2 shows that a subject's interpretation of a cue was judged *accurate* if he assigned it a negative weight and it had any negative weight (-1, -2, or -3) on the matrix, and the same was true for assignment of positive weights. The accuracy of interpretation score was a percentage: number of correct interpretations divided by total number of interpretations. Since clinical problem solving is comprised of data acquisition, hypothesis generation, and cue interpretation, it was considered probable that this vari-

Table 3.2 Accuracy of interpretation of cues by participating physicians. A = accurate interpretation, O = overinterpretation, M = misinterpretation, and U = underinterpretation.

Doctor's interpretation	Cue-hypothesis matrix		
	+1, +2, +3	Zero	-1, -2, -3
Positive	A	O	M
Noncontributory	U	A	U
Negative	M	O	A

able would make an important contribution to any judgments about subjects' problem-solving skills.

(m) *Modal interpretive error.* We also speculated that the specific type of error committed would help differentiate the more skillful from the less skillful diagnostician. Accordingly, the most frequent type of interpretive error made by each participant was noted. A subject *overinterpreted* a cue if he assigned a positive or negative weight to a cue that was given a "zero" weight on the cue-hypothesis matrix. *Underinterpretation* was the assignment of a "zero" weight to a cue in the presence of either a positive or a negative weight on that matrix. *Misinterpretation* was the assignment of a weight to a cue opposite to that provided in the cue-hypothesis matrix.

(n) *Accuracy of formulation.*

(o) *Accuracy of outcome.* This pair of variables answered two questions: Did the subject generate the accurate solution hypothesis(es)? Was it retained? Both variables were scored dichotomously. One index of clinical problem-solving skills is accuracy in decision making. Although a problem solver should not be judged solely on the accuracy of solution, it is an important factor. Furthermore, the frequency with which a problem is solved acts as an index of its difficulty. Distinguishing between accuracy of formulation and accuracy of outcome clarifies different reasons for errors of outcome and their relation to other aspects of performance. This topic will be discussed in the next chapter.

Methodological Problems

Construction of the Cue-Hypothesis Matrix

The analyses of acquisition of critical findings, of accuracy of interpretation, of modal interpretive error, and finally of the modeling of hypothesis evaluation will all hinge on comparing the participating clinician's performance with the entries in the appropriate cue-hypothesis matrix. Yet each matrix is the product of the thinking of one or two expert clinicians. Was this procedure justified?

It would have been preferable to have these matrices be the product of extensive deliberation among many clinicians, but this was impossible because of the small number of physicians at Michigan State University at the time the matrices were developed.

Nevertheless, we do not believe that the matrices are substantially in error. After all, the task for the rater was not to decide which data ought to be collected and which omitted in the workup. Consensus among even expert physicians on this task repeatedly has been found to be weak. The task was to evaluate the significance of any particular finding, assuming it had been elicited, not to judge whether it should have been obtained. Discussions of the developed matrices with other clinicians have led us to the view that while some entries would probably have been changed had there been deliberation by a committee of experts, the overall pattern of weights conformed to generally held expert medical opinion.

In conclusion, our judgment is that the matrices are useful in their present form, particularly since one of our aims is to demonstrate an approach to evaluating clinical competence rather than to develop definitive scoring keys for three specific problems.

Introspection as a Research Technique

Using introspective evidence from the problem solver to help elucidate steps by which a problem is solved has a long history in psychological research (Claparède, 1934; Duncker, 1945; de Groot, 1965; Newell and Simon, 1972). The meaning of such testimony nevertheless has been a perennially troublesome issue in the history of psychology (Neisser, 1968; Hebb, 1974; Radford, 1974).

In the present research two related questions had to be considered: In reviewing a videotape, to what degree was the subject's retrospective account of what he was thinking at time t distorted or confounded by his knowledge of the data subsequently available, his interpretation of those data, and, indeed, his final resolution of the problem? If retrospective distortion occurred, could it be consistently identified and controlled, or at least discounted?

These questions get to the heart of the problem of using verbal reports in the study of problem-solving strategies. We cannot ever be certain that all instances of retrospective distortion are identified. However, a number of heuristic principles were established to alert us to the occurrence of retrospective distortion and to correct the interpretation. The basic judgmental principles are that each formulation must be consistent with the data base existing at the time, and that stimulated-recall accounts of reasoning must be consistent with accounts provided by the ongoing thinking aloud (episodic review). Where retrospective distortion is identified by conflict between testimony from the episodic-review and stimulated-recall segments, the general principle is to give greater credence to episodic review. Similarly, if a physician were to state in stimulated recall that his thinking at a particular point was supported by cues that had not yet been obtained, this is clear evidence of distortion and the testimony is ignored. Where two recall statements are inconsistent, we accepted the one which is more consistent with the episodic review or is more conservative.

We believe that with these principles a conservative line of interpretation of the stimulated-recall segments was consistently adopted. The vast majority of recall protocols were consistent with the testimony provided in the episodic review. The use of verbalization as a means of having a subject explicate his strategy proved generally to be very satisfactory. We found that the subject's account of his strategy was usually consistent with his behavior. Further exploration of this issue is found in Chapters 7 through 10, each of which deals with verbalization as part of the research method.

Summary

A method has been presented for observing the work of physicians who are solving diagnostic problems by means of actors who play patient roles in a setting that closely resembles the physician's office. The method provides freedom for the physician to interact with the patient as he chooses. The quantity and sequence of data collection are controlled largely by the participant, with minimal cuing provided by the case materials. The physician's thought processes are studied by analysis of transcription of the workup, the thinking-aloud comments of the physician, and additional comments obtained during stimulated-recall review of the videotapes of each workup. Three problems were designed in this format.

The scoring system developed to analyze these protocols has the task of reducing an extremely complex interaction to a set of manageable variables that makes sense in terms of both clinical medicine and cognitive psychology. The fundamental units of protocol analysis are information search units, cues, and hypotheses. Information search units tabulate the data-gathering behavior of the physician; cues are the data obtained; and hypotheses are the formulations of possible solutions to the problem. A matrix of cues and hypotheses was constructed to represent the appropriate cue weightings for each hypothesis, as determined by an expert. The analysis of each protocol initially examined the following variables: total number of information search units, point at which the first hypothesis was generated, number of hypotheses active one-quarter and one-half of the way through each workup, total number of hypotheses generated, number of hypotheses retained at conclusion of workup, number and percent of cues acquired, number and percent of critical findings obtained, efficiency, accuracy of interpretation, modal interpretive error, accuracy of formulation, and accuracy of outcome.

Some methodological problems associated with the scoring system have been discussed, as well as the use of introspection as a research technique.

4 / High-Fidelity Simulation: Results

The analyses reported in this chapter are based on a series of three simulated medical problems worked up by a sample of twenty-four physicians. Considerable pilot testing with these simulations was necessary before they were ready for use, and the pilot testing itself led to the formulation of some preliminary notions about the processes of medical thinking. Thus, what began as a plan for hypothesis-free observation soon became transformed into a plan for observation and analysis guided by a conceptual framework that identified certain elements as important. The Medical Inquiry Project then became partly hypothetico-deductive, much as we shall claim medical problem solving itself is. The scoring variables described in Chapter 3 focus on certain aspects of medical problem solving, particularly the processes of hypothesis generation and evaluation. Before proceeding to the substance of the chapter, let us review the main points emerging from the pilot work as they provide context for the material that follows.

A Model of Medical Inquiry

Our preliminary formulation of the process of medical inquiry (Elstein et al., 1972) stated that physicians generate specific diagnostic hypotheses well before most of the data have been obtained in a particular case. As we shall see, this is only partly correct: early hypothesis generation remains a feature of the theory of medical inquiry, but our views about specificity have changed. Provisional hypotheses are generated out of the physician's background knowledge of medicine by an associative process that links the problematic aspects of the case to long-term memory. It was quickly recognized that a sharp distinction between the content of medical knowledge and the processes of medical problem solving was not going to be particularly fruitful, for the process operations can only be performed upon some content, and that content must include materials stored in memory as well as those obtained from the patient via data-collection procedures.

It is even more critical, however, to explain why early hypothesis generation was so commonly observed in the pilot study that it became a central concept in our thinking and in the manual for protocol analysis. We have already touched on this point in the literature review in Chapter 2. The generation of hypotheses and utilization of a hypothetico-deductive method seem to be a nearly universal characteristic of human thinking in complex, poorly defined environments. Work in the psychology of memory and thinking has suggested why this is so: the problem must be represented cognitively in the mind of the problem solver. While rational problem solving is characterized by a high degree of adaptation of this representation to the demands of the problem, there are limits to human capacity both in working memory and in respect to the number of operations that can be performed simultaneously (Simon, 1969; Newell and Simon, 1972).

The function of early hypotheses, therefore, is to limit the size of the space that must be searched for solutions to the problem. Some way of progressively constraining the size of the search space must be found or else a clinical workup could never end in the time that is actually available. Many classical studies in the problem-solving literature employ a paradigm in which the problem solver begins from a known point and searches for the most appropriate or legal route to a specified goal. The cryptarithmetic problems studied by Bartlett (1958) and by Newell and Simon (1972) are fine examples. In contrast, the problem solver working in an open system, of whom the physician is a good exemplar, must begin from a known starting point—in clinical work, the chief complaint—and move to an as yet unknown terminal point, a diagnostic classification or treatment decision. Cognitive strain is high under such conditions. A useful and frequently employed technique for dealing with the demands of reasoning within an open system is to transform the system cognitively into a series of hypothetical closed systems, which can be explored either serially or simultaneously. The problem solver generates a small number of probable terminal points and then proceeds in the inquiry to test the appropriateness of various routes to the hypothesized terminal points. By restating this framework in more specifically medical terms, we can clarify our approach to the task of analyzing the data.

A physician's observable activity in working up a patient consists in questions asked to collect data, including the physical examination and routine or special laboratory procedures that may be ordered as well as the tactics of interviewing and history taking. Information search units encompass all of these activities. Acquiring cues, clinical findings, or data is thus the observable component of medical reasoning. The pilot studies disclosed that in addition to asking questions, physicians generate hypotheses and interpret data in the light of these hypotheses as the workup proceeds. This set of hypotheses defines the problem space of possible solutions for the diagnostic problem. Data subsequently collected are used to evaluate the hypotheses and, if necessary, to formulate or generate new ones and thereby modify the problem space. Each hypothesis implies a list of probable features. In cue interpretation some of the data obtained are evaluated by their correspondence to, or departure from, the specifications of these lists; some are simply ignored or treated as noncontributory.

In our earliest article on this subject (Elstein et al., 1972) we offered some speculations about the principles used in retrieving hypotheses from memory in medical problem solving. They were identified then as probability, seriousness, treatability, and novelty. More will be said about this topic in the next section, where cognitive features of the problems are discussed, and again in Chapter 7, which reports in detail on the initial problem formulations of a group of experienced physicians. The pilot theory of medical inquiry was silent on the subject of hypothesis evaluation, the problem of how choices are made between alternatives; the topic will be discussed later in this chapter.

A general psychological model of diagnostic inquiry can thus be built around four major activities: cue acquisition, hypothesis generation, cue interpretation, and hypothesis evaluation.

The reader should bear these four cognitive processes in mind as the analysis unfolds in the following pages. The variables deal with each of these phases. In particular, evidence will be presented on the following questions:

(a) How are medical diagnostic problems solved?
(b) What processes characterize the thinking of expert physicians as contrasted with nonexperts?

(c) What processes distinguish accurate from inaccurate diagnostic outcome?
(d) How early are preliminary diagnostic hypotheses generated, and how extensive a data base is needed?
(e) What decision rules are used to confirm hypotheses or eliminate them?
(f) What are the most common errors in diagnostic reasoning?

As the analysis of data proceeds, it will be helpful to keep these questions in mind.

The next section deals with the medical and cognitive aspects of the three sample problems. This section, and indeed the entire chapter, was written with a multidisciplinary audience in mind. We shall present the medical content of each simulation in a manner that we hope will be understandable to psychologists and educators and will not seem unduly oversimplified to physicians. We shall try likewise to discuss the cognitive processes and the statistical analysis in a style that will be comprehensible to physicians and will not talk down to educators and psychologists. Still, no one reader may find all the material relevant. The following outline sketches the shape of the discussion:

(a) Medical content and cognitive organization of simulations:
Simulation 1
Simulation 2
Simulation 3
(b) Statistical summary of results on twelve dependent variables
(c) Detailed results on five selected dependent variables:
Criterial versus noncriterial physicians
Accurate versus inaccurate physicians
(d) Hypothesis evaluation: modeling diagnostic judgments
(e) Possible errors in solving diagnostic problems
(f) Summary:
The psychology of medical reasoning
Criterial and noncriterial physicians
Critique of the scoring system.

Medical Content and Cognitive Organization

In this section the medical content of each problem will be summarized and its cognitive organization analyzed. Attention will be directed chiefly to the major hypotheses generated, the types of hypotheses (general or specific), their structural relations, and the relevant data sources. These accounts may be compared to Feinstein's (1973a, 1973b) analysis of diagnostic reasoning from a logical, rather than a psychological, standpoint. Our concern here is with the structure of the problem, how it is grasped by the clinician, and the limits on the physician's adaptive capability. The process of reaching a diagnostic decision and the more common errors will be analyzed separately.

Simulation 1

This problem involved a female college student, age about twenty, with three main complaints—extreme fatigue and excessive sleeping, poor appetite, and severe headache. Further history disclosed mild chills and fever with general aching of about five days' duration. The picture is complicated somewhat by the absence of a report of sore throat, despite physical findings consistent with an inflamed, painful throat. On physical examination the tonsils are found to to be enlarged and covered with exudate; the white of the eyeball is somewhat yellow; the anterior cervical lymph nodes and spleen are palpable. Some type of infection is implied, and a mild jaundice must also be accounted for.[1]

A detailed list of the most frequently considered hypotheses generated in this case and the number of physicians who considered each is provided in Table 4.1. The initial hypotheses are most commonly general (for instance, infection). Subsequent hypotheses fall mainly into four categories of infections:

(a) General, nonspecific infections, including "infection," influenza, viral illness, and viral respiratory infection. Generated early, these hypotheses account for most of the initial complaints. While excessive sleeping might point to disturbance of the central nervous system (CNS), most of our subjects argued that

---

[1] Nonmedical readers need not be worried if the implications of each cue are not clear. The point is that some explanation must be found for each abnormal finding. The problem solver's task is to work out a defensible explanation that also can lead to remedial action, if possible, and if not, to offer comfort, support, and reassurance to the patient.

Table 4.1 Number of subjects (physicians) who considered major hypotheses at selected points in the workup of simulation 1.

Hypothesis[a]	Total at any point	As first hypothesis	At quarter mark	At halfway mark	At conclusion
Infection[b]	21	14	15	19	5
Infectious mononucleosis	20	2	9	15	20
Infectious hepatitis	18	5	9	11	5
Hemolytic anemia	17				
Hereditary spherocytic anemia	10				8
Viral illness or viral respiratory infection	8		4	6	1
Meningitis	7		5	4	0
Anemia	6			3	
Influenza	4		3	1	0
Encephalitis	4		2	3	0
Leukemia	4			1	0
Lymphoma	4		0	0	1

[a] Twelve hypotheses in addition to those listed were each considered by one or two subjects at some point in the problem.
[b] Includes acute febrile illness, viral illness, bacterial infection, and viral respiratory infection.

flu-like illnesses are often associated with feelings of exhaustion and prolonged sleeping. As more data become available, the general category is reformulated into more specific hypotheses.

(b) Central nervous system infections, including meningitis and encephalitis. These hypotheses, which attempt to account especially for severe headaches and excessive sleeping, are considered in the first half of the workup. Subsequent support is lacking and they are rejected as the workup proceeds.

(c) Infectious mononucleosis. This hypothesis is entertained early by slightly less than half the subjects, and the number increases steadily as the problem moves along. It is an association not only to the complaints but also to the patient's age and occupation.

(d) Infectious hepatitis is considered early, along with infectious mononucleosis, but support diminishes in the laboratory phase of the workup.

Regardless of which of these hypotheses are considered, the laboratory tests open up a new phase of the inquiry. All physicians ordered a routine complete blood count and differential. A low hemoglobin (9.7 mg%) and a low red-cell count are reported. Anemia is clearly a finding to be pursued, and the problem now shifts to the differential diagnosis of anemia and its relation to the infectious process already identified. This exploration was conducted to varying degrees of depth by the physicians, those more expert in hematology considering more possibilities and ordering a more thorough set of laboratory tests. The number of physicians who will independently pursue the differential diagnosis of anemia compared with the number who will seek consultation or refer the problem to a specialist is likely to vary from one sample to another, since these numbers will depend upon the physicians' assessments of their own competence in the domain, the availability of specialists, and the expectation of one's local medical reference group that a consultant be called for this problem. In our sample all but one of the physicians explicitly generated at least one anemia hypothesis. Even he mentioned hemolytic anemia once, ordered a Coomb's test,[2] and noted that it was negative. It is difficult to see why he would have done this were hemo-

---

[2] A positive Coomb's test indicates that red cells have become immune to, or have developed an antibody response to, some substance in the bloodstream. This immune response predisposes red cells to destruction (hemolysis).

lytic anemia not being considered, but his protocol is not entirely clear on this point.

It seems reasonable to conclude that given the cue of low hemoglobin, any physician ought to be able to identify anemia and have a plan either for workup or consultation. The more difficult question, perhaps, is when to order a complete blood count and so obtain the needed cue. In our sample this question was answered by treating the complete blood count (CBC) as a routine datum to be obtained with all new patients to search for problems and to establish a data base. In general, the problem is one of balancing a routine workup to search for potential problems with a workup focused to test existing formulations.

The problem space of simulation 1 is the set of possible diagnostic solutions to the problem. There are two major areas of problem formulation, infection and anemia. Part of the complexity of this problem consists in recognizing two separate problem areas. Most of the inaccurate diagnoses came about as a result of linking anemia to infection, however it was diagnosed, and not considering anemia as a separate problem. As in many other studies of problem solving, we find that multiple-solution problems are more difficult to solve than single-solution problems. Feinstein (1973b) claims that patients with multiple diseases are inadequately handled by statistical models of diagnosis. Our data suggest that clinical logic also has difficulty with disorders such as anemia that may arise from a variety of linked or unrelated entities. The problem in either instance is when to cluster probabilistic cues and when to treat them as implying distinct causes. A statistical model need not necessarily be inferior for this task.

In the representation in Figure 4.1 more specific diagnoses are nested under general categories. The earliest hypothesis of fourteen out of twenty-one physicians was very general, such as infection or acute febrile illness. As more data became available, the problem formulation became more specific. The pattern is similar with anemia. First the general diagnosis is made, and then more specific classification is achieved via laboratory tests. Tree structures for infection and for anemia effectively represent this problem space. On the whole, physicians in this case moved from general to specific formulations.

Simulation 2

This case involved a white, male college student in his early twenties who complains of growing weakness and exhaustion. In

Figure 4.1 Cognitive organization of simulation 1.

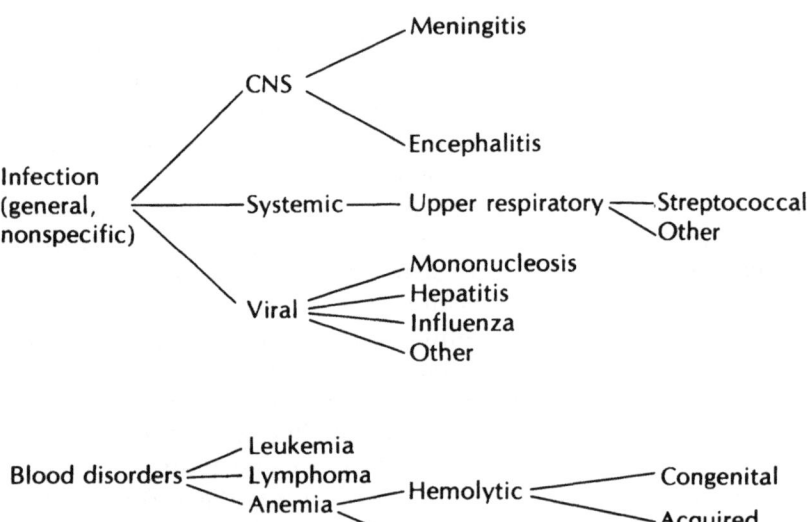

the history it emerges that these symptoms were preceded by severe cramping and diarrhea of several months' duration. Further inquiry discloses that he has lost about thirty pounds in spite of continued high food intake. Shortness of breath and some chest pain on mild exertion, such as climbing stairs, are also reported. The difficulty of diagnosis is increased by the absence of gross blood in the stool, a point which nearly all physicians ask about.

A gastrointestinal problem of some sort or an endocrine problem is implied by the initial history. Table 4.2 presents the hypotheses considered most frequently. A psychogenic problem (irritable bowel syndrome) is suggested by the age and college status of the patient as well as his initial complaints, but is ruled out by the subsequent history of substantial weight loss as well as positive laboratory and X-ray findings. Ulcerative colitis and regional enteritis (Crohn's disease, ileitis, or granulomatous colitis) are initiated by the complaints of cramping and diarrhea, and supported by the subsequent workup. Hypoglycemia is suggested by weakness and exhaustion, but is ruled out when other causes for those complaints become clear. Hyperthyroidism is initiated chiefly by the report of weight loss in spite of normal or increased food intake, but is not confirmed by thyroid function tests. When

Table 4.2 Number of subjects (physicians) who considered major hypotheses at selected points in the workup of simulation 2.

Hypothesis[a]	Total at any point	As first hypothesis	At quarter mark	At halfway mark	At conclusion
Ulcerative colitis	20	9	13	17	18
Anemia	15	1	2	3	6
Regional enteritis (and Crohn's disease)	13	5	8	9	2
Hyperthyroidism	13	1	3	8	
Granulomatous colitis	10		2	2	7
Malabsorption syndrome	9		3	4	1
Psychogenic problem	7	4	5	2	0
Amebiasis	7		4	4	1
Ileitis	6		1	2	1
Ulcer	5			2	
Carcinoid syndrome	5			3	1
Diabetes	5			1	
Whipple's disease	4		1	3	1
Hypoglycemia	4		1	4	

[a] Twenty-one hypotheses in addition to those listed were each considered by one to three subjects at some point in the problem.

Figure 4.2   Cognitive organization of simulation 2.

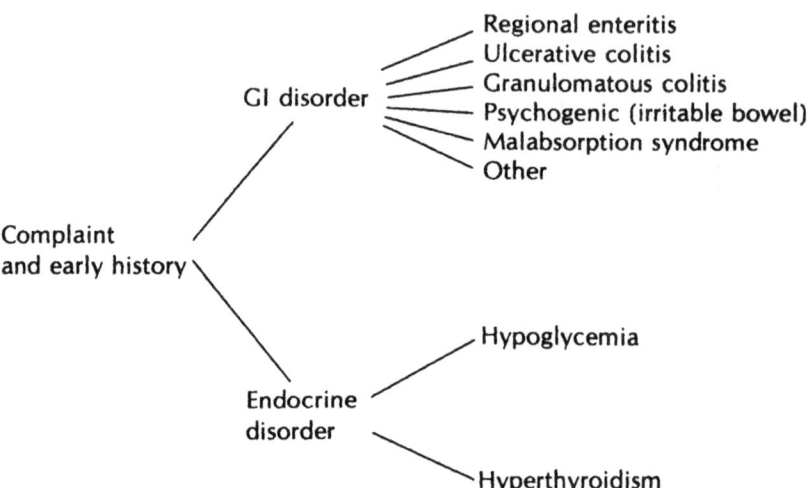

anemia is identified as a separate problem, it is assumed to be secondary to the gastrointestinal disease that has caused blood loss, a view supported by the laboratory finding of occult blood in the feces.

In contrast to simulation 1, this problem is not characterized by an orderly progression from general to specific hypotheses. The earliest hypotheses are generally quite specific, as shown in Table 4.2, and the problem structure is that of multiple competing hypotheses at a roughly similar level of specificity (Figure 4.2). Hypotheses are gradually eliminated by the failure to find confirmatory data and by the accumulation of support for other hypotheses. For example, hyperthyroidism is ruled out by a normal PBI (protein-bound iodine, a test of thyroid function) as well as by finding occult blood in the feces. The case narrows eventually to a choice between ulcerative colitis and regional enteritis (or variants such as regional ileitis, Crohn's disease, or granulomatous colitis). Sigmoidoscopy[3] and a lower gastrointestinal X-ray series (barium enema) are decisive diagnostic procedures. Most of the physicians relied upon the radiologist's report, but the gastroenterologists preferred to read the films themselves. In

[3] Visual examination of a portion of the colon by means of an instrument that illuminates the tissue.

either case the workup rapidly leads to a relatively small set of hypotheses with the ultimate diagnostic decisions resting on selected physical findings and results of special tests. Accurate problem solving in this case thus depends on generating an adequate set of hypotheses; recognizing what data are needed to confirm or rule out each alternative, a matter of retrieving knowledge from memory; and obtaining these data and interpreting them accurately.

The structure of the problem space—multiple competing hypotheses—makes it possible to test several hypotheses at once by the same set of data. The difficulty of the problem is not increased by adding many alternative diagnoses, though skilled internists can certainly do that. The difficulty is rather a function of the ambiguity of symptoms and the absence of typical findings. For example, early diagnosis would be facilitated if the patient had reported gross blood in the stool. Once a pyschogenic disturbance is ruled out, usually by the evidence of severe weight loss, the search is located within the gastrointestinal or endocrine domains, with the latter finding no confirmation in subsequent laboratory studies.

Simulation 3

In this case an unmarried female, age twenty-one, is brought to the emergency room in the morning with acute paralysis in both legs. She had gone to bed the previous evening apparently well. The patient is extremely upset by the sudden loss of motion and is agitated and crying. The chief complaint and her dramatic agitation lead to the common early hypothesis of conversion hysteria. Early in the encounter the patient repeatedly asks question like, "What is wrong with me? Will the paralysis spread? How long will I be like this? What do you think is going on?" The physician's initial problem is to calm the patient sufficiently so that some history can be obtained and a physical examination performed. The available history includes the experience for the past two weeks of a transient, peculiar sensation on the right side of the patient's body. When she took a bath or shower, she also noticed that her body did not feel the same on both sides. Two or three days prior to admission to the emergency room she began to experience intense urinary urgency. Four weeks earlier she had become suddenly blind in one eye, but this symptom passed; it is not reported spontaneously unless particular inquiries are made into previous sensory deficits. The social history is that the patient is single, has a boyfriend with whom she has been sexually intimate, and her menstrual period is two weeks overdue.

On physical examination, the available findings[4] include a positive bilateral Babinski sign; weakness of left arm, hand, and fingers; and complete loss of sensation and voluntary motion from the waist down, with sensation preserved in the saddle area. Temperature sense is lost to T2 bilaterally, deep pain lost to T3 on the right and to T4 on the left, vibration lost to T9, and touch lost to T10. Weakness of the abdominal muscles may be inferred when the patient cannot sit up without assistance and cannot maintain a sitting position without support.

The case history is fairly typical for multiple sclerosis, since there are transient multiple sensory and motor losses that cannot be neurologically accounted for by one lesion. For those physicians who had retained a working knowledge of neurological disease, it was not an especially difficult diagnostic problem. The case became difficult for those physicians who closed prematurely on the earliest hypothesis, conversion hysteria, and who therefore either did not obtain or did not correctly interpret the evidence that pointed away from psychiatric and toward neurological illness. Moreover, the case was emotionally demanding. The simulated patient was the only one of the three who was agitated and upset; her manner was sometimes perceived as uncooperative and overly demanding. History taking was difficult because of the patient's anxious condition. Furthermore, a variety of symptoms and findings were not linked in her mind, so she did not spontaneously report the findings that a knowledgeable physician could connect. A great deal of specific questioning was required. The patient responded poorly to nonleading questions and relatively well to directive questions, although some clinicians tried to deal with her agitation by using nonleading questions to encourage her to tell her own story. It was difficult for some physicians to establish effective rapport with her.

As the diagnosis was suspected or became clear, several were

---

[4] This paragraph describes in technical medical language a variety of neurological abnormalities including sensory and motor losses. The pattern of losses is inconsistent with a single location for the lesion and consistent with multiple sites. The letter-number codes (T2, T3) identify the vertebra at which normal function is restored, for example, thoracic vertebra #2. Babinski's sign is an abnormal fanning of the toes when the sole of the foot is stroked and indicates some type of lower motor neuron lesion.

distressed by the patient's illness, because they knew that no accepted treatment has a definitive effect on its course. What to tell the patient and how to comfort her thus became a major problem. Rapport issues are a significant component of the doctor-patient relationship and impinge upon the patient's immediate and longer-term satisfaction with a given physician. However, these issues did not appear to have any substantial impact on the processes of gathering data, formulating hypotheses, and drawing diagnostic conclusions. Facility in these areas appeared to be more related to experience and practice in neurological problems.

Table 4.3 presents the hypotheses considered most frequently at several points in this case. Conversion hysteria, a specific formulation of psychiatric illness, was the first hypothesis of twenty out of twenty-three physicians. It accounts for the chief complaint, paralysis of the legs, prior to the discovery of positive neurological findings. For many physicians in the sample, the hypothesis was also suggested by the patient's agitated, "hysterical" manner. They did not recall or did not know that patients with conversion reactions are more typically described in psychiatric literature as calm and relatively undisturbed by their symptoms. A plausible psychogenic justification for the patient's ailment often was located in the possibility that she was pregnant. Multiple sclerosis, the other popular alternative, was usually not generated until later in the workup when evidence was uncovered of multiple sensory losses that could not be explained by one lesion. The discovery of transient blindness in one eye was frequently the critical stimulus for the hypothesis—anecdotal evidence for the critical role that may be played by a single cue in hypothesis generation. Multiple sclerosis is also somewhat more frequent in pregnant women. Provided that multiple sclerosis was generated, the cognitive structure of the problem (Figure 4.3) became that of multiple competing hypotheses: most of the evidence positive for multiple sclerosis is also negative for hysteria. More general hypotheses such as trauma, upper motor neuron lesion, or tumor had scattered support, but most of the information search dealt with testing specific alternatives.

Psychology of Early Hypothesis Generation

Each of these problems illustrates that early hypothesis generation is a typical feature of medical inquiry. In some cases an early hypothesis is progressively refined and revised with increasing

Table 4.3 Number of subjects (physicians) who considered major hypotheses at selected points in the workup of simulation 3.

Hypothesis[a]	Total at any point	As first hypothesis	At quarter mark	At halfway mark	At conclusion
Hysteria (conversion)	22	20	18	17	10
Multiple sclerosis	16		7	12	16
Guillain-Barré syndrome	9	1	5	3	2
Spinal cord tumor, abcess, or lesion	6				2
CNS infection (other than polio)	6		1	3	3
Tumor (other than cord or un-specified)	5	1	2	3	2
Polio	4		0	1	1
Trauma	4	1	1	1	1
Upper motor neuron lesion	4				3

[a] Twelve hypotheses in addition to those listed were each considered by one to three subjects at some point in the problem.

Figure 4.3 Cognitive organization of simulation 3.

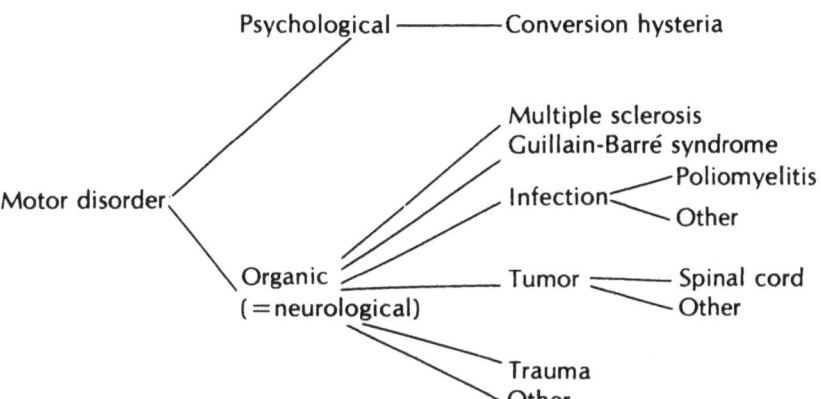

specificity. For example, physicians move from the general disorder "anemia" to a more particular etiologic classification, such as "hemolytic anemia." In other cases the existence of a general category such as "gastrointestinal problem" may be logically necessary, but the working categories of the physician seem to be more specific practically from the outset. A less experienced clinician or a medical student might move through the more general categories more explicitly and slowly.

The number of hypotheses generated and assessed in each problem appears to far exceed the usually accepted capacity of working memory. However, memory capacity can be substantially augmented by testing hypotheses hierarchically (Chapter 7). Besides, as long as one hypothesis replaces another and evaluation proceeds sequentially, the principle of a limit on working memory is not violated; indeed, it is exemplified.

In our preliminary work (Elstein et al., 1972) early generation of specific hypotheses was identified as a critical feature of a new theory of medical inquiry. As a generalization, that statement is clearly in error. The structure of medical problems is varied and complex. Some are handled by generating specific hypotheses early, others by a more regular progression from general to specific. The consistent finding is that some hypotheses are always generated early and that medical diagnosis does not proceed in a strictly inductive fashion. Hypothetico-deductive processes are ubiquitous in solving complex problems. Information-processing theories of problem solving may be viewed as hypothesis-testing theories (Thomas, 1974). Feinstein's (1973b) analysis of diagnostic reasoning as a series of intermediate decisions is also consistent with this view. He pointed out that some diagnostic decisions are reached by an orderly progression through stations, while in other cases a diagnostician may move directly to a terminal point. We conclude that both the route and the nature of the end point are determined more by the structure of the task than by the problem solver's preferences or cognitive style.

Hypothesis generation involves retrieval from memory, a process that is studied in more detail in Chapter 7. Clinicians generally identify incidence or probability as the major heuristic principle guiding the retrieval process. It is conceivable, however, that some hypotheses are more salient and more easily recalled for reasons other than frequency. For example, recent exposure to a rare case may influence salience, which is then translated into an elevated estimate of probability. More recent events tend to be recalled more easily and judged more likely than instances from the more distant past (Tversky and Kahneman, 1974).

A different bias produced by availability relates to utility: the probability of a medical complication or unfavorable outcome might be estimated by the ease with which it can be imagined, not by its true rate of occurrence. Subjective estimates of the probability of an undesirable event could be correlated with estimates of its hazard or potential loss (utility), while an analytic treatment of this problem would seek independent estimates of the two parameters. Ease of recall is not the only heuristic principle used in estimating probability. The similarity between a cluster of cues and recognized clinical descriptions is also used, an instance of representativeness (Kahneman and Tversky, 1972).

There have been very few studies dealing with the accuracy of clinicians' estimates of disease base rates or of the degree of association between a sign or symptom and a disease (Gustafson et al., 1971; Leaper et al., 1972). Nevertheless, it is possible that even substantial errors in estimates of disease base rates do not make much difference in clinical medicine, since typically so many data are collected and evaluated. Lusted (1968) suggested that where large numbers of data are gathered for a diagnostic judgment, the prior estimate of the base rate of any disease will be so greatly revised that the initial accuracy is relatively unimportant. The effects of errors in base rates, or clinicians' insensitivity to base rates, upon the cost of diagnostic workups have not been extensively studied.

Statistical Summary of Twelve Dependent Variables

Thus far we have discussed cognitive aspects of medical problem solving by reference to three problems studied in some detail. It is now time to take up the second question on our list, "What processes characterize the thinking of expert physicians as contrasted with nonexperts?" Basically, we shall be testing for statistically significant differences between two groups. We shall approach this topic first by analyzing the three problems statistically and looking for evidence of consistency among physicians across problems.

Table 4.4 presents the means and standard deviations of the continuous dependent variables for each simulation, calculated over the entire sample of physicians who worked each problem. Fewer than twenty-four workups are available for each simulation because of occasional equipment malfunctions during the workup or, rarely, because time pressures and conflicts made it impossible to schedule a subject for all three simulations.

Cue Acquisition

The length of workups, as measured by the number of information search units, varies considerably both across and within simulations. A certain portion of each workup is assumed to be devoted to a routine search for additional problems or cues. Variations in the thoroughness of this search can produce variations in the number of information search units without similar variation in the number of pertinent data collected. By contrast, then, the number of pertinent data collected varies much less. The mean percentage of cues acquired ranges from a low of 46.5 on simulation 3 to a high of 57.4 on simulation 1. The mean percentage of critical findings acquired varies from 45.0 on simulation 3 to 66.6 on simulation 1. Subsequent analyses will investigate the relation of thoroughness of data collection to successful medical problem solving. For now, it may be observed simply that the number of data acquired by experienced physicians, even under conditions of minimal time pressure, averages about 50 percent of the defined data base of presumably relevant cues.

The correlation between the variables percentage of cues acquired and percentage of critical findings acquired is always high; .75 in simulation 1, .90 in simulation 2, and .69 in simulation 3. It appears that the physicians generally did not focus data collection

Table 4.4 Means and standard deviations (in parentheses) of the dependent variables in each of the three simulations.

Variable	Simulation 1 ($n=21$)	Simulation 2 ($n=22$)	Simulation 3 ($n=23$)
1. Total information search units	147.6 (51.0)	203.4 (86.9)	210.7 (65.3)
2. Point of generation of first hypothesis	13.9 (19.0)	20.8 (17.8)	7.4 (14.9)
3. Number of hypotheses active one-quarter through workup	2.3 (1.4)	2.4 (1.7)	2.0 (1.1)
4. Number of hypotheses active halfway through workup	2.8 (1.4)	3.6 (2.0)	2.2 (1.2)
5. Total number of hypotheses generated	6.7 (2.0)	7.0 (2.2)	4.2 (2.0)
6. Number of hypotheses retained	2.9 (1.3)	2.0 (1.4)	2.1 (1.2)
7. Percentage of cues acquired	57.4 (6.4)	47.1 (8.0)	46.5 (9.6)
8. Number of cues acquired	52.1 (5.9)	52.3 (8.8)	32.7 (5.1)
9. Number of critical findings acquired	66.6 (8.8)	51.8 (7.8)	45.0 (10.5)
10. Percentage of critical findings acquired	32.9 (4.3)	24.1 (3.6)	18.5 (4.9)
11. Efficiency	46.8 (7.0)	32.4 (9.1)	46.4 (9.0)
12. Accuracy of interpretation	62.4 (9.7)	74.6 (16.0)	64.3 (16.7)

on critical findings in preference to other cues in the cases. Several processes seem to be at work here. First, there are data of general usefulness that are collected even though they do not bear on the hypotheses that will turn out to be of critical importance. In a setting with no time constraints there is no need to focus exclusively on data relevant to the immediately presenting problem, and several clinicians conducted very wide-ranging inquiries. Second, as will be discussed in more detail later, the physicians tended not to employ the distinction between cues and critical findings, and instead used a three-point system for weighting all cues. Third, as a case unfolds, hypotheses may become more focused and permit greater concentration on critical findings. For example, there is an orderly plan for the differential diagnosis of anemia which, if followed to the end, will yield a large number of critical findings in a focused and concentrated fashion. But in the early stages of this case, there is little to suggest that this subroutine should be implemented. Anemia is not identified as a problem until partway through the workup. Finally, the cue list itself was selective and did not include noncontributory normal findings.

Early Hypothesis Generation

The scores on variable 2, point of generation of first hypothesis, support the proposition that hypotheses are generated early, well before data collection is far advanced. Even under the strict rules set out for determining when the first hypothesis was generated, it appears that hypothesis generation begins about 10 percent of the way through a workup.

Two additional measures of early hypothesis generation support this statement. Consider first how many potentially relevant data each physician had obtained prior to generating this first hypothesis: a relevant datum was defined as any cue that had at least one nonzero entry in the cue-hypothesis matrix of weights. These cues should have some weight in evaluating at least one of the hypotheses in the matrix. The median numbers of nonzero cues obtained by each physician prior to generating the first hypothesis were four, five, and three cues in simulations 1, 2, and 3, respectively. These cues were either available on the summary sheets of basic data presented to the physician as he entered the room to meet the patient or were obtained in the early minutes of history taking and observation.

How much time was needed to generate the first hypothesis?

The first five minutes of running time on each videotape, including any thinking-aloud episodes, were watched and any scorable hypothesis generation was noted. The number of physicians generating at least one hypothesis in the first five minutes was 20 in simulation 1, 18 in simulation 2, and 23 in simulation 3. Hypothesis generation was most delayed in simulation 2, but even there over 80 percent of the sample had at least one hypothesis within five minutes. In sum, the evidence for early hypothesis generation is so consistent that it remains a major feature of our theory of medical problem solving.

Memory Capacity and Hypotheses

Variables 3 through 6 deal with the number of hypotheses under consideration at various points in the workup. There is remarkable consistency across problems: the means range between 2 and 4, the standard deviations between 1 and 2. On all three simulations the mean number of hypotheses considered at any one time remains relatively constant through various points of the problem even to the conclusion. Regarding the earlier phases of the inquiry, this finding shows that when a hypothesis is rejected, its place is usually taken by another or by a reformulation of the rejected hypothesis, so that premature closure is prevented. The function of hypotheses as organizers of data in short-term memory is suggested by the fact that the values obtained for number of hypotheses active one-quarter of the way through workup and number of hypotheses active halfway through workup are both on the order of the values for the number of chunks of complex material that can be retained at once in memory (Simon, 1974). The number of hypotheses retained at the conclusion of the workup reflects also the stringent rules employed for determining when a hypothesis had been terminated. One consequence of these rules is that a hypothesis was classified as "under consideration" unless it was explicitly terminated at the conclusion of a workup. This means that the values for hypotheses retained are an upper limit. It is quite probable that many of the physicians had in fact rejected a number of hypotheses carried on the books as under consideration.

The total number of hypotheses considered in any problem averaged between 4 and 7 (variable 5). Storage capacity can be increased by a nesting strategy or by sequential reformulation. Fewer than five hypotheses may be considered either because of deficiencies of knowledge in an area or a lack of complexity of the problem.

Problem Specificity

The dependent variables presented in Table 4.4 measure several aspects of the medical inquiry process: hypothesis generation, cue acquisition, and cue interpretation. These operations are necessarily involved in all medical inquiries. Yet our original intent was to distinguish criterial from noncriterial physicians on the basis of differences in aspects of the problem-solving process. A first step toward this aim was to analyze the data for evidence of intraindividual consistency across problems using correlation technique. Table 4.5 provides no evidence of statistically significant intraindividual consistency on any of these dependent measures across problems. Remarkably, not even one of thirty-six correlations reached significance at the .05 level, a finding that could have been attributed to chance alone. Table 4.5 thus suggests that intraindividual consistency on any of the dependent variables is weak and that scores on the variables are influenced much more by the structure of the problem and the individual clinician's understanding of its task demands than by consistency in individual problem-solving style.

Table 4.5 Stability of dependent variables across simulations, as indicated by product-moment correlations *r* between simulations 1 and 2, 1 and 3, and 2 and 3.

Variable	$r_{1,2}$ (n=20)	$r_{1,3}$ (n=20)	$r_{2,3}$ (n=21)
Total information search units	.19	.27	.35
Point of generation of first hypothesis	.35	.16	.03
Number of hypotheses active one-quarter through workup	.19	-.16	.02
Number of hypotheses active halfway through workup	-.02	.07	.05
Total number of hypotheses generated	-.22	-.23	.31
Number of hypotheses retained	-.26	-.03	.13
Percentage of cues acquired	.33	.06	.20
Number of cues acquired	.39	-.18	.17
Percentage of critical findings acquired	.27	-.09	.27
Number of critical findings	.24	-.07	.15
Efficiency	.36	.19	-.12
Accuracy of interpretation	.32	-.37	-.35

Further implications of this table will be discussed in detail subsequently. For now, let us simply point out that: (a) there is a high degree of content specificity in the process of solving medical problems; (b) it will therefore be difficult to predict from a physician's performance on one problem his performance on a new problem in a different domain; (c) content specificity implies that excellence in medical problem solving is content dependent as well as process dependent; and (d) assessing clinical competence is complex, and multiple measures will be required.

Results on Five Selected Dependent Variables

The analysis of differences between criterial and noncriterial physicians in terms of process measures of medical problem solving was carried one step farther, using five variables selected from Table 4.4: point of generation of first hypothesis, total number of hypotheses generated, percentage of cues acquired, efficiency, and accuracy of interpretation.

Rationale for Selection

These variables were selected by a combination of theory and cluster analyses of the correlations among scores on the twelve continuous variables, computed separately for each problem. The cluster analysis was corroborated by factor analysis. Both techniques identified essentially the same groups. The selection of variables to represent each cluster was based on the model of medical inquiry developed in the study. Cue acquisition variables are efficiency and percentage of cues acquired, cue interpretation is represented by accuracy of interpretation, and hypothesis generation is represented by point of generation of first hypothesis and total number of hypotheses generated. The correlation matrices are presented in Table 4.6.

Univariate analyses of variance were performed on each of these dependent variables, for each simulation separately, and then for the grand means over all three simulations. For this final set of analyses the sample comprised only those physicians for whom data were available on all three problems. Multivariate analysis of variance was considered, but not performed because it was not known how to order the variables.

Table 4.6 Correlations of dependent variables for simulations 1, 2, and 3.

	N ISUS	ISU/H₁	H/25% ISUS	H/50% ISUS	H_{TOT}	H_{RET}	%CUES	NCUES	%CF	NCF	EFF	ACC INT
Simulation 1 (n = 21):												
N ISUS	1.00											
ISU/H₁	-0.11	1.00										
H/25% ISUS	.23	-0.46	1.00									
H/50% ISUS	.22	-.44	0.84	1.00								
H_{TOT}	.30	-.14	.57	0.70	1.00							
H_{RET}	.19	.03	.23	.34	0.20	1.00						
%CUES	.60	-.17	.48	.36	.42	0.10	1.00					
NCUES	.60	-.11	.39	.28	.36	.09	0.96	1.00				
%CF	.40	-.21	.20	.18	.18	-.04	.75	0.79	1.00			
NCF	.41	-.21	.17	.15	.18	-.07	.75	.80	1.00	1.00		
EFF	.15	-.25	.19	.46	.57	.18	.10	.14	0.34	0.36	1.00	
ACC INT	.18	-.01	.13	.28	.06	.56	.23	.14	.19	.16	0.12	1.00
Simulation 2 (n = 22):												
N ISUS	1.00											
ISU/H₁	0.36	1.00										
H/25% ISUS	.48	-0.27	1.00									
H/50% ISUS	.48	-.68	0.87	1.00								
H_{TOT}	.13	-.26	.71	0.63	1.00							
H_{RET}	.12	-.11	.09	.02	0.25	1.00						
%CUES	.55	.20	.54	.55	.45	0.24	1.00					
NCUES	.55	.21	.54	.56	.44	.23	0.91	1.00				
%CF	.46	.24	.50	.50	.56	.17	.90	0.91	1.00			
NCF	.49	.24	.54	.53	.57	.15	.90	.91	0.99	1.00		
EFF	-.13	-.28	.31	.27	.54	-.09	.15	.15	.28	0.29	1.00	
ACC INT	-.17	-.44	.15	.05	.02	.22	-.24	-.24	-.29	-.26	0.11	1.00
Simulation 3 (n = 23):												
N ISUS	1.00											
ISU/H₁	-0.16	1.00										
H/25% ISUS	.27	-0.46	1.00									
H/50% ISUS	.29	-.39	0.79	1.00								
H_{TOT}	.03	-.22	.57	0.47	1.00							
H_{RET}	-.12	.25	.17	-.05	0.49	1.00						
%CUES	.49	-.32	.48	.38	.27	0.02	1.00					
NCUES	.56	.05	.37	.39	.29	.03	0.89	1.00				
%CF	.25	.01	.29	.07	.45	.43	.69	0.70	1.00			
NCF	.14	.08	.26	.02	.58	.49	.46	.55	0.92	1.00		
EFF	.03	.09	.23	.08	.07	-.08	.05	.21	.26	0.27	1.00	
ACC INT	.01	.08	.05	.16	-.16	.47	.28	.24	-.02	-.16	0.10	1.00

KEY

N ISUS = total information search units.
ISU/H₁ = point of generation of first hypothesis.
H/25% ISUS = number of hypotheses active one-quarter through workup.
H/50% ISUS = number of hypotheses active halfway through workup.
H_{TOT} = total number of hypotheses generated.
H_{RET} = number of hypotheses retained.
%CUES = percentage of cues acquired.
NCUES = number of cues acquired.
%CF = percentage of critical findings acquired.
NCF = number of critical findings acquired.
EFF = efficiency.
ACC INT = accuracy of interpretation.

Criterial versus Noncriterial Groups

Criterial and noncriterial group means on the selected variables, by simulation and averaged across simulations, are shown in Table 4.7.

The results of the analyses are presented in Table 4.8. None of the differences between groups are statistically significant at the .05 level, except that criterial physicians ask more questions prior to generating a first hypothesis on simulation 2. The extent of differences fluctuates widely across problems, as shown by shifts in the observed means. This is another indication of problem specificity in measures of problem-solving process. There is considerable variation within each group, and poor discrimination between the performances of criterial and noncriterial groups. One might identify a trend in the difference in accuracy of interpretation, where scores are averaged across simulations ($p = .07$). Certainly the means all tend in this direction, but intragroup variation or unreliability of measurement wash out intergroup effects. Even if this finding were clearly significant statistically, accuracy of interpretation is as much a matter of memory organization as it is of problem-solving strategy. Moreover, this variable turns out to be even more strongly related to accuracy of diagnosis.

The findings are consistent with the notion that performance on medical problems is highly problem specific and that process measures do not especially reflect underlying individual consistency in approach to problems.

To explore this question one step further, we asked about the degree to which scores on the problems could be generalized to other problems. The correlations in Table 4.5 had already suggested that intraindividual consistency was low. A generalizability analysis (Hoyt, 1941; modified by Allal for a repeated-measures design) was performed with respect to group differences and within-group variability. Statistically speaking, the question is whether scores on the three simulations could reasonably be regarded as repeated measures of the same processes. Is there enough consistency across problems to give confidence that the problems could be treated as items selected from a larger pool of all possible medical problems? To what degree are we entitled to generalize from scores on these problems, treated as test items, to the larger domain of behavior that the test presumably samples? Table 4.9 shows clearly that, with respect to the distinction

Table 4.7 Criterial (C) and noncriterial (NC) group means (M) and standard deviations (SD) on selected dependent variables: by simulation, and average across simulations.

Variable		Simulation 1		Simulation 2		Simulation 3		Average[a]	
		C (n = 14)	NC (n = 7)	C (n = 15)	NC (n = 7)	C (n = 17)	NC (n = 6)	C (n = 13)	NC (n = 6)
Point of generation of first hypothesis	M	16.86	5.86	26.73	8.14	8.06	5.50	15.18	6.78
	SD	21.62	4.82	16.16	12.40	16.59	5.22	9.44	7.47
Total number of hypotheses generated	M	7.00	5.71	6.73	6.86	3.94	5.00	5.95	5.78
	SD	2.04	1.28	2.14	2.64	1.63	2.38	1.09	1.34
Percentage of cues acquired	M	57.50	56.57	48.53	44.14	46.82	45.50	50.62	47.56
	SD	6.23	6.54	8.25	5.72	10.07	6.78	4.95	2.99
Efficiency	M	48.64	43.00	32.60	31.86	45.82	50.00	42.80	41.67
	SD	0.48	6.05	7.48	11.31	8.58	7.42	6.13	2.98
Accuracy of interpretation	M	65.14	58.14	75.13	73.43	65.41	61.17	70.08	64.50
	SD	7.97	10.59	13.83	19.00	15.40	18.29	6.27	8.26

[a] Figures in this column are derived only from physicians who completed all three simulations.

Table 4.8 Univariate analyses of variance: criterial versus noncriterial group means on selected dependent variables.

Variable	Source of variation	df	MS	F	p
Simulation 1:					
ISU/H_1	Between	1	366.10	1.01	.33
	Within	19	361.74		
	Total	20			
H_{TOT}	Between	1	4.67	1.14	.30
	Within	19	4.11		
	Total	20			
% CUES	Between	1	0.21	0.00	.95
	Within	19	43.10		
	Total	20			
EFF	Between	1	141.17	3.18	.09
	Within	19	44.43		
	Total	20			
ACC INT	Between	1	309.43	3.74	.07
	Within	19	82.72		
	Total	20			
Simulation 2:					
ISU/H_1	Between	1	1,539.83	6.03	.02
	Within	20	255.27		
	Total	21			
H_{TOT}	Between	1	3.91	0.79	.39
	Within	20	4.95		
	Total	21			
% CUES	Between	1	13.26	0.20	.66
	Within	20	66.37		
	Total	21			
EFF	Between	1	0.50	0.00	.94
	Within	20	86.83		
	Total	21			
ACC INT	Between	1	48.00	0.10	.68
	Within	20	268.07		
	Total	21			

Variable	Source of Variation	df	MS	F	p
Simulation 3:					
ISU/H_1	Between	1	29.04	0.13	.73
	Within	21	230.69		
	Total	22			
H_{TOT}	Between	1	4.97	1.32	.26
	Within	21	3.76		
	Total	22			
% CUES	Between	1	7.77	0.08	.78
	Within	21	95.24		
	Total	22			
EFF	Between	1	24.35	0.29	.60
	Within	21	85.25		
	Total	22			
ACC INT	Between	1	79.92	0.28	.60
	Within	21	287.57		
	Total	22			
Average across simulations:					
ISU/H_1	Between	1	231.51	2.91	.11
	Within	17	79.58		
	Total	18			
H_{TOT}	Between	1	0.11	0.08	.79
	Within	17	1.40		
	Total	18			
% CUES	Between	1	31.71	1.55	.23
	Within	17	20.41		
	Total	18			
EFF	Between	1	11.62	0.39	.54
	Within	17	29.93		
	Total	18			
ACC INT	Between	1	157.53	3.63	.07
	Within	17	43.44		
	Total	18			

ISU/H_1 = point of generation of first hypothesis.
H_{TOT} = total number of hypotheses generated.
% CUES = percentage of cues acquired.
EFF = efficiency.
ACC INT = accuracy of interpretation.

Table 4.9 Consistency of criterial and noncriterial physicians across three simulations.

Variable	$MS_{S:G}$	$MS_{SM:G}$	$MS_{S:G} - MS_{SM:G}$	Generalizability coefficient
1. Total information search units	7,912.52	2,284.22	5,628.30	.71
2. Point of generation of first hypothesis	239.21	166.16	73.05	.31
3. Number of hypotheses active one-quarter through workup	2.09	2.03	0.06	.03
4. Number of hypotheses active halfway through workup	2.61	2.33	0.28	.11
5. Total number of hypotheses generated	4.22	4.40	-0.18	-.04
6. Number of hypotheses retained	1.58	1.68	-0.10	-.06
7. Number of cues acquired	61.36	49.15	12.12	.20
8. Percentage of cues acquired	39.81	31.86	7.95	.20
9. Number of critical findings acquired	89.96	73.94	16.02	.18
10. Percentage of critical findings acquired	20.32	17.09	3.23	.16
11. Efficiency	89.97	69.10	20.87	.23
12. Accuracy of interpretation	130.57	241.20	-110.63	.85

$MS_{S:G}$ = mean square for subjects within groups.
$MS_{SM:G}$ = mean square for subjects by repeated measures within groups.
Generalizability coefficient = $(MS_{S:G} - MS_{SM:G}) / MS_{S:G}$.

between criterial and noncriterial physicians, generalizability is very low. Once again, the behavior of the groups is not consistent across problems except on length of workup. The argument for problem specificity in medical inquiry, for its dependence on understanding the content and particular demands of the task, is substantially strengthened.

Thus far it has been shown that early hypothesis generation and a limit on the number of hypotheses that can be evaluated concurrently are two general features of the problem-solving process. Criterial and noncriterial physicians could not be clearly differentiated on a variety of process measures. Physician performance varied from problem to problem, and the intraindividual consistencies that could distinguish criterial from noncriterial physicians did not materialize. Instead, problem-related variation loomed large, a finding further confirmed when generalizability coefficients were computed and examined. These results imply that diagnostic competence is not a unidimensional construct that can be measured with a small sample of test items. When one looks at the number of problems that have been used in many assessments of problem-solving capability in medical examinations, one sees that this is not an obvious, predictable conclusion.

Accurate versus Inaccurate Groups

The analysis next turned to another question: with respect to the selected dependent variables, what differences in problem-solving process could be found between those physicians who accurately solved the problems and those who did not? First, it was determined that splitting the subjects along the accurate/inaccurate dimension would not be a straightforward replication of the analysis of criterial/noncriterial physicians. Table 4.10

Table 4.10   Comparison of criterial versus noncriterial groups on accuracy of outcome (across three simulations).

Outcome	Criterial	Noncriterial	Total
Accurate on all three simulations	6	2	8
Inaccurate on one or more simulations	7	4	11

$\chi^2 = 0.26$, ns.

presents the relationship between these two classifications by comparing criterial and noncriterial physicans on accuracy of outcome. It is apparent that the two dimensions are independent; criterial physicians are not significantly more accurate than the noncriterial group. This statistical independence justified analysis of process differences associated with diagnostic outcome.

Table 4.11 presents the means of the five selected dependent variables for accurate and inaccurate groups. The accurate group for each simulation comprised those clinicians who made the correct diagnosis and, naturally, varied from one problem to another. Across all three simulations, the accurate group was composed of those who reached a correct diagnosis on all three problems, and the inaccurate group, those who made an inaccurate diagnosis on at least one simulation.

Univariate analyses of variance are summarized in Table 4.12. The significance level of the differences again varies substantially from problem to problem; once more, the influence of content on the process measures and possibly the unreliability of measurement are highlighted. However, when the scores were averaged over three problems, significant differences were found on two variables. The accurate group was more thorough in cue acquisition and more accurate in cue interpretation. Since the inaccurate group contained no one who erred on all three cases, the importance of these differences is emphasized. The variables are statistically independent of each other (Table 4.6). The correlation between percentage of cues acquired and accuracy of interpretation is .23 for case 1, −.24 for case 2, and .28 for case 3—none of which approaches statistical significance. Since cue acquisition and accuracy of cue interpretation are statistically independent, their retention as two separate stages in the model of medical reasoning is justified.

To summarize, statistical analysis of five selected dependent variables failed to disclose any significant differences between criterial and noncriterial physicians. However, when the data were reanalyzed in terms of an accurate/inaccurate dimension, it was found that diagnostic accuracy was associated with a higher percentage of cue acquisition and greater accuracy of cue interpretation. These findings are not an artifact of correlated scores.

Table 4.11 Accurate (A) and inaccurate (IA) group means (M) and standard deviations (SD) on selected dependent variables: by simulation, and average across simulations.

Variable		Simulation 1		Simulation 2		Simulation 3		Average[b]	
		A (n = 14)	IA[a] (n = 7)	A (n = 17)	IA (n = 5)	A (n = 16)	IA (n = 7)	A (n = 8)	IA (n = 11)
Point of generation of first hypothesis	M	14.79	10.00	17.82	31.00	3.19	17.00	9.87	14.39
	SD	22.61	9.27	15.31	23.59	4.15	24.79	5.80	11.42
Total number of hypotheses generated	M	6.71	6.29	6.82	6.60	4.69	3.14	5.88	5.91
	SD	2.09	1.80	2.48	2.19	2.12	0.90	1.04	1.26
Percentage of cues acquired	M	58.36	54.86	47.35	46.40	50.75	39.57	52.33	47.70
	SD	7.41	3.58	8.88	4.34	7.94	12.23	3.52	4.36
Efficiency	M	47.21	45.86	32.82	30.80	48.75	45.57	42.54	42.36
	SD	6.84	7.90	9.20	9.58	8.87	9.43	3.64	6.38
Accuracy of interpretation	M	63.43	64.43	77.18	64.20	66.00	60.43	70.00	67.30
	SD	9.41	7.48	14.03	21.06	16.42	17.90	5.70	8.10

[a] Simulation 1 was a complex problem with two diagnoses. Subjects in this group arrived at only one.
[b] Figures in this column are derived only from physicians who completed all three simulations. Accurate group includes those who made an accurate diagnosis on all three simulations; inaccurate group includes those who reached an inaccurate diagnosis on one or more of the three simulations.

Table 4.12 Univariate analyses of variance: accurate versus inaccurate group means on selected dependent variables.

Variable	Source of variation	df	MS	F	p
Simulation 1:					
ISU/H_1	Between	1	32.60	0.09	.77
	Within	19	379.33		
	Total	20			
H_{TOT}	Between	1	0.10	0.02	.88
	Within	19	4.35		
	Total	20			
% CUES	Between	1	36.21	0.88	.36
	Within	19	41.21		
	Total	20			
EFF	Between	1	6.88	0.13	.72
	Within	19	51.49		
	Total	20			
ACC INT	Between	1	42.00	0.43	.52
	Within	19	96.80		
	Total	20			
Simulation 2:					
ISU/H_1	Between	1	670.80	2.25	.15
	Within	20	298.72		
	Total	21			
H_{TOT}	Between	1	0.81	0.16	.69
	Within	20	5.11		
	Total	21			
% CUES	Between	1	3.51	0.05	.82
	Within	20	66.85		
	Total	21			
EFF	Between	1	15.82	0.18	.67
	Within	20	86.06		
	Total	21			
ACC INT	Between	1	698.64	2.97	.10
	Within	20	235.53		
	Total	21			

Variable	Source of variation	df	MS	F	p
Simulation 3:					
ISU/H_1	Between	1	929.04	4.95	.04
	Within	21	187.83		
	Total	22			
H_{TOT}	Between	1	11.62	3.38	.08
	Within	21	3.44		
	Total	22			
% CUES	Between	1	480.03	6.60	.02
	Within	21	72.75		
	Total	22			
EFF	Between	1	7.50	0.09	.77
	Within	21	85.06		
	Total	22			
ACC INT	Between	1	151.16	0.53	.47
	Within	21	284.18		
	Total	22			
Average across simulations:					
ISU/H_1	Between	1	17.87	0.19	.67
	Within	17	92.15		
	Total	18			
H_{TOT}	Between	1	0.59	0.43	.52
	Within	17	1.38		
	Total	18			
% CUES	Between	1	81.20	4.64	.05
	Within	17	17.50		
	Total	18			
EFF	Between	1	8.36	0.28	.61
	Within	17	30.12		
	Total	18			
ACC INT	Between	1	185.65	4.44	.05
	Within	17	41.78		
	Total	18			

ISU/H_1 = point of generation of first hypothesis.
H_{TOT} = total number of hypotheses generated.
% CUES = percentage of cues acquired.
EFF = efficiency.
ACC INT = accuracy of interpretation.

Hypothesis Evaluation: Modeling Medical Judgment

We have now completed our discussion of cue acquisition, hypothesis generation, and cue interpretation as these relate to discriminating between criterial and noncriterial physicians and between accurate and inaccurate diagnosticians. We turn to the final phase of the model of medical inquiry, hypothesis evaluation—the stage of a medical workup where a choice or decision is made among diagnostic alternatives. In the psychological literature this topic is often treated under the rubric of "judgment." Whether the process is conceptualized as "choice," "judgment," or "decision making," a major concern of psychologists and educators has been to identify the rules or processes that account for these decisions. Psychologists have dealt with these processes as part of the discipline's concern with explaining an important aspect of human behavior, rational thought. Educators have sought to have the processes made explicit so that they could be more easily learned.

Describing Diagnostic Decisions

Our search for a model that describes what physicians do, rather than one that prescribes what they ought to do, began with the observation that in all the protocols clinicians were consistently able to rank hypotheses in terms of some combination of probability, seriousness, and treatability, but were unwilling or unable to assign greater numerical precision to their categorical rankings. Attempts to obtain estimates of the odds or probability assigned to each hypothesis, or likelihood ratios, or estimates of the correlations between cues and hypotheses were all unsuccessful. On the other hand, the clinicians spontaneously weighted cues as positive, negative, or noncontributory for each hypothesis. It was reasonable to conclude that neither a Bayesian decision model nor a lens model were in fact used by clinicians untrained in these approaches, but that a version of the cue weights tabled in the cue-hypotheses matrices was employed. The problem then became, how can these cue weights be combined so as to reproduce the diagnostic decisions reached by the sample of clinicians? If a combination of separate cue weights could be found that did reproduce their judgments, the judgmental rule would have been modeled.

Since more complex rules should not be invoked unless simpler ones prove inadequate, we began by testing the sufficiency of linear combinations of cue weights. The seven-point scale of the cue-hypothesis matrix would have been used exclusively, except that the protocols indicated that the clinicians themselves generally used a three-point scale in weighting cues. Therefore, both three-point and seven-point scales were employed, and one aspect of the analysis asked which was more accurate in reproducing the diagnostic decisions actually reached. Wherever possible, the weights assigned to cues were obtained from each physician's comments while thinking aloud and later reviewing his workup. Where an obtained cue was not explicitly interpreted by the physician, the weight assigned was taken from the cue-hypothesis matrix, a technique that in effect assumes the cue would have been interpreted correctly.

Three linear models for combining clinical data were tested by comparing decisions reached by the models with the diagnostic judgments of the physicians. The models were the following: (a) choose the hypothesis supported by the most positive cues; (b) reject the hypothesis for which the most negative cues have been acquired; (c) choose the hypothesis that has the preponderance of evidence favoring it. In more quantitative terms, model 1 states that the maximum sum of positive cues predicts which hypothesis will be retained, model 2 states that the maximum sum of negative cues predicts which hypothesis will be rejected, and model 3 implies that the maximum difference of positive cues minus negative cues predicts which hypothesis will be retained. Two seriously considered hypotheses were defined for each clinician as the hypothesis each retained as the final diagnosis and the alternative considered longest before it was rejected. The means and ranges of the numbers of cues used in the calculations are shown in Table 4.13.

Table 4.14 presents the number of accurate predictions for the three cases using the three models. Data are tabulated separately for the seven-point as well as three-point (unit) scale. Entries in cells denote numbers of outcomes accurately predicted. The accuracy of prediction of the seven-point and three-point scales is essentially equivalent for all three cases. Major differences in accuracy of prediction occur when different models are applied. With any of the three models prediction was best for simulation 3, intermediate for simulation 1, and poorest (about 50 percent at best) for simulation 2. Of the three judgmental rules tested, basing decisions on negative weights only was the poorest predictor, especially in simulation 2. The other two models, based wholly or

Table 4.13   Positive and negative cues available for predicting physicians' decisions. M = mean; R = range.

Cue value		Accurate hypothesis +	Accurate hypothesis −	Inaccurate hypothesis +	Inaccurate hypothesis −
Simulation 1;	M	15.89	7.42	14.21	9.32
$n = 19$	R	7-23	5-16	7-19	4-14
Simulation 2;	M	24.85	9.10	21.10	6.15
$n = 20$	R	19-31	4-15	3-35	0-11
Simulation 3;	M	14.53	2.13	5.67	6.60
$n = 15$	R	5-21	0-12	2-9	0-12

partially on positive weights, did an average to good job depending on the problem. Specifically, model 3 had more hits on simulation 1, and the two models performed equivalently on simulation 3.

These results are interesting for several reasons. First, the seven-point scale is no better for predicting physicians' decisions than a simpler three-point scale. Although it might seem that the interpretation of diagnostic cues and the evaluation of hypotheses are complex enough to warrant assigning differential weights or even probability values to the relation of cues and hypotheses, the data do not suggest that physicians make such assignments. Whether decisions might be improved by more precise scaling is another question.

Our goal was to describe medical reasoning, not to develop a normative rule. The results imply that if the task confronting the physician is to select one diagnosis from among several hypotheses without stating how much more likely it is than any other alternative, then a rough scale of likelihoods, such as a three-point scale, is sufficient. The "pro," "con," and "does not help" formulation does at least as good a job of describing information-processing behavior as does a more complex differential weighting system.

Second, the model that is based on negatively weighted cues performs less accurately than the other two. Many psychological studies, particularly in the area of concept acquisition (Bruner, Goodnow, and Austin, 1956; Bourne, 1966; Wason, 1968) have suggested that subjects do not process negative information as

Table 4.14 Prediction of physician decisions by three models of decision making. Entries in cells are the number of times physician's diagnosis was predicted. Number of possible predictions is the n for each case.

	Model 1		Model 2		Model 3	
Simulation	7-point scale	3-point scale	7-point scale	3-point scale	7-point scale	3-point scale
1—hematology; n = 19	11	14	12	11	14	16
2—gastroenterology; n = 20	10	12	2	4	8	10
3—neurology; n = 15	14	13	12	11	13	13
Total 54	35	39	26	26	35	39

well as positive information. Although the present results suggest that subjects do not process negative cues efficiently, the diagnostic alternatives chosen for analysis were generated reasonably early in the workup and retained as contenders throughout the problem. Studies are currently planned to look carefully at the processing of cues relevant to shorter-lived hypotheses generated and dropped in the course of a workup. Perhaps negative information plays a more significant role than presently recognized in eliminating these alternatives.

Improving Diagnostic Decisions

Since none of the three models accurately predicted actual clinical decisions on simulation 2, we wondered whether all the models were inappropriate for this case or whether for unknown reasons the physicians had not employed a useful decision rule. The circumstance that the models did not predict actual decisions made it possible to ask whether any model could have predicted accurate decisions, had it in fact been utilized. The inquiry moved then from the description of diagnostic judgment with a linear rule to asking whether the same linear rule could be used to improve diagnostic accuracy, a procedure known as bootstrapping (Slovic and Lichtenstein, 1971). A similar concern with systematic application of rules and procedures to increase clinical accuracy is found in studies of psychological diagnosis (Goldberg, 1970), computer-assisted diagnosis (de Dombal and Horrocks, 1974), and ambulatory-care protocols (Sox, Sox, and Tompkins, 1973; Sherman and Komaroff, 1974).

The three models already described were tested to determine if any was useful in helping to make more accurate diagnostic decisions. What should a physician do when seriously considering two alternative hypotheses, one of which is probably the accurate solution to the problem? Should he (a) retain the hypothesis with the greater sum of positive weights on cues elicited, (b) reject the hypothesis with the most negative evidence, or (c) retain the hypothesis with the greater difference between positive and negative cues elicited? The means and ranges of the number of cues used in these calculations are presented in Table 4.15, and the results of this analysis are shown in Table 4.16.

Fewer cases appear in Table 4.16 than in Table 4.14 because only those clinicians who entertained the accurate hypothesis are included in the analysis. Entries in the cells represent numbers of physicians. To simplify the presentation, results of predictions based on negative cues only (model 2) have been omitted because they were so poor. Once again, the seven-point scale provides no greater power in predicting the accurate diagnosis. The second combination rule in Table 4.16 appears slightly superior to the first, though the samples were so small that no statistical tests were performed.

Table 4.15 Positive and negative cues available for predicting accurate outcomes. M = mean; R = range.

Cue value		Accurate hypothesis		Inaccurate hypothesis	
		+	−	+	−
Simulation 1;	M	15.64	6.36	14.00	9.43
$n=14$	R	7-20	5-8	7-19	4-14
Simulation 2;	M	27.67	6.27	23.22	8.60
$n=15$	R	21-35	4-11	11-29	0-15
Simulation 3;	M	16.00	0.92	6.00	5.92
$n=12$	R	11-21	0-3	2-9	0-12

Table 4.16 Prediction of accurate diagnosis by two models of decision making. Entries in cells are the number of times the correct diagnosis was predicted.

Simulation	Model 1		Model 3	
	7-point scale	3-point scale	7-point scale	3-point scale
1—hematology; accurate hypothesis considered by 14 physicians	8	10	11	13
2—gastroenterology; accurate hypothesis considered by 15 physicians	14	12	15	13
3—neurology; accurate hypothesis considered by 12 physicians	12	12	12	12
Total 41	34	34	38	38

The errors made by both combination rules in simulation 1 are instructive about the limitations of the model and where it fails to represent the physician's cognitive processes. The rule to work only with positive cues and ignore negative cues most frequently errs by predicting infection instead of infectious mononucleosis. These were the two most commonly generated hypotheses in this problem, and infection was usually generated quite early, before mononucleosis. When infectious mononucleosis was generated, infection often was not dropped. Thus, infection became the alternative hypothesis for the analysis. Since mononucleosis is an infectious disease, it is automatically a subset of the infection category, not a mutually exclusive alternative. Many cues positive for mononucleosis are also positive for infection. The models often chose the hypothesis that had the most positive cues and was retained the longest, namely infection, in preference to a more specific diagnosis. Model 3 did slightly better in predicting the accurate outcome for this case, but is still subject to the same error. Both models can be improved in this case by specifying that alternative hypotheses must be at the same level of specificity and not nested one as a subset of the other. This revision is equivalent to making the decision model more sequential so that once infection is established, it cannot compete with a specific infection.

It was earlier noted that for simulation 2 no model did very well in predicting actual diagnostic decisions and that both models 1 and 3 did much better in predicting the correct decision, at least for those physicians who generated the accurate hypothesis, than they did in predicting the decisions actually made. This problem and the data in Tables 4.15 and 4.16 were reviewed with the consulting gastroenterologist who had developed the cue-hypothesis matrix for this problem. We observed that most physicians who diagnosed Crohn's disease (regional enteritis) were themselves gastroenterologists, while none of the physicians who diagnosed ulcerative colitis were. Indeed, until the situation was reviewed it was believed that ulcerative colitis was the correct diagnosis, and we were perplexed by the apparent error of the gastroenterologists in the sample. Upon review, it was concluded that this is an often controversial and arguable issue (Cook and Dixon, 1973) and that nongastroenterologists had guided themselves largely by a radiological interpretation with which our consultant did not entirely agree. The gastroenterologists, on the other hand, had read the films independently and their interpretations concurred closely with those of the consulting gastroenterologist. Although physicians diagnosing ulcerative colitis tended to be more accurate in interpreting single cues (Table 4.11), here was a case where this advantage was offset by overreliance on one arguable interpretation. In simulation 2, then, most physicians did not diagnose by assigning equal weights to all the relevant evidence collected and adding, for if each had done so he would have arrived at the decision reached by model 3 and by the gastroenterologists. The decisions generally were made by attending to a small data set that was interpreted by another physician. The capacity of the model to predict the correct diagnosis, given the physician's own data base, highlights the distinction between knowledge of a set of symptom-disease relations as measured by the accuracy of interpretation score and the ability to apply this knowledge in judgment.

It cannot be concluded that the gastroenterologists employed a linear additive model, for it is likely that their information processing was also sequentially organized and that their advantage lay in interpreting the X-ray films independently. Thus, to the extent that a linear model resulted in increased diagnostic accuracy without changes in the data base, its adequacy as an account of human performance may be questioned, although its ability to better that performance may be welcomed. A systematized procedure or algorithm for data collection and decision making may be used deliberately to improve diagnostic decisions and may be the optimal path when the decision maker is not a specialist in a domain. An additive rule helps reduce reliance on single cues, erroneous observations, or misinterpretations.

Relation to Bayes' Theorem

The subject of this discussion is model 3, since it alone uses all of the evidence available. This model is a system for revising opinion in the light of evidence that does not require explicit statement of the prior probability of each hypothesis. Although a physician could probably say that A is more likely than B, even this is not required. The model in effect assumes that all hypotheses considered have an equal prior probability. While this assumption is almost never correct, it may well be a satisfactory working assumption in medicine, since the extensive collection of data minimizes the importance of prior probabilities. It does not assume that the hypotheses being evaluated are exclusive and exhaustive, although a more complete list of alternatives is better than an impoverished one. It does not require estimates of $P(S|D)$ beyond a three-point weight. In these ways the model makes weaker assumptions about the data and the decision maker than does decision analysis (Lusted, 1968; Raiffa, 1968; McNeil, Keeler, and Adelstein, 1975). The model uses what physicians know, and does not ask the medical decision maker to estimate precisely that which clinicians generally have such difficulty estimating, the base rates of various diseases (beyond categorizations, such as "X is frequent" or "Y is rarely seen") and the probability of observing a particular cue or finding given that a disease is present, $P(S|D)$. The system lacks the precision of decision analysis; however, it may be good enough "for all practical purposes" until objective data for $P(Disease)$ and $P(Symptom|Disease)$ are available.

Other Judgmental Rules

The models for hypothesis evaluation examined in this chapter are not an exhaustive catalog of the rules or heuristics used by physicians to make diagnostic judgments. For example, different principles are probably employed in testing hypotheses that are considered only briefly. In at least some of these instances, it appears that rejection is based on the absence of one or more distinctive features. The rule may be stated generally as, "If feature A is absent, it cannot be diagnosis X."

Other diagnostic strategies are implied by the very definition of a disease, as these are formulated in various sources. Rules like "At least three out of the following five features must be present to make a diagnosis of Y," or "X is diagnosed if and only if all of the following features are present," imply list-matching or pattern-matching procedures that emphasize acquisition of cues, assume little or no problem in making reliable observations, and de-emphasize the role of complex judgmental or decision procedures. As generally taught, these rules do not provide statistical information on the number of patients who are ultimately diagnosed as cases of Y with four features, or which set of three is the best, or what the false positive and false negative rates are with different combinations of cues. Rules of this class are variations of what Tversky (1972) called "elimination by aspects." In medicine, inclusion by aspects can be used to "rule in" and elimination by aspects "rules out." These rules substitute the representativeness of a case to its presumed population for probability estimates. Often these estimates will be accurate for all practical purposes, but diagnostic errors may occur. The rules have the useful psychological property of reducing cognitive strain by enabling the decision maker to focus attention on a small set of features out of a much larger data base and by emphasizing cue acquisition rather than hypothesis evaluation. By reasoning from considerations of working memory capacity, we may estimate that the number of features incorporated in these decision rules rarely exceeds four or five.

The psychological basis for the structural characteristics of these rules is clear enough. Unfortunately this seems to be about as far as cognitive psychology can take us at the moment. A set of generalizations that indicates when each rule is, or should be, employed is not yet formulated. How does a physician know when to select one rule and not another? That question seems to be still tied up in the specifics of each medical problem—and in the physician's prior knowledge.

Errors

In the previous section the topic of improving diagnostic judgment by systematic application of certain rules for combining evidence was explored. It was shown that at least some diagnostic errors come about because of mistakes in cue integration, not because of errors in cue acquisition. This provides a convenient transition to the next topic, the analysis of errors. We shall consider errors both in cue interpretation and in diagnosis.

Errors in Cue Interpretation

Three types of errors in cue interpretation were defined in Chapter 3: overinterpretation, underinterpretation, and misinterpretation. Table 4.17 summarizes the distribution of physicians by the most common error each made. The modal interpretive error by far is overinterpretation: that is, the most common mistake is treating noncontributory cues as relevant to a particular hypothesis. From the point of view of a cognitive theory of medical judgment this makes sense: clinicians are trying to reduce uncertainty and complexity by assimilating data to existing schemata. The more noncontributory data there are, the greater the necessity for additional hypotheses and a concomitant increase in the complexity of the problem. Complexity is reduced by storing as many cues as possible within existing rubrics rather than remembering them as "unaccounted for" or creating new clusters.

This interpretation should be viewed cautiously. It is possible, of course, that the interpretations used as the standard for judging the sample are overly conservative. Further investigations readily suggest themselves; as a start, a test of the data against standards developed by more than a single physician.

Inaccurate Diagnosis

Let us now consider some factors associated with inaccurate diagnosis. Material already presented will be summarized and further analyses provided. Our conclusions must be tentative indeed, for we are dealing with small samples of cases and physicians and with a limited number of errors.

Table 4.17 Distribution of errors in cue interpretation. All significance tests are X^2 with 3 df. Entries in cells are numbers of persons, not of errors.

Simulation	No errors	Overinterpretation	Underinterpretation	Misinterpretation	p
1	0	18	1	2	< .01
2	6	11	1	4	< .02
3	3	12	5	3	< .03

THOROUGHNESS. Thoroughness of data collection is frequently identified as a cardinal virtue in medical practice. Conversely, mistakes are often attributed to errors of omission in data collection, that is, insufficient thoroughness. For example, studies of patient-care protocols frequently point to increments in data collection, especially history and physical examination, as evidence for the beneficial effect of this innovation (see Grimm et al., 1975). Our data (Tables 4.11 and 4.12) have shown that overall diagnostic accuracy is weakly associated with greater thoroughness as measured by percentage of cues acquired. Diagnostic accuracy was unrelated to efficiency, the percentage of cues obtained related to all hypotheses considered by the physician, although more efficient workups will undoubtedly cost less, especially where laboratory tests are ordered.

One additional question can be asked of the data: can inaccurate outcomes be attributed to failure to collect sufficient data relevant to the correct diagnostic hypothesis? To judge from the three problems studied, the answer appears to be "sometimes" or "yes, but not always." In the hematology problem (simulation 1) physicians diagnosing both infectious mononucleosis and hereditary spherocytic anemia tended to be somewhat more thorough in collecting data relevant to these two hypotheses than those who accepted only one alternative ($p < .10$ for a one-tailed test). Again, in the neurological problem (simulation 3) those diagnosing multiple sclerosis collected significantly more data relevant to this hypothesis than those diagnosing a psychogenic problem ($p < .05$, one-tailed test). However, this pattern was not observed in the gastrointestinal problem (simulation 2), where there were no significant differences in relevant thoroughness between accurate and inaccurate groups. The proper rules for interpreting and combining data are the information-processing issue in this case, not data collection.

HYPOTHESIS EVALUATION. The previous discussion of modeling diagnostic judgment is relevant here. An increase in diagnostic accuracy was noted in simulation 2 when a linear decision rule was systematically employed. It appears, therefore, that the errors in this case were not a result of mistakes in cue acquisition. Further, Tables 4.11 and 4.12 show that cue acquisition was equivalent among those who diagnosed ulcerative colitis and those who diagnosed regional enteritis. Differences in judgment arise from cue interpretation and integration into a decision, not from differences in thoroughness.

A systematic linear additive rule, such as a regression equation or one using equal unit weights, has the additional virtue of being reasonably resistant to errors in observation, recording, or interpretation of single cues. Since a diagnostic decision is made by summing over all relevant cues, the likelihood that a single error could lead to an incorrect decision is substantially reduced. This additive strategy is particularly useful, then, whenever a probability distribution on diagnostic states is converted to dichotomous decisions based on a cutoff point (Gettys, Kelly and Peterson, 1973; de Dombal and Horrocks, 1974).

We have already suggested that an adaptive system for medical diagnosis would be somewhat resistant, although not immune, to errors in cue interpretation. Earlier it was seen that accuracy of cue interpretation did not discriminate between accurate and inaccurate subjects on any one case, but that taken as a whole over three cases, accurate diagnosis was associated with more accurate cue interpretation. We wondered whether an analysis of interpretive accuracy with respect to the correct hypothesis would illuminate this matter further, since it could be argued that accurate physicians make fewer errors in interpreting particularly crucial data but are not more accurate overall. In other words, can inaccurate diagnostic outcomes be attributed to misinterpretation of cues particularly relevant to the correct diagnostic hypothesis?

To answer this question, misinterpretations of cues relevant to the correct diagnoses were counted for each case. In the hematology problem, correct diagnosis of both diseases was associated with significantly fewer misinterpretations ($p < .05$). Physicians who made a diagnosis of regional enteritis misinterpreted fewer cues relevant to this alternative than did those who diagnosed ulcerative colitis ($p < .05$). However, in the neurology problem, the relation between diagnostic accuracy and number of misinterpretations was not statistically significant. Over all three problems accurate diagnosis was associated with fewer misinterpretations ($p < .05$). The results are consistent with those of Gill and associates (1973), who found that errors in data acquisition were not as important a source of diagnostic error as mistakes in processes that we would call cue interpretation and hypothesis evaluation.

HYPOTHESIS GENERATION. In addition to cue acquisition and cue interpretation, the model of medical inquiry directs attention to hypothesis generation as a significant element in diagnosis. The meaning of the cues obtained is not self-evident or attained purely by inductive methods. Rather, clusters of cues serve as the starting points for generating preliminary formulations. Later decisions are concerned with selecting among alternatives. Clearly, a correct selection (accurate diagnosis) is not possible without first generating the correct alternative (accurate formulation). On the other hand, accurate formulation does not guarantee accurate diagnosis, since the correct formulation may be rejected.

Table 4.18 summarizes these issues for the three problems analyzed in this chapter. Simulation 3 best exemplifies error caused by faulty problem formulation. All seven physicians who made a diagnostic error failed to generate the correct formulation as a hypothesis. Premature closure on an incorrect alternative led to their ignoring contradictory evidence. All the physicians who generated the correct hypothesis retained it. This case clearly illustrates a situation where correct outcome depends on correct formulation. Simulation 1 had two correct diagnoses, a solution reached by fourteen out of twenty-one physicians. The remaining seven physicians reached only partially accurate solutions, in that they diagnosed only one disease. How were these seven diagnostic errors made? In two instances the formulation was only partially accurate and one of the correct hypotheses was never gen-

Table 4.18 Analysis of hypothesis generation and diagnostic accuracy. Entries in cells are the numbers of physicians who arrived at the specified formulation.

Simulation	Accuracy of formulation		
	Fully accurate	Partially accurate[a]	Inaccurate
1	19	2	0
2	20	0	2
3	16	0	7
	Accuracy of outcome		
1	14	7	0
2	17	0	5
3	16	0	7

[a] Simulation 1 was a complex problem with two accurate diagnostic outcomes. A partially accurate formulation and/or solution implies that one but not both of the appropriate diagnostic hypotheses was generated or generated and retained.

erated. In the other five cases both correct hypotheses were generated but only one was retained. Most errors in this problem, therefore, are the result of a faulty combination rule, incorrect evaluation of alternatives, or an erroneous tendency to find a parsimonious explanation for complexity; they are not the result of failures in hypothesis generation.

Other Errors

Based on collateral observations of the difficulties of medical students in tackling simulated and actual patient problems, additional errors have been identified.

EXCESSIVE DATA COLLECTION. In the case of this error, the patient is implicitly assumed to have multiple problems. The hypotheses generated are representative of several problem areas instead of being competing alternatives within the same domain. Each accounts for a small cluster of findings with insufficient attention paid to parsimonious organization into a unifying diagnostic concept. An extreme form of this error is to use each new cue to generate a new hypothesis; given the probabilistic relation between symptoms and diseases, it is an almost certain way to guarantee failure to close. This strategy may be taught and employed as a corrective to an inappropriate search for diagnostic unity when a patient indeed has multiple problems. A heuristic principle for this potential dilemma is to consider the probability of each alternative formulation. The joint probability of two or more relatively common problems may well exceed the probability of a single unifying but rare ailment. On the other hand, the base rates of certain unifying formulations may be greater than the joint probability of two or more symptom clusters considered as independent entities.

UNINTERPRETED CUES. Even experienced physicians will not formally and systematically interpret all the data collected in the light of the expectations implied by a list of hypotheses. However, there must be a lower limit to data collection without data utilization. The data must be interpreted to evaluate hypotheses, to determine whether there is enough evidence to rule in or rule out particular alternatives and to assess whether new hypotheses should be formulated. The deductive process is not automatic, even though experienced practitioners can make it seem to be.

Correlates of Medical Problem-Solving Performance

A small battery of tests was administered to assess the relation between the processes of clinical reasoning and selected personality characteristics, including one measure of logical reasoning. The tests included three logical problems developed by Rimoldi and his associates (Erdmann, 1964), the dogmatism scale (Rokeach, 1960), the flexibility scale of the California Psychological Inventory (Gough, 1957), a complexity scale developed by Barron (1967) and published as a scale of the Omnibus Personality Inventory (1968), and a measure of cognitive complexity developed by Bieri and colleagues (1966).

The first relationships evaluated were between the personality variables and the capacity to interpret medical data from many standpoints. Flexibility of interpretation was measured by four clinical process variables related to hypothesis generation: number of hypotheses considered one-fourth and halfway through the workup, total number of hypotheses generated, and point of generating the first hypothesis. Correlations between these scores and the personality variables described were computed. The association between personality variables and clinical problem-solving measures was inconsistent at best. The statistically significant correlations were divided between those that could be interpreted as supporting a positive relationship between the two sets of variables and those that could not. On the whole, the correlations reflected chiefly that clinicians are not consistent across problems. Case specificity precludes finding significant stylistic consistency with small samples of physicians and problems.

There were no statistically significant correlations between measures of logical problem solving and clinical problem solving. Here it should be emphasized that the logical problems used were by design highly formal and lacked much meaningful semantic content, while clinical problems have a strong content component. Furthermore, clinical tasks depend upon probabilistic inference and logical problems do not. It may be suggested that the psychology of problem solving is more complex than has been suspected: different operations are appropriate for different tasks, and mastery of one set of operations does not necessarily imply mastery of another. Similar views have been expressed by Wason and Johnson-Laird (1972) and Dawes (1975).

It seems fair to say that in searching for personality correlates of medical problem-solving behavior, the existence of general problem-solving dispositions was taken for granted. The research task was, in a sense, to demonstrate scientifically what everyone intuitively knows. Lack of dogmatism or a preference for complexity were assumed to be personality traits that were sufficiently stable and enduring to express themselves both in scales measuring the characteristic and in rational thought processes in clinical medicine. It was precisely this common-sense wisdom that was not confirmed.

At least one study has reported significant correlations between personality scores and ratings of clinical performance by peers and supervisors (Kegel-Flom, 1975). Clinical performance was not directly assessed in that study, however; it should be noted that indirect ratings are subject to a number of distorting effects in the direction of greater consistency and higher intercorrelations than are found when behavior is directly observed and rated (Shweder, 1975).

Summary

Having now completed our analyses of the high-fidelity simulations, let us review the ground that has been covered. We shall first recapitulate the major findings, placing them in the context of cognitive psychology, then consider the implications of the failure to discriminate between criterial and noncriterial physicians, and conclude with a brief evaluation of the research method and scoring system.

The Psychology of Medical Reasoning

Diagnostic problems are solved through a process of hypothesis generation and verification. Hypotheses are consistently generated early in a workup when only a very limited data base has been obtained. While any early formulation may be revised or discarded if subsequent data fail to confirm it, there is a high probability that at least some of the formulations of experienced physicians will be correct. Hypotheses serve as organizing rubrics in working memory. They help to overcome limitations of memory capacity and serve to narrow the size of the problem space that must be searched for solution. Since it would be impossible to conduct an efficient inquiry without some hypothetical goal that would tell the inquirer when to stop, hypotheses serve to transform an open medical problem (What is the patient's illness?) into a set of closed problems (Bartlett, 1958) that are much easier to solve (Is the illness *X*? or *Y*? or *Z*?). Means-ends analysis (Newell and Simon, 1972) is used to reduce the difference between end points and the state of affairs existing at any time. As data are collected, they are used first to generate preliminary hypotheses, then to evaluate these periodically, and if necessary, to reformulate or generate new hypotheses and thereby modify the problem space. In this way erroneous or impossible end points can be eliminated by a process of successive approximations. The general model of medical inquiry encompasses four major processes—cue acquisition, hypothesis generation, cue interpretation, and hypothesis evaluation or judgment. Thoroughness of cue acquisition and accuracy of cue interpretation are statistically independent.

Hypotheses imply that certain findings may be observed if the hypothesis is true. Thus, a hypothesis can be tested, and the workup consists partly in a guided search for other findings implied by each hypothesis. Anticipations direct problem-solving behavior, as de Groot (1965) noted. We were unable to distinguish reliably between hypothesis-testing questions and questions asked routinely, although the distinction seems clear enough to any clinician reading a protocol. The problem is that any question may be either. We speculate that the so-called routine question in a workup is really aimed at testing particular hypotheses or at least determining whether further inquiry into a particular hypothesis is warranted.

In the process of cue interpretation, data are evaluated in terms of their fit to the anticipated findings. Our results indicate that this evaluation is ordinarily conducted by weighting each interpreted finding on a three-point scale. A cue may be positive, noncontributory, or negative with respect to a particular hypothesis. There are undoubtedly instances where a particular diagnosis is confirmed or ruled out by the presence or absence of a particular pathognomonic cue. But the physicians studied in this research did not appear to employ this weighting scheme—at least not for the cases analyzed. A three-point weighting scheme fitted the data as well as a seven-point system. Diagnostic accuracy is related to both thoroughness of cue acquisition and accuracy of cue interpretation, although these two variables are themselves uncorrelated.

In the analysis of hypothesis evaluation or judgment, an effort was made to discover the rule or model used by physicians to make diagnostic decisions. The majority of judgments in this study were accounted for by either of two rules: (a) select the hypothesis with the maximum number of positive cues, or (b) select the hypothesis with the maximum difference of positive cues minus negative cues. In one problem systematic application of these rules led to increased diagnostic accuracy, which suggested that some physicians had not used the rules when they would have been appropriate. This finding further implied that some diagnostic errors occur because of mistakes in combining evidence, while others may result from misinterpretations of single cues. Other diagnostic errors come about when the appropriate data are not collected (cue-acquisition problems) and when mistakes are made in the definition of the problem space because of faulty hypothesis generation.

The data thus indicate that diagnostic problems are solved by a hypothetico-deductive method. A purely inductive method of gathering data until a solution spontaneously emerges is never employed. It is unlikely that it would be successful if it were employed, because the size of the search space would be so enormous that a problem could never be finished in a reasonable time. Experienced physicians have therefore learned not to use this method. Evidence will be presented later to show that medical students also use a process of hypothesis generation and verification.

The principle of early hypothesis generation does not mean that hypotheses must not be revised or that new ones ought not be generated later in the problem. It means simply that the first diagnostic hypotheses are generated early. The choice of these hypotheses is not arbitrary or random. They are generated typically by associations from clusters of a few cues. Each hypothesis accounts for some, but usually not all, of the initial data base. If all of the data could be accounted for, the case might not be experienced as a problem at all. Each problem's list of hypotheses includes both frequently occurring diseases and serious possibilities. The roles of probability and utility in hypothesis generation and judgment are still unclear and might profitably be studied by lower-fidelity simulation. Nowick (1976) suggests that hypothesis generation is mediated largely by availability of concepts to recall, a finding consistent with the associative mechanisms described.

The number of hypotheses considered at any one time is limited and rarely exceeds five. There are numerous instances in the protocols where one hypothesis is reformulated so that the total number under consideration is unchanged; this suggests that a limitation on working memory capacity, noted in many other investigations, is manifest in medical problem solving.

A move from more general to more specific hypotheses was not consistently observed. This pattern, reported by Kleinmuntz (1968) in a study of neurological diagnosis, was observed in our problems in the differential diagnosis of anemia but not in the gastroenterological problem nor the neurological problem. (The physicians in Kleinmuntz's study were neurologists, however, which may account for the difference in results.) In some cases the early hypotheses are rather general and imply some additional steps before the problem is transformed by reformulation into more specific hypotheses. In other cases the early data base permits relatively specific hypotheses to be generated. It was *not* observed that some physicians consistently move from general to specific while others gamble on specific alternatives at the outset. The strategy chosen appears to depend largely on the content of the problem and the physician's understanding of it.

It may be observed that this description of medical problem solving is a description of a set of cognitive operations that involve considerations of memory organization, decision making, and probability estimation. Hypothesis generation involves retrieving a limited number of hypotheses from long-term memory and setting them up as a problem space. Cue acquisition depends heavily but not exclusively on routinized knowledge of history taking and physical examination, which permits a physician to select smoothly from the battery of questions and maneuvers stored in memory. Cue interpretation and hypothesis evaluation are likewise acquired processes stored in memory until needed. This is to be expected in developing a theory of problem solving in which prior experience of the problem solver is called upon to aid in finding a solution. The emphasis of the theory is upon learning, generalization, and transfer, not upon innate capacities or personality dispositions of the problem solver. At the same time, the requisite skills stored in memory are not measured by examinations that emphasize recall of specific facts.

Criterial and Noncriterial Physicians

Our inquiry began, however, with the aim of discriminating between criterial and noncriterial physicians in terms of their cognitive processes. This search was largely unsuccessful, though some suggestive trends were found. Specifically, criterial physicians were found to ask more questions prior to generating a first hypothesis, to collect a few more data, and to interpret their data slightly more accurately. None of these trends was statistically significant, but all were in the same direction over three problems studied.

There are several possible explanations for the failure to discriminate between expert and nonexpert physicians. Conceiving of the problems as test items, it can be argued that they were poor items, or that there were not enough items, or that there were no real differences between groups tested. Let us take up each of these possibilities in turn.

POOR ITEMS. The difficulty raised by this objection may be viewed by looking at the complementary question, "What makes a medical problem good in the sense that it would be suitable for a test?" One criterion is that it is fairly representative of the competencies to be assessed. Our problems were chosen with little reference to their content, since it was assumed initially that a common problem-solving approach could be detected in the solution of any medical problem. We did not determine systematically that hematology should be assessed and that the particular case developed was the best available for assessing problem solving in hematology. Retrospectively it may be argued that the items were poor, although it is doubtful that this objection would have been raised if the results had distinguished more clearly between criterial and noncriterial physicians. Had differences been found, it is unlikely that they would have been dismissed as inconsequential because the problems were too artificial. The items may also be poor in the sense of being too easy or too hard; still, more difficult problems would have been rightly criticized as too exotic, and easier items would only increase the problem of discriminating between the groups. There is one sense in which the items are clearly good, not poor, and that is in face validity. Our efforts at making the items "good" were directed at the fidelity of the simulation. Representative sampling of the domain and broad content validity were traded for problem-specific content validity. This tradeoff led to the second possible objection, too few items.

NOT ENOUGH ITEMS. The statistical power of a test to detect a difference between groups is related to test length. By attempting to distinguish between two groups using only three cases that serve in effect as test items, the likelihood of a type 2 error is increased, as a small sample invariably requires a greater difference to reach statistical significance. The failure to discriminate between criterial (expert) and noncriterial (nonexpert) physicians may be the result of a lack of statistical power in the study. Improved sampling by increase in the number of problems each physician worked would reduce errors of measurement and increase the power of any statistical test employed.

This argument may be couched in more clinical terms: suppose the difference between an expert diagnostician and an average physician is about 15 percent—that the average physician solves 75 to 80 percent of the problems encountered, while an expert solves 90 to 95 percent. This difference is real enough in clinical terms, but is not likely to be evident over samples of three cases or even six, though it might well be demonstrable over fifty to one hundred cases or with very difficult cases. Similarly, the differences between groups might be clear if the groups were larger.

This argument is unassailable. All that can be said is that this limitation on the results is inherent in the method selected to study physician performance. High-fidelity simulation requires a great deal of time; given the realities of the work schedule of the physician, it is unlikely that high-fidelity simulation studies with more than three cases will ever be feasible unless the sampling time is extended, not concentrated in two days. More cases in a lower-fidelity format will be needed to sample medical reasoning more extensively within a realistic, practical time frame. However, the problem was not fully appreciated when this study was designed. It was explicitly assumed that differences between physicians would be sufficiently large to be detectable with small samples of problems and physicians, and that differences in strategy would be evident even if differences in diagnostic outcome were not. The major problem of research on clinical judgment, as we saw it then, was the face validity and content validity of the materials used, not generalizability; so high-fidelity simulation of a small group of problems was chosen. The choice of method was criticized early by Kenneth Hammond (personal communication, 1970) from a classic Brunswikian standpoint. He argued that situations vary more than persons, that the task demands of medical problems are more likely to vary than the cognitive processes of the physicians who solve them, and that a better strategy would be to study fewer physicians with more cases in a representative design. The merit of his criticisms was not fully appreciated. Certainly, there is room for additional studies of clinical judgment that will meet the methodological difficulties of the present investigation.

We were not alone in the view that differences between criterial and noncriterial physicians were so marked that they could be assessed validly with a limited number of cases, a corollary of the doctrine that problem-solving excellence is not case specific. In a study begun somewhat after the Medical Inquiry Project and conducted quite independently of it, Hoffman (1974) assessed a computer-based examination system for the American Board of Internal Medicine. He studied two groups that could reasonably be assumed to differ more than those in our study. The first consisted of successful Board candidates and a group of house officers, not yet certified, who had been rated by their superiors as outstanding clinicians. His noncriterial group was composed of physicians who had failed the oral examination of the American Board of Internal Medicine three times. A series of four computerized problems failed to discriminate between these groups for much the same reasons as discussed here: physician performance on the problems was so highly variable that it was not possible to predict any individual's performance from one problem to another.

INSUFFICIENT VARIABILITY IN SAMPLE. The participating physicians were all volunteers, and nonrandom factors influenced their decisions to participate. There is some anecdotal evidence in our files which suggests that several physicians who perceived themselves to be the weakest and the strongest excluded themselves. If their self-perceptions are accurate, the sample lacked sufficient variability. A group of largely homogeneous physicians may have been studied, and there were not clearly different levels of competence to discriminate.

It can also be argued that the skill with which a physician works in an area depends upon mastery of both the general problem-solving heuristics described in the model of medical inquiry and knowledge within a specific domain. Since each physician in the sample had a minimum of seven years of postresidency experience, it is possible that the groups were essentially equivalent with respect to mastery of problem-solving heuristics and differed only with respect to knowledge of content.

WHAT IS A "GOOD" PHYSICIAN? The term *criterial* has many meanings when applied to physicians, and our raters may have had different qualities in mind when they made their global judgments. A good physician may be defined as one who is (a) technically proficient, as in surgery, *or* (b) makes accurate diagnoses in particularly difficult cases, *or* (c) is skilled in treating and managing multiple-problem patients, *or* (d) has a high level of interpersonal skill and rapport with patients, *or* (e) achieves patient compliance where others fail, *or* (f) has a high level of expertise in a complex and difficult area, *or* (g) is a devoted and respected teacher. Any single individual may of course combine several of these attributes, but it might be sufficient to have only one or two to be called a good physician. The reader can probably provide additional definitions.

Our results are, however, consistent with other studies that were able to sample the range of physician competence more adequately. Hoffman's (1974) study of the computer-based examination system for recertification of internists and unpublished data from the certification examination of the Canadian College of Family Physicians both show that performance varies more as a function of the problem than as a function of the intellectual processes thought to cut across problems. These studies support the conclusion that our results do not depend primarily on psychological features of the sample.

In our estimation, the single most critical factor in the nondiscrimination of criterial and noncriterial physicians is the phenomenon of case specificity of performance. Intraindividual consistency on a variety of process measures was very low. The performance of individual physicians varies considerably from case to case. Thus it is difficult to speak of good physicians without specifying the domain of problems for which they are good.

Although criterial and noncriterial physicians could not be clearly distinguished, it was possible to identify process variables associated with accurate and inaccurate diagnostic outcomes. In general, accurate diagnosis is associated with greater thoroughness of cue acquisition and greater accuracy in cue interpretation. Information-processing errors that may lead to mistakes in diagnosis have been discussed.

Critique of the Scoring System

At the beginning of Chapter 3, four principles that guided the formulation of the scoring system were identified. As the conclusion of the present chapter, let us review the extent to which these criteria were met.

The first principle was objectivity and reliability of the scoring categories. Very satisfactory reliabilities were achieved for the categories that were analyzed intensively. We were unable to obtain adequate consistency in judging whether an information search unit was hypothesis testing or routine, and whether a question was leading or nonleading (closed or open). Some potentially significant aspects of the data-collection process consequently were neglected.

Task relevance was the second principle. The scoring system does emphasize critical and relevant elements of medical problem solving by focusing attention on cue acquisition, cue interpretation, hypothesis generation, and hypothesis evaluation. The types of questions asked are relatively slighted because satisfactory reliability in judging categories of questions could not be obtained.

The third principle was theoretical relevance. We believe that it has been adequately demonstrated that scores generated out of a process-tracing approach to medical problem solving can relate this activity to problem solving in other domains and to contemporary cognitive psychology.

Discriminant validity was the fourth principle. We have already discussed a number of reasons why criterial and noncriterial physicians were not differentiated. Thus the scores generated do not distinguish effectively between clearly different levels of overall clinical competence, but at least some do distinguish the cognitive processes associated with accurate and inaccurate diagnosticians. Given the wide range of meaning that can be assigned to the concept *good physician,* it seems advisable for future inquiries to focus on more specific properties and not on the general construct.

5 / Patient-Management Problems

In this chapter we present an analysis of the performance of fifteen out of twenty-four physician subjects on four paper-and-pencil simulations called patient-management problems (PMPs). We begin with a discussion of the general nature of these problems and the scoring scheme developed for them; an in-depth analysis of physician performance on each problem follows. Overall performance on these problems and its relation to performance on high-fidelity simulations are the concluding topics.

Method

Each patient-management problem is designed to simulate certain aspects of the physician-patient encounter, notably diagnosis and management. The encounters are collapsed over time, so that events that in reality could spread over weeks or even months are dealt with in a problem whose duration may be thirty to forty-five minutes. The interpersonal skills of the physician, the degree to which he communicates effectively with a patient, and the degree to which a patient feels satisfied with the encounter are assessed only indirectly. The focus, rather, is on the cognitive formulation, appraisal, and management of problems by the physician and the provision of a vehicle by which the adequacy of medical problem solving in the cognitive domain may be evaluated.

Each problem begins with a brief verbal description of the patient's problem. The introductions range in length from five to fifteen typewritten lines and present a minimum to a moderate amount of information about the case. The examinee must then decide how to approach the patient, that is, what if any further workup is indicated at this point. The decision is recorded in two ways: by entering the choice in an answer booklet (a page of which is reproduced as Appendix A), and then by erasing the opaque overlay on a specially constructed answer sheet and finding an instruction that directs the examinee to the section designated by that choice. In the section chosen, the clinician is confronted with a long list of possible questions that will yield further information about the patient. As many procedures may be selected as seem appropriate in light of the specific circumstances. Choices are again recorded by entering them in the answer booklet and then by erasing the appropriate portion of the overlay to find the result of those choices presented in verbal or visual form. On the basis of these new data, decisions are made on the next step to be taken.

Three of the four problems used in this study contain several sections, some of which are not appropriate for optimal management of the patient. The sections are arranged in scrambled order. At the end of each section of questions, the physician is again faced with a list of choices concerning what, if any, data to obtain next or whether to move now to the treatment or management options. The decision is indicated, as before, by erasing the appropriate portion of the overlay sheet and finding directions to the next section. The clinician's choices determine the sequence of sections. Once a section is entered, however, all of the options available within it are visible and may serve as cues for choices. For example, as Appendix A shows, a wide range of questions is offered for the physical examination. The clinician chooses which of these to ask, and there may be a sizable cuing effect.

Modifications of the Format

For purposes of this study certain modifications were made in the format of each problem.

MODIFICATIONS IN RECORDING OF RESPONSE CHOICES. A section of a PMP contains a number of possible options. Rubbing out the opaque overlay on the answer sheets indicates only which options were chosen, not the order of choice. Yet the sequential character of data gathering is an important feature of the medical problem-solving process. In an attempt to gather data on this point, physicians were instructed to record the *sequence* of their choices within each section in the answer booklet. Most found this instruction an unreasonable constraint on their behavior and neglected it. Although they agreed that the data would actually be gathered sequentially, some found that having to record choices in this way in an answer booklet was artificial and impeded the flow of thought. Others argued that sequence was immaterial for some questions, as long as they were asked, but was crucial for other questions. For these reasons data about sequence within each section are not available from a sufficient number of physicians to provide material for analysis. A computer-based simulation that automatically recorded sequence could provide a more accurate record with less burden on the examinee.

MODIFICATIONS IN TYPES OF RESPONSES. In pilot testing the high-fidelity simulations, we became aware of the role of preliminary hypotheses in guiding acquisition of clinical data. The traditional PMP scoring scheme takes this variable into account implicitly, but we wished to be explicit about it. Therefore, space was provided at the end of each section of a problem for the physician to list the diagnostic alternatives being considered at that point. In three out of four problems space was also provided at the end of the brief introduction, before the physician exercised any options, for listing any diagnostic hypotheses that might have been generated at that early point in the problem. In fifty-nine out of sixty instances (fifteen physicians and four problems) these spaces were used.

Each physician was also asked to indicate degree of certainty about each diagnostic hypothesis by assigning a percentage to each possibility (dividing one hundred points among the alternatives). We wanted to obtain an estimate from each physician of his subjective probability for each diagnostic hypothesis at several points in the problem, and to see how these probabilities changed as data were collected. However, most of the physicians simply ignored this instruction. When we reviewed their behavior with them, they stated that hypotheses are roughly rank ordered, but they were very uncomfortable about assigning percentages, numerical probabilities, or odds to their rank-ordered hypotheses. Consequently, the impact of the data on subjective probabilities could not be analyzed. As a result of the format modifications, however, we were able to examine a list of hypotheses generated at each point, the number of physicians who generated these hypotheses, and the way in which the lists gradually narrowed as a solution was approached.

Subjects

Fifteen of the twenty-four physicians who participated in the Medical Inquiry Project worked these problems. This group had been in practice an average of nineteen years. The other nine did not participate in this aspect of the project because by the time these four problems became available, several of the physicians had completed their participation in our study. The problem materials were sent to these physicians by mail with accompanying letters and follow-up phone calls. The return rate was very poor, however—largely, we believe, because of the extremely busy schedule of most practicing physicians. Although some booklets were returned by mail, most respondents completed them during their visit to our laboratory. In one instance of absentee assessment, unclear instructions or confusion over format made a problem unusable. Otherwise, a complete data set is available.

Scoring

To score the PMPs a system similar to that used by the University of Illinois was developed. (The Illinois scoring method is discussed in Chapter 9 and is presented briefly in Appendix C.) Since we wished to assess the relation between the cues obtained and diagnostic hypotheses, part of our analysis rests on an evaluation of all cues available in the PMP. A cue-hypothesis matrix for each PMP was constructed along the lines described in Chapter 3. The hypotheses entered were those most frequently generated by the fifteen physicians, plus some others needed to indicate the broad range of possibilities evoked by the introduction. The matrices were evaluated by physicians who specialized in the areas covered by each problem—hematology, gastroenterology, or vascular surgery. Each cue (an option in a section) was evaluated in terms of its usefulness for each hypothesis on a seven-point scale. Cues weighted ± 2 or ± 3 were designated "critical findings" because presumably they should help most in decision making.

The high-fidelity simulations focused on the diagnostic phase of patient care. So that the analysis of the PMPs could be as consistent with the analysis of those simulations as possible, we stressed the process of reaching a diagnosis and not the physician's handling of the management sections of these problems. Consequently the cue-hypothesis matrices were constructed only for the workup sections of the problems—history, physical examination, and laboratory tests. We shall, nonetheless, comment upon erroneous treatment decisions and their relation to diagnostic hypotheses and to data collection.

The in-depth analysis of each problem centers around four quantitative variables: (a) number of hypotheses generated, (b) percentage of cues acquired, (c) percentage of critical findings acquired, and (d) efficiency. The number of hypotheses generated at various points in each of the problems was determined by counting the physician's list of alternative formulations. Unlike the analysis of the high-fidelity simulations, there was no need for a detailed set of rules to establish what constituted a hypothesis. Hypotheses were the formulations of the problem that physicians wrote in the spaces provided. The remaining three variables are defined as in Chapter 3:

$$\text{percentage of cues acquired} = \frac{\text{number of cues selected}}{\text{total cues available}} \times 100,$$

$$\text{percentage of critical findings acquired} = \frac{\text{number of critical findings selected}}{\text{total critical findings available}} \times 100,$$

and efficiency = percentage of cues selected that are critical findings for at least one hypothesis generated.

The analysis of each problem begins with some general remarks about the problem's structure and the routes commonly used through it. The hypotheses considered and the final diagnoses are then summarized. Last, patterns of data acquisition and the relation between data collection, hypothesis generation, and diagnostic accuracy are discussed.

Patient-Management Problem 1

Structure of the Problem

The introduction to this problem is quite substantial (nearly fourteen typewritten lines) and includes salient history, summary of a physical examination, and some laboratory findings from an initial workup of the case. Space is provided to list hypotheses only once, after the introduction. There is one section for further data collection which consists of thirty items (three pertaining to more detailed history and twenty-seven to laboratory tests). Options are selected from this section and there is no branching. The final diagnosis is then entered. The only possible route through the problem is shown in Figure 5.1.

Figure 5.1 Route of workup of patient-management problem 1.

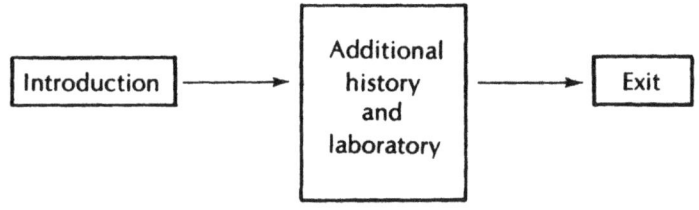

Hypothesis Generation

Basically, three types of hypotheses were generated:

(a) *Hemolytic anemia.* All fifteen physicians generated one or more hemolytic anemia hypotheses. For 40 percent ($n = 6$), the correct diagnosis of congenital spherocytic anemia was included among the hemolytic anemia hypotheses generated. For 80 percent ($n = 12$), the most popular "distractor," sickle cell anemia, was included among the hemolytic anemia hypotheses generated.

(b) *Other anemia hypotheses.* Fifty-three percent ($n = 8$) generated one or more hypotheses pertaining to some other type of anemia (that is, acquired red cell aplasia, anemia due to blood loss, or nutritional deficiency anemia).

(c) *Nonanemia hypotheses.* In addition to anemia hypotheses, 33 percent ($n = 5$) of the clinicians generated one or more hypotheses pertaining to other disease entities (such as leukemia/lymphoma, infectious mononucleosis, nephritis, and porphyria).

Statistical Summary

Number of hypotheses listed:
 Mean = 3.7
 Standard deviation = 1.3
 Range = 2–6
 Percentage of physicians generating 4 ± 1 hypotheses = 73.

Diagnosis

Sixty percent ($n = 9$) of the physicians arrived at the correct diagnosis, congenital spherocytic anemia. A few specified a red cell crisis phase of this type of anemia. Of the remaining six physicians, five arrived at a diagnosis of anemia (congenital hemolytic anemia or acquired red cell aplasia), and one made a diagnosis of lead poisoning. Examination of the relation between each physician's list of preliminary hypotheses and final diagnosis indicated that if the correct diagnosis was among the hypotheses a physician generated, it was invariably retained as the final diagnosis. However, if the correct diagnosis was not included in the initial set of hypotheses, the physician failed to arrive at the correct diagnosis by means of further data collection in six out of nine instances (Table 5.1).

Hypothesis Generation, Accuracy of Diagnosis, and Data Acquisition

Table 5.1 also indicates that all physicians who generated the accurate hypothesis at the start of the problem retained it as the correct diagnosis and did this with more efficient, less thorough data acquisition than those who did not generate the appropriate formulation until the end of the problem. If a subject failed to generate the correct hypothesis among his early alternatives, more thorough data collection enabled him to arrive at the correct hypothesis, but less thorough search did not. In this problem, therefore, thorough data collection will direct the physician to a formulation not suggested by earlier data.

Table 5.1 Relation of data acquisition to diagnostic accuracy on patient-management problem 1.

Variable	Group A ($n = 6$)		Group B ($n = 3$)		Group C ($n = 6$)	
	Mean	Range	Mean	Range	Mean	Range
Cues acquired	26	13-37	80	66-100	37	23-50
Critical findings acquired	40	21-58	91	84-100	54	37-68
Efficiency	82	60-100	48	33-55	63	53-71

Group A: correct diagnosis; list of initial hypotheses included the correct diagnosis.

Group B: correct diagnosis; initial hypotheses did not include the correct diagnosis.

Group C: incorrect diagnosis; initial hypotheses did not include the correct diagnosis.

Patient-Management Problem 2

Structure of the Problem

The problem solver is presented with six typewritten lines of introduction to the problem (primarily history of the chief complaint). Any of several workup (history, physical, or lab) or management options can then be selected. As indicated in Figure 5.2, no physician chose to begin treatment on the basis of the introduction; all chose to conduct a complete workup before making a management decision. After completion of the workup, only four eventually chose surgical management, although that is the recommended action. Two of the four chose the surgical procedure recommended for this problem, but this may be of minor relevance, since a surgeon would ordinarily make the decision after referral. In this PMP the option of consultation with or referral to a surgeon was not available, as it is in PMP 3.

Hypothesis Generation

Each clinician was asked to list diagnostic hypotheses at four points in the workup: after reading the introduction, at the end of the history, at the end of the physical, and at the end of the lab (which is also the end of the workup portion of the PMP).

Figure 5.2   Routes chosen for workup and management of patient-management problem 2.

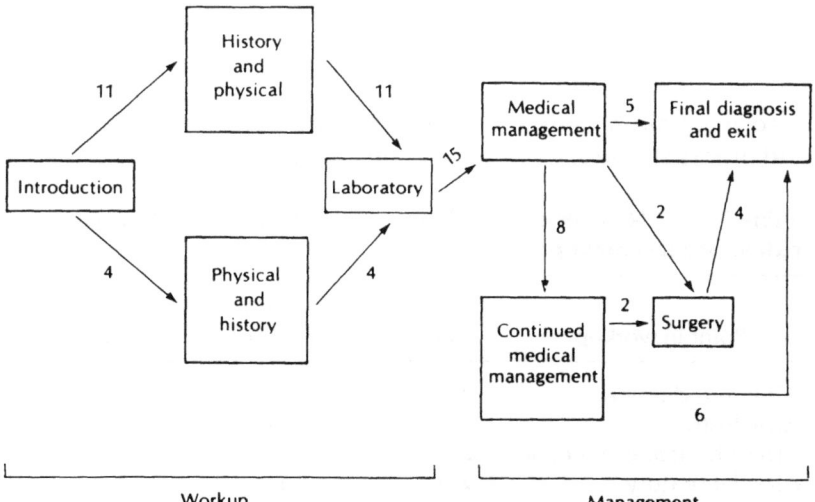

The following categories of hypotheses were generated:

(a) *Peptic ulcer.* All fifteen physicians generated some sort of peptic ulcer hypothesis after reading the introduction. Eleven (73 percent) generated the hypothesis of peptic ulcer *with* complication (obstruction and/or perforation) at some point during the workup. This hypothesis is one component of the correct diagnosis.

(b) *Gallbladder disease.* Fourteen physicians (93 percent) generated a gallbladder hypothesis at some point in the workup; twelve of the fourteen generated it after reading the introduction.

(c) *Pancreatitis.* This hypothesis was considered by all physicians but one at some point in the workup; twelve of the fourteen generated it after reading the introduction.

(d) *Diabetic acidosis.* Fourteen physicians had generated this hypothesis by the end of the workup. Four (27 percent) listed it after the physical; the other ten generated it after the lab (that is, at the end of the workup). This formulation is the second component of the correct diagnosis.

(e) *Other.* Nine clinicians (60 percent) generated one or more other hypotheses.

In sum, almost every subject generated four types of hypotheses: peptic ulcer, gallbladder disease, pancreatitis, and diabetic acidosis. The means and standard deviations of the number of hypotheses considered at various points (Table 5.2) again fall nicely within the estimated capacity of the size of working memory (Simon, 1974).

Diagnosis

To maintain a degree of comparability between this problem and others studied, this analysis considers the diagnostic possibil-

Table 5.2 Number of hypotheses at various points in the workup of patient-management problem 2.

Point in workup	Mean	Standard deviation	Range
After introduction	3.7	1.25	2-7
After history	2.7	0.93	1-5
After physical examination	2.6	1.02	1-5
After laboratory	2.6	1.14	1-5

Table 5.3 Diagnostic formulations at end of workup of patient-management problem 2.

Diagnosis	Physicians making diagnosis	
	Number	Percent
Peptic ulcer	10	67
Peptic ulcer with complication	7	47
Gallbladder disease	3	20
Pancreatitis	7	47
Diabetic acidosis	14	93
Other	5	33

ities listed after the laboratory studies (at the end of the diagnostic workup) as the diagnosis, rather than the final diagnosis listed after various management options had been selected.

The diagnostic possibilities considered at the end of the workup are shown in Table 5.3.

Hypothesis Generation, Accuracy of Diagnosis, and Data Acquisition

The correct diagnosis involved two components, peptic ulcer and diabetic acidosis. Interestingly, the former hypothesis was always generated very early but was rejected by five of fifteen physicians, while the latter was generated late by all but one and was retained by all who generated it. It is worthwhile to determine the way data-acquisition behavior may be related to these outcomes. The first question is, how does the data acquisition of the physicians who retained the hypothesis of peptic ulcer differ from that of the five who generated but failed to retain this hypothesis?

All the physicians had entertained a peptic ulcer hypothesis at some point in the workup, but only ten (67 percent) retained this hypothesis at the end of the workup. On the other hand, fourteen had arrived at the hypothesis of diabetic acidosis by the end of the diagnostic workup. The number who listed both components of the correct diagnosis at the end of the workup is relatively low:

(a) Peptic ulcer and diabetic acidosis were listed by ten physicians (67 percent);

Table 5.4   Relation of data acquisition to diagnostic accuracy on patient-management problem 2.

	Group A (n = 10)		Group B (n = 5)	
Variable	Mean	Range	Mean	Range
Cues acquired	24	21-52	31	16-55
Critical findings acquired	50	34-70	46	24-78
Efficiency	45	37-53	43	24-55
Relevant critical findings[a]	67	42-100	58	16-100

Group A: physicians who retained peptic ulcer hypothesis.
Group B: physicians who generated but failed to retain peptic ulcer hypothesis.
[a] Percent of critical findings selected relevant to peptic ulcer (out of 19 available).

(b) Seven of these diagnosed peptic ulcer *with complication* and diabetic acidosis.

Table 5.4 presents the mean scores on three data-acquisition variables and the mean scores on one additional variable pertaining to this question—the percentage of relevant critical findings. This last tabulation shows the percentage of the nineteen critical findings relevant to peptic ulcer (with or without complication) that was selected by each group of physicians. Examination of this table reveals very little difference on the three general data-acquisition variables between physicians who retained the hypothesis of peptic ulcer and those who did not. Thus it does not appear to be possible to attribute differences in diagnostic outcome to differences in thoroughness or efficiency of data acquisition.

Moreover, when the performance of the two groups is examined with respect to a more specific variable, relevant critical findings, only a very moderate mean difference is found (67 vs 58 percent). Examination of individual scores on this variable reveals that two of the five clinicians who did not retain the peptic ulcer hypothesis had very low scores (16 and 26 percent), two had very high scores (95 and 100 percent), and one had an intermediate score (53 percent). With regard to the two with low scores, it is possible that failure to elicit sufficient data relevant to the hypothesis of peptic ulcer was responsible for rejection of the hypothesis. The scores of the other three physicians, however, make it evident that failure to retain the hypothesis of peptic ulcer cannot be solely attributed to failure to elicit sufficient relevant data. Given this finding, it may be hypothesized that failure to retain the formulation of peptic ulcer may result from inadequacies in the process of data interpretation, rather than in the process of data acquisition per se. Unfortunately, the PMP format did not permit us to investigate the process of data interpretation.

Our second question is, given the finding that the hypothesis of diabetic acidosis was never considered early in the workup (after the introduction or the history), how did the data acquisition lead all but one physician to generate and retain this hypothesis as part of the diagnosis? To answer this question, the selection of critical findings relevant to diabetic acidosis was examined.

Four physicians generated the hypothesis of diabetic acidosis at the end of the physical examination. This section included two critical findings relevant to diabetic acidosis, and one or both were selected by all four physicians. Three of the four physicians selected critical findings that were also relevant to *another* hypothesis generated earlier in the workup. Ten clinicians generated the hypothesis of diabetic acidosis at the end of the lab. Thus, by the end of the workup, a total of fourteen physicians had generated (and all retained) the hypothesis of diabetic acidosis. The lab section included three critical findings relevant to diabetic acidosis *only*. All fourteen selected at least two out of the three critical findings relevant to *both* diabetic acidosis and pancreatitis. Seven also selected one of the two critical findings relevant to diabetic acidosis only.

The only physician who never generated the hypothesis of diabetic acidosis was working with the pancreatitis possibility from the start. He elicited two of three cues highly indicative of diabetic acidosis, but still did not generate that hypothesis. This particular subject may not have processed these cues, so attached was he to the pancreatitis hypothesis. A more likely explanation is that he interpreted these cues as supportive of his working hypothesis of pancreatitis. In fact, these signs (elevated blood sugar and presence of acetone in urine) are present in some cases of pancreatitis.

A number of routes for generating the hypothesis of diabetic acidosis are suggested. First, data may have been selected that were relevant to another active hypothesis and at the same time provided the basis for thinking of diabetic acidosis. An associative mechanism from one or more areas to a competing hypothesis is thus implied. Second, some clinicians evaluated the patient for possible surgery and in pursuing this goal, elicited data that revealed the presence of diabetes. These findings suggest that most successful physicians can generate multiple hypotheses and flexibly process cues that are relevant to them. At times this mechanism does not work, and a physician becomes wedded to one hypothesis, which leads to gathering and interpreting data as supporting it. Lack of practice or ineptness at generating multiple diagnostic hypotheses can lead a physician down a garden path toward diagnostic error.

Patient-Management Problem 3

Structure of the Problem

The problem begins with an introduction of eight typewritten lines, which include an intern's admitting diagnosis of "low back pain, possible disc" and a letter from a referring physician. The letter concludes with the referring physician's diagnosis, herniated disc. In contrast to the other three PMPs, no space is provided at the end of the introduction to list hypotheses; the end of the history is the first point where they can be listed. The history section is divided into eight subsections, seven of which are labeled and may provide additional cues about relevant areas of inquiry. As shown in Figure 5.3, all physicians moved through history, physical examination, and laboratory workup in that order. There is, however, considerable variation in the amount of data selected in each section. Management plans also diverge: ten ordered some type of consultation, usually surgical; two tried medical management; one referred immediately to a vascular surgeon; and one discharged the patient while waiting to consider vascular surgery.

Treatment decisions followed from and were justified by the diagnosis (disc, malingering, or arthritis). Management results were of little effect in altering opinions expressed at the end of the diagnostic section: at the start of the management sections, ten clinicians were on routes that would eventually lead the patient to a vascular surgeon, and four were on routes that would probably not lead to surgery. At the end of the management sections, these four had not changed their minds.

Figure 5.3 Routes chosen for workup and management of patient-management problem 3.

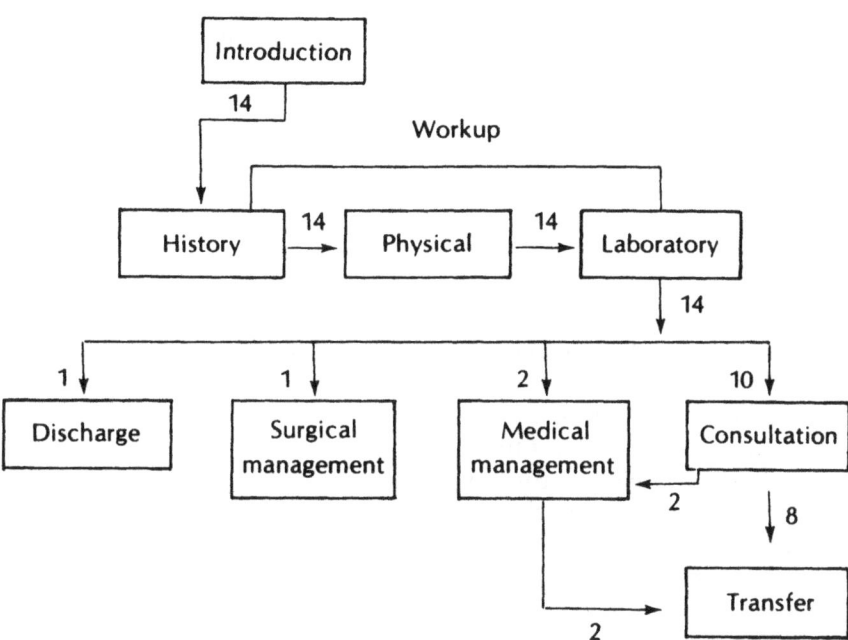

NOTES:

1. Only 14 physicians are included in the chart. One did not complete the problem (after history and physical, he listed diagnosis and stopped).
2. The chart portrays only the *major* options selected at the end of the workup.

Hypothesis Generation

All physicians were asked to list diagnostic hypotheses at three points: after the history, after the physical examination, and after the laboratory (which is the end of the diagnostic section). Fourteen are included in this part of the analysis, since one failed to list hypotheses for the problem.

The major types of diagnostic hypotheses entertained were:

(a) *Lumbar disc.* Thirteen of fourteen physicians (93 percent) listed this hypothesis at the end of the history section. It was generated, therefore, either from the data obtained in the history or from the suggestions planted in the introduction.

(b) *Peripheral vascular insufficiency or occlusion.* Eleven (79 percent) generated this hypothesis at some point in the problem;

seven of these listed it immediately after the history. This hypothesis is the correct diagnosis.

(c) *Arthritis*. Three (21 percent) generated this hypothesis. One listed it first after the history, one after the laboratory work, and one after the management section.

(d) *Malingering*. This hypothesis was mentioned by two clinicians (14 percent), both after the physical examination.

(e) *Other*. Miscellaneous hypotheses were listed by twelve physicians. Each was considered for only one or two sections of the problem and was entertained by too few physicians to be tabulated.

In summary, almost every subject generated two types of hypotheses: a disc problem and a peripheral vascular insufficiency or occlusion problem. The hypotheses of arthritis and malingering were generated by a few physicians and were the basis of management errors. Other miscellaneous hypotheses were generated by twelve of the fourteen clinicians, but were rejected in the course of the workup and did not enter into the management decision making.

Basic statistics on hypothesis generation are presented in Table 5.5.

On the average, fewer hypotheses were listed at the earliest point in this problem than in any other; this may be the result of a number of features of the problem itself. First, the earliest point for listing hypotheses is after the history; the data elicited in this stage probably permitted some convergence by rejection of less supported hypotheses. Second, the introduction to this problem is the only one to offer another physician's diagnostic opinion and it is given twice, in the intern's admitting diagnosis ("possible disc") and again in the referring physician's letter ("my diagnosis is herniated disc"); the orientation created by these instructions

Table 5.5 Number of hypotheses at various points in the workup of patient-management problem 3.

Point in workup	Mean	Standard deviation	Range
After history	2.50	0.54	1-4
After physical examination	2.00	1.14	1-4
After laboratory	1.79	0.45	1-3

may have decreased the number of alternatives considered. Third, it is possible that low-back-pain situations do not have as many potential etiologies as the other problems studied; the smaller number of hypotheses generated may thus reflect the complexity of the task environment. The available data do not permit a choice among these alternatives or statistical assignment of portions of the variance in number of hypotheses to each possible cause. But it does seem clear that variations in the number of hypotheses generated may be produced by variations in the amount of information provided before hypotheses are listed, the presence or absence of misleading expectations (Einstellung), and other psychological characteristics of the problem solver, and the complexity of the task environment itself. A more precise unraveling of the respective contribution of these three components awaits further research.

Diagnosis

The diagnostic possibilities listed at the end of the diagnostic workup are summarized in Table 5.6.

Eleven physicians arrived at the correct diagnosis. Of these, four were still entertaining other hypotheses at the close, while seven had narrowed their search and evaluation down to one. Four did not arrive at the correct diagnosis at the end of the laboratory section. Their diagnostic alternatives at that point were disc and arthritis, disc and malingering, disc and diabetes, and malingering.

Table 5.6 Diagnostic formulations at end of workup of patient-management problem 3.

Diagnosis	Physicians making diagnosis	
	Number	Percent
Peripheral vascular insufficiency or occlusion	11	79
Lumbar disc	5	36
Arthritis	2	14
Malingering	2	14
Other	3	21

Table 5.7 Relation of data acquisition to diagnostic accuracy on patient-management problem 3.

Variable	Group A (n = 11)		Group B (n = 4)	
	Mean	Range	Mean	Range
Cues acquired	27	10-51	20	13-28
Critical findings acquired	62	44-80	47	36-56
Efficiency	20	14-34	20	13-34
Relevant critical findings[a]	90	71-100	36	14-43

Group A: physicians who generated and retained vascular hypothesis.
Group B: physicians who did not generate vascular hypothesis.
[a] Percentage of critical findings relevant to vascular insufficiency and/or occlusion selected (out of 7 available).

Hypothesis Generation, Accuracy of Diagnosis, and Data Acquisition

All physicians who generated peripheral vascular insufficiency and/or occlusion as a diagnostic hypothesis retained it as their final diagnosis. All of the physicians who reached another conclusion never considered peripheral vascular insufficiency and/or occlusion as an alternative. Table 5.7 shows that the physicians who made the correct diagnosis tended to obtain more data than physicians whose outcome was incorrect. In this problem differences in diagnostic outcome may be attributable to variation in thoroughness of data acquisition. Herniated lumbar disc was the alternative most frequently considered by the physicians who ultimately made the correct diagnosis, and they were able to rule out this hypothesis as they proceeded through the problem. The physicians who erroneously made a final diagnosis of herniated lumbar disc tended to restrict acquiring cues, particularly those that would have helped reject the erroneous hypothesis.

This interpretation is substantiated by the following facts. In the entire problem seven critical findings were available relevant to vascular insufficiency and/or occlusion. The eleven physicians who correctly reached that diagnosis obtained an average of 6.3 of these cues (range 5 to 7). The four who did not arrive at the correct diagnosis acquired an average of 2.5 of these relevant critical findings (range 1 to 3). It seems reasonable to infer that the initial expectations of the four in error led them to restrict their data collection and to exclude those cues which would have assisted them in arriving at the correct diagnosis.

To summarize: in PMP 3, physicians who did not make the correct diagnosis generally gathered fewer data than those who reached the correct solution. Moreover, the correct solution was not explicitly rejected; it was never adequately considered. Erring physicians were misled into premature closure by some traps set in the introduction to the problem. It will be recalled that in the opening statement of the problem, the suggestion is twice made that the patient has a disc problem. Three of the four physicians who did not reach the correct conclusion made a diagnosis of a disc problem, a clear example of the effect of suggestions upon thought processes (Maier, 1942; Luchins and Luchins, 1950).

This pattern of error in part resembles the behavior of the physician in PMP 2 who did not generate diabetic acidosis but perseverated with the erroneous hypothesis of pancreatitis. Similarly, it was shown in PMP 1 that more thorough data acquistion could lead to new formulations. The lack of relationship between data acquisition and the fate of the peptic ulcer hypothesis in PMP 2 is all the more striking. What is the cause of the observed variation in the relation of data collection to hypothesis generation? Is it differences in the structure of the problem? Or in the mental representations of the problem solvers? Or is it these elements interacting with others not yet identified? These are unanswered questions.

Patient-Management Problem 4

Structure of the Problem

The problem begins with a five-line introduction that presents the age and sex of the patient, and a brief statement of the chief complaint. Following this introduction the physician is offered an opportunity to list diagnostic hypotheses. The format is similar to that of PMPs 1 and 2, but in PMP 4 even less information is provided prior to the request for preliminary hypotheses. After listing preliminary hypotheses, the physician can choose one of several workup options. All of the physicians studied selected the option of history and physical examination followed by laboratory. In PMP 4, unlike PMPs 2 and 3, history and physical examina-

Figure 5.4 **Routes chosen for workup and management of patient-management problem 4.**

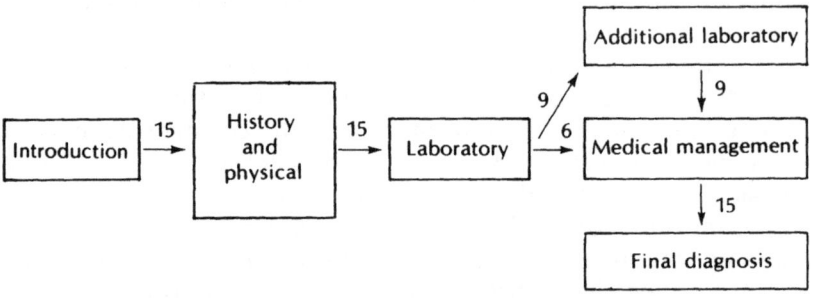

tion are offered in the same section rather than in separate sections the order of which might be varied.

Figure 5.4 indicates that after some preliminary lab work, physicians have the option of ordering additional laboratory studies or proceeding directly to medical management. The first alternative was selected by nine physicians who subsequently went on to management, while six proceeded directly to management. All physicians reached the same diagnosis and chose the same management option.

Hypothesis Generation

Pernicious anemia. This hypothesis was generated by all fifteen clinicians. Eleven generated it after the introduction and prior to the history and physical, the remaining four after the history and physical examination. Pernicious anema with degeneration of the spinal cord was also considered by four. This variant takes into account and explains the particular cortical symptoms (forgetfulness, lack of alertness) noted in the patient. Pernicious anemia, either with or without spinal cord degeneration, was the correct diagnosis.

Carcinoma. This hypothesis was generated by twelve physicians (80 percent). Four listed this formulation after the introduction, prior to any history taking or physical examination.

Cerebral arteriosclerotic disease. This was generated by five physicians (33 percent). Four listed it after the introduction, prior to any history taking or physical examination.

Table 5.8 Number of hypotheses at various points in the workup of patient-management problem 4.

Point in workup	Mean	Standard deviation	Range
After introduction	3.2	1.2	2-6
After history and physical examination	1.9	1.0	1-4
After laboratory	1.5	1.0	1-3
After additional laboratory	1.2	0.3	1-2

Folic acid deficiency. This hypothesis was generated by four respondents (27 percent), three after the preliminary laboratory work, the fourth even later.

Other. Twelve respondents (80 percent) entertained one or more hypotheses other than the four major ones listed above. But each of these other hypotheses was mentioned by only one or two physicians and was usually listed for only one section of the problem.

In summary, three out of the four hypotheses most frequently entertained in this problem were generated very early in the problem, directly after a brief preliminary introduction and before any history or physical examination data had been obtained.

Table 5.8 indicates that approximately 4 ± 2 hypotheses are entertained very early in the problem based on minimal information and that there is rapid convergence toward the diagnostic solution as additional information is selected.

Diagnosis

The diagnostic possibilities listed at the end of the workup, but before therapy had been begun, are summarized in Table 5.9.

From the standpoint of outcomes this problem is the easiest in the series, as shown by the fact that it is the only problem correctly solved by all fifteen physicians. Analysis of the weights assigned to the cues by our consultant hematologist discloses that pernicious anemia is the only hypothesis listed that is in any way supported by the data. Little support is provided for other alternatives, and only three cues (out of ninety-two) point away from pernicious anemia to even the slightest degree. It is easy to see how even minimal data collection would permit confirmation of the hypothesis. One might conclude either that the diagnosis of

Table 5.9 Diagnostic formulations at end of workup of patient-management problem 4.

	Physicians making diagnosis	
Diagnosis	Number	Percent
Pernicious anemia	15	100
Pernicious anemia with degeneration of spinal cord	4	27
Other hypotheses in addition to pernicious anemia	2	13
Carcinoma	1	7
Folic acid deficiency	1	7

pernicious anemia generally is simple or that this situation did not offer enough distractions and challenges to experienced physicians. If difficulty of a medical problem can be gauged by the number of reasonable alternative hypotheses supported by the data, then PMP 4 was not a difficult problem.

Thorough data acquision apparently bears little relation to accuracy of solution in this problem. An extremely thorough physician is not rewarded with a better grasp of the situation, nor is one who is efficient and limited in data collection penalized. The correct hypothesis is generated early, and a correct diagnosis can be reached even with great variation of data acquisition. Although the University of Illinois scoring key indicates that most of the data in the history and physical examination sections are desirable or necessary in this problem, relatively few data are in fact needed by experienced physicians for a solution. The problem appears to be one in which a relatively small amount of the information recommended can confirm an early hypothesis. Not all medical problems are of this sort, since not all can be formulated so specifically with extremely limited data and have specific diagnostic tests to confirm early hunches. But when this combination occurs, limited and focused data collection appears to be an efficient approach to problem solving.

Consistency among Problems

A major aim of our research has been to identify those heuristics used consistently by expert clinicians to solve diagnostic problems. It was hoped that physicians would display the operation of these heuristics by employing consistent strategies over a range of problems. To facilitate the search for evidence of heuristics, a number of assumptions were made. First, it was assumed that the use of any heuristic would be expressed in the four basic variables quantified. This, of course, implied that any heuristic used that could not be expressed with these variables would probably not be perceived by the researchers. A second assumption was that, since any heuristics could be applied uniformly across problems, a small number of problems would allow subjects to use these heuristics in a way that could be grasped by the researchers. Our search for consistently applied heuristics was therefore confined to four problems and four quantitative variables. Consistency of performance across these four problems on one or a combination of the variables would have been evidence for use of a heuristic. The fact that no such consistency was seen, again emphasizes the significance of case specificity.

Table 5.10 presents the intercorrelation across the four PMPs of the four variables used in our analysis. Number of hypotheses (d) refers to the number listed by each subject at the first point in the problem where lists were obtained. The correlation matrices reveal the degree of intraindividual consistency in data acquisition and hypothesis testing. It may be seen that only three of twenty-four correlations in the four tables exceed .51, the lowest degree

Table 5.10 Correlations of four process variables across four patient-management problems.

(a) Cue acquisition				(b) Critical findings			
Problem	1	2	3	Problem	1	2	3
2	.01			2	.26		
3	.16	.01		3	.14	.29	
4	.65[a]	.17	.55[a]	4	.44	.41	.63[a]

(c) Efficiency				(d) Number of hypotheses			
Problem	1	2	3	Problem	1	2	3
2	-.05			2	-.03		
3	-.09	-.11		3	.08	-.04	
4	.37	.04	-.03	4	.31	.33	-.24

[a] $p < .05$.

of association that may be considered significantly different from zero (5-percent level). There is obviously little evidence here of intraindividual consistency in data gathering and hypothesis generation. In analyzing the PMPs, we found that rates of data acquisition and hypothesis generation varied considerably within each problem. It appears that this variation is not the result of physicians' consistently applying different strategies, but that the strategy itself changes, depending on the problem. Thus an underlying principle like "branch and screen" will lead to workups of different length depending upon how much branching and screening is required in a particular task environment.

Analysis of Errors

Each problem was correctly solved by the majority of the physicians. Four solved all four problems, seven solved three problems, three solved two, and one solved only one problem. Thoroughness and efficiency of data collection associated with accurate problem formulation varied widely. A qualitative analysis of the reasoning involved in inaccurate solutions was more helpful than further statistical analysis in understanding varying approaches to each problem.

Inaccurate Hypothesis Generation

One type of error that was common to two problems points up the importance of generating accurate diagnostic hypotheses before initiating management. PMPs 2 and 3 offer extensive management options. PMP 2 has a complex diagnostic solution. In both problems subjects who were not considering accurate diagnoses before initiating management chose inappropriate management procedures and did not revise their diagnoses as a result of the patient's response to management. These observations cause us to emphasize again the importance of correct diagnosis in those medical problems where choice of treatment depends on the diagnosis. (Many problems, especially in surgery, are not of this type.)

Some errors in hypothesis generation illustrate the Einstellung effect of Gestalt psychology (Maier, 1942). In PMP 3, early suggestion of a herniated lumbar disc led some physicians to neglect collecting data that could have pointed them to alternative hypotheses. They were apparently led to premature closure on an attractive but incorrect alternative and failed to gather information that would have helped to solve the problem.

Errors in Evaluation of Hypotheses

Rejecting an accurate hypotheses once it had been generated occurred in more than one problem and was particularly noticeable in PMP 2, a problem with two solutions. Five physicians did not retain the hypothesis of peptic ulcer, which all had generated. Two were very thorough in data collection, two collected data skimpily, and one occupied an intermediate position. The unsuccessful problem solvers were quite comparable in thoroughness to those who solved the problem. Rejection of the hypothesis cannot be attributed solely to failure to elicit sufficient data relevant to it.

The rejection of a correct alternative in a two-formulation problem strongly suggests that these physicians were striving for a parsimonious solution and were attempting to understand the case as an instance of one disease. To evaluate and retain two diagnostic hypotheses is a difficult conceptual task, since there is a strong tendency to find one formulation to account for the maximum number of data. The problem-oriented approach might be particularly useful in helping physicians as well as students to avoid this type of error. Since this approach emphasizes formulation of problems at a level for which there is sufficient justification in the data base, the formulation of two separate problems would be facilitated in this instance. Furthermore, careful assessment of each problem would assist the problem solver in keeping them separate and encourage the development of an evaluation and treatment plan for each.

Misinterpretation of Data

The third and last type of error is that caused by misinterpretation of cues. An example occurred in PMP 1, when one physician interpreted a normal serum lead value as elevated and made a diagnosis of lead poisoning based on this erroneous interpretation.

Comparisons with High-Fidelity Simulations

Performance on the PMPs can be compared to that on the high-fidelity simulations along several dimensions: relations of certain quantitative variables to accuracy of diagnostic outcome, consistency across problems, and types of errors made.

Quantitative Variables

In these data percentage of cues acquired and percentage of critical findings acquired are uniformly highly correlated, as was also found with the high-fidelity simulations. This may be largely a result of the part-whole relationship of the two variables. On the other hand, the relation between thoroughness of data collection and efficiency is generally negative for PMPs, while for high-fidelity simulations it is much less clearly defined and ranges from essentially zero to low positive. Given the definitions of the variables, this appears to indicate much less hypothesis-focused inquiry in the high-fidelity simulations than in the PMPs. These variations may be partly attributable to artifacts of the scoring system, as we have seen that the percentage of items needed for solution of a PMP varies across problems, or to varying degrees of difficulty in the two types of simulations. It is also possible that this phenomenon is caused in part by the cuing available in the PMPs, the argument being that if a subject is considering one or several hypotheses and can select from a list of items to test those hypotheses, it is easier to focus inquiry on the hypotheses than when the hypothesis-focused items have to be generated internally.

Interproblem Consistencies

It has been noted that a physician's approach is not consistent across problems. Despite a widely held expectation that there should be an identifiable approach to problem solving that would differentiate good problem solvers from poor ones, such a behavior pattern has not emerged in our studies, nor was any particular behavior pattern identifiable with (or idiosyncratic to) an individual. Consistency of problem-solving approach tends to be associated with the problems themselves. That is, the problem (or task) is structured into a problem space that is the primary determinant of the approach to the task. This suggests, again, that rather than searching for a general trait called clinical competence or general problem-solving ability, we should pursue the issue of problem-solving strategy *with respect to specific problems*. Perhaps dimensions or distinctive features of problems can be identified so that classes of problems may be formed that will lead eventually to a problem taxonomy. One dimension to be considered in any taxonomy is problem difficulty.

In the absence of such a taxonomy, extensive sampling of a variety of clinical situations is needed to draw valid conclusions about a physician's or a student's competence. Until the characteristics that make problems unique are identified, the variance contributed to a set of observations by specific characteristics of problems must be treated as error. The magnitude of this source of error may be reduced by observing a large sample and a broad spectrum of behavior.

Diagnosis and Management

In the high-fidelity simulations participants were instructed to arrive at a diagnosis, but were not required to generate a treatment plan. Some did so spontaneously; for these, data on the diagnosis/management relationship are available. In both the high-fidelity simulations and the PMPs, failure to generate an accurate diagnosis was always accompanied by failure to formulate a proper management plan. Even an adverse patient response to inappropriate management did not stimulate the physician to generate an accurate diagnosis if it had not already been formulated. On the other hand, those who had arrived at the correct diagnosis were much more likely to formulate an appropriate management plan. True, not all of these physicians developed the optimal plan, but having a correct diagnosis was a significant help toward planning for proper patient management.

Errors in Reasoning Process

To obtain a better idea of the possibilities of error in medical reasoning, we compare here the types of errors made on PMPs with those discussed in Chapter 4.

Failure to generate the accurate hypothesis is one type of error. If that formulation was not reached before management was initiated in the PMPs, then the correct diagnosis was never generated. In some cases the correct hypothesis was not considered, despite accumulation of considerable data to support it.

On the other hand, generating the accurate hypothesis does not guarantee its retention. This is particularly true in complex problems that have more than one solution (PMP 2 and simulation 1, for example). In these problems an apparent tendency toward parsimony led some physicians to assign all of the data to one diagnostic formulation, or to redefine the second hypothesis so it could be a subset of the first. In simulation 1, anemia could be viewed as secondary to mononucleosis rather than being pursued and defined as a completely separate problem. A similar phenomenon occurred in PMP 2, where all respondents generated a peptic ulcer hypothesis early in the workup, but five had rejected it by the end of the workup.

A third possible error is erroneous assessment of the likelihood of competing hypotheses. In problems where the hypothesis pool could be reduced to two or three competing hypotheses (such as PMP 3 and simulation 2), the accurate hypothesis may have been dropped despite supporting evidence, because of inaccurate prior probabilities. Since data on subjective probabilities of hypotheses are unavailable, no firm conclusions can be drawn about this potential basis for error.

None of these errors was common in the group studied. Yet where each occurs, it is characteristic of a certain type of problem. The complex problem with multiple solutions and the strategy of multiple competing hypotheses both are vulnerable to certain types of error. That is, errors are associated with particular types of problem structures and with particular heuristics.

Comparison with University of Illinois Scoring System

Table 5.11 presents correlations among the three measures of data acquisition used in the present analysis and four measures of data acquisition developed by the University of Illinois for scoring PMPs. Material for this analysis was obtained by scoring the PMPs completed by our subjects according to the Illinois scoring scheme.

Table 5.11 shows that the Illinois efficiency index is negatively correlated with our thoroughness measures except in PMP 4. On the other hand, the proficiency index correlates positively with cues acquired and critical findings acquired across all four PMPs; this demonstrates that proficiency, as defined by the Center for Educational Development, contains a large component of thoroughness. The Inquiry Project's efficiency measure is an assessment of the proportion of findings obtained by a physician that were positive for at least one generated hypothesis. It is thus a measure of how high-yield or hypothesis-focused the data gathering was. This variable is negatively correlated with errors of commission in PMP 1. In PMP 4, it correlates positively with errors

Table 5.11 Correlations of Medical Inquiry Project and University of Illinois scores on diagnostic portions of each PMP. EI = efficiency index; OM = errors of omission; COM = errors of commission; and PI = proficiency index.

Variable	EI	OM	COM	PI
PMP 1				
Cues acquired	-.71[a]	-.78[a]	.90[a]	.56[b]
Critical findings	-.67[a]	-.77[a]	.80[a]	.59[a]
Efficiency	.45	.36	-.67[a]	-.14
PMP 2				
Cues acquired	-.60[a]	-.88[a]	.61[a]	.79[a]
Critical findings	-.60[a]	-.89[a]	.58[b]	.81[a]
Efficiency	-.05	-.08	-.30	.16
PMP 3				
Cues acquired	-.55[b]	-.87[a]	-.06	.86[a]
Critical findings	-.26	-.94[a]	.00	-.93[a]
Efficiency	.23	.36	.13	-.37
PMP 4				
Cues acquired	-.07	-.99[a]	-.31	.98[a]
Critical findings	.04	-.93[a]	-.40	.94[a]
Efficiency	.19	.71[a]	-.13	-.70[a]

[a] $p < .01$.
[b] $p < .05$.

of omission and negatively with proficiency. Overall, the absence of consistent correlations implies that the Illinois scoring scheme tends not to assess hypothesis-testing activity.

In PMP 4, efficiency is positively correlated with errors of omission and negatively correlated with proficiency. This problem could be adequately solved by a much more focused workup than was recommended by the Illinois standardization group. As expected, errors of omission are negatively correlated with cues acquired and critical findings acquired over all PMPs. The more data one elicits, the less likely one is to omit positively weighted items.

The relation among errors of commission, cues acquired, and critical findings acquired is not so consistent. This is probably a result of the lack of a consistent proportional relationship between items in each category. Using the Medical Inquiry Project scoring system, the items designated as cues vary with each problem. The potential determinants of the efficiency score not only vary with each problem but also with each subject. Similarly, in the Illinois system each problem has varying percentages of items to be avoided and the problems thus require varying amounts of selectivity. From a psychometric perspective, then, the penalty for guessing not only varies with each problem, but in some instances with each subject.

For example, to calculate the proficiency index, one subtracts the negatively weighted selections from the positively weighted ones and divides by the maximum possible score. The subject's proficiency index is this quotient times 100. PMP 1 comprises a total of 30 items, 15 of which are positive, 9 negative, and 6 of which have zero weights. In this problem, then, the probability of selecting a positive item by guessing randomly is .50 while that of selecting a negative item is .30. On the other hand, PMP 2 consists of 134 scorable items (51 positive, 20 negative, and 63 zero). Here the probability of selecting a positive item by chance is .38, while the probability of randomly selecting a negative item is only .15. Thus the potential penalty for guessing is much lower on PMP 2 than on PMP 1. We are not suggesting that anyone who takes these problems seriously will select items at random, but it is of interest to note that in any testing situation where a small number of these problems is used, the contributions of these unintended (and controlled) variations may be considerable.

Conclusion

Four patient-management problems have been discussed and the results compared to those on the high-fidelity simulations. Several points may be noted:

(a) Intraindividual consistency across problems is low. It appears that the problem solver's representation of the task environment strongly determines how the problem is attacked.

(b) Despite differences caused by format, some comparable problem situations are found in both high-fidelity simulations and PMPs. This comparability is encouraging for creators of lower-fidelity simulations, since it seems to indicate that certain aspects of performance on the lower-fidelity simulation may be generalized to high-fidelity simulation and perhaps to a real world environment.

(c) Errors made when attempting diagnostic problems can be identified and related to basic psychological processes. These errors should be more clearly defined so they can serve as a focus for training and evaluation of students in problem solving.

This and other analyses (see Chapters 7, 8, and 9) imply that the structure of the task environment governs problem-solving behavior far more strongly than the contribution of individual differences. Although we have repeatedly qualified our interpretations by noting that the task environment is structured by the problem solver into a psychological problem space, different task environments have a similar effect on a broad spectrum of problem solvers. In one sense, learning medicine means learning to interpret certain problems as one's teachers do. Problem spaces are not arbitrary constructions; among people who are knowledgeable about a class of problems, they are structured in predictable ways, adapted to the task.

6 / Fixed-Order Problems

This chapter describes a study of medical reasoning that used simulated medical problems in which the physician had no control over quantity or sequence of data available. This constraint moved the study one more step from medical reality, but it had certain important advantages for the Medical Inquiry Project. The problems analyzed here are the only *medical* problems in our entire battery in which all clinicians worked with precisely the same data in the same order; they are therefore called fixed-order problems. Even more significantly, they were designed to embody a set of specific structural dimensions and are the only medical problems in the battery where certain problem-structure variables were systematically varied.

Generation of multiple hypotheses via association of a small number of cues with patterns stored in memory, early hypothesis generation, and utilization of cues to test hypotheses in a hypothetico-deductive manner were all observed in pilot testing of high-fidelity simulations. At first, we wished to know whether these phenomena could be observed and measured in less elaborate settings to facilitate further investigations. As our understanding of medical problem solving broadened, it was increasingly recognized that the structure of the problem itself may interact with the physician's internalized strategies to produce the behavior observed. We wished to learn more about these effects. This study, therefore, had two major objectives: (a) to explore the potential of relatively low-fidelity simulations for making inexpensive but extensive observations of medical problem solving; and (b) to begin systematic study of the effects of variations in problem structure on a number of parameters central to the diagnostic process.

Method

Problems

Twenty-two of the twenty-four physicians of the project sample completed four fixed-order problems. In each, data were presented on six cards, with approximately two cues added per card, so that at the sixth card all cues were available for a problem. The cards were always presented in the same order. The four problems were administered to each physician individually by a member of the project staff. Each participant was instructed to think aloud after reading each card and to focus his commentary on the hypotheses being entertained and the cues associated with them. The card most recently presented was always in the subject's view, so that memory was not a factor in the experiment. All responses were tape-recorded and subsequently transcribed for analysis.

Each problem was structurally unique. Problem structure was varied along two dimensions, diagnostic specificity and cue consistency. Two cases were designed to converge on a single diagnosis, whereas in the other two several cues could reasonably be applied to more than one diagnosis. Further, in two problems *all* cues were consistent with one diagnosis, while in the other two not all cues could be so clustered. Since problem 2 lacks both cue consistency and diagnostic specificity, it should be the most "problematic" of the cases, the most difficult problem "to make sense of." In cognitive terms, problem 4 is the most simply structured; as the data unfold, they are consistent with, and converge upon, a single diagnosis. Problems 1 and 3 occupy intermediate positions. In problem 3, the data converged on a single diagnosis, but not all the cues were consistent with the textbook description of the disease. In problem 1, the cues were consistent with a single diagnosis, but general enough to point to other diagnoses. Data consistent with all were provided; hence the cues did not converge on a single diagnosis, but could apply, if properly clustered, to several diagnoses. Figure 6.1 presents these relationships.

Variables

Six measures were devised to assess the effect of the structure of the problem on both criterial and noncriterial groups of physicians:

Figure 6.1 Structural attributes of fixed-order problems.

	DIAGNOSTIC SPECIFICITY	
CUE CONSISTENCY	High	Low
High	*Problem 4* All data are consistent with and increasingly specific for a single diagnosis. Clustering easy.	*Problem 1* One or more diagnoses possible, given cues; all cues are consistent with a single diagnosis, but general enough to point to other diagnoses.
Low	*Problem 3* Majority of cues converge on a single diagnosis, but not all cues are consistent with it.	*Problem 2* No clear clustering. Cues do not converge on a single diagnosis, and do not even cluster clearly on two or three. Maximum noise, minimum signal.

Number of hypotheses
Number of serious hypotheses
Maximum number of cues associated with a hypothesis
Mean number of cues associated with a hypothesis
Number of early hypotheses
Number of cues utilized to generate hypotheses.

Number of hypotheses. This means the total number of hypotheses mentioned by a physician across all cards of a problem. Once a given hypothesis was mentioned, say at card 2 of a problem, it was not counted again if repeated on the same card or on a subsequent card.

Number of serious hypotheses. A hypothesis was defined as serious either if it was mentioned on at least two cards or if at least four cues were associated with it. Any hypothesis was counted only once in each problem.

Maximum number of cues associated with a hypothesis. This variable is most easily defined by example. If cues 2, 3, and 4 were associated with hypothesis *X* on card 3, cue 5 was associated with *X* on card 6, and no other cues were related to this hypothesis, the score for maximum cues associated would be 4. Once a given cue is associated with a given hypothesis, it is not counted again for that hypothesis. For example, if cues 2, 3, and 4 were associated with hypothesis *X* on card 3, and cue 3 mentioned again with *X* on card 6, the score on maximum cues associated would be 3.

Mean number of cues associated with a hypothesis. Varying numbers of cues were associated with each hypothesis by the different subjects. The mean was computed for each subject on each problem by dividing the total number of cues associated with his hypotheses by the total number of hypotheses generated.

Number of early hypotheses. A hypothesis was defined as early if it was mentioned on card 1 or card 2 for any problem. As above, a repetition of a given hypothesis within the same card or on a subsequent card was not counted.

Number of cues utilized to generate hypotheses. Each problem had a limited number of cues in its data base. The cues utilized score is the number of cues that were used at least once.

For each problem, all hypotheses were identified, categorized, and coded. In addition, each cue mentioned in association with a hypothesis was coded.

Reliability measures were obtained to assess the accuracy of the coding of both the hypotheses and the cues associated with them. For problem 1, four protocols were randomly selected and coded independently by three coders. The reliability was measured by the ratio of coding agreements to the total number of coding decisions (Holsti, 1969). In problems 2, 3, and 4, two coders used two randomly selected protocols to assess reliability.

Table 6.1 Mean intercoder agreement on coding hypotheses and cues.

	Problem			
Variable	1	2	3	4
Hypotheses	.88	.84	.90	.92
Cues	.80	.82	.82	.91

Table 6.1 summarizes the reliability of the coding scheme. With a sufficiently high degree of intercoder agreement established, all protocols were coded and the scores on each of the six variables for each problem were computed.

Results

A repeated-measures analysis of variance was performed on each variable. Each analysis included "group" (criterial versus noncriterial physicians) as an independent variable and "problem" as the repeated-measures dimension. In order to maintain an overall alpha level of about .06 for the entire set of six analyses of variance, the .01 level of statistical significance was generally adopted for each problem. One analysis where a significance level of .025 was found will be discussed later. Scheffé post hoc comparisons were performed on each variable where significant differences were found, to identify the sources of the difference. Because of the pilot character of this study and the small sample size, the .05 level of significance was generally used in these post hoc comparisons. Basic statistical data and analyses of variance are presented in Tables 6.2 to 6.9.

Table 6.2 **Means and standard deviations (in parentheses) on six dependent variables, by problem.**

	Problem			
Variable	1	2	3	4
Number of hypotheses	14.50 (6.06)	9.59 (5.33)	13.05 (5.27)	12.82 (4.97)
Number of serious hypotheses	5.91 (2.77)	1.68 (1.62)	4.41 (2.59)	4.05 (1.98)
Maximum cues associated	6.00 (1.56)	3.86 (1.29)	5.14 (1.35)	5.64 (2.85)
Mean cues associated	2.24 (0.76)	1.90 (0.50)	2.45 (0.41)	1.41 (0.81)
Number of early hypotheses	4.50 (2.50)	3.18 (3.07)	3.45 (2.44)	4.41 (2.85)
Number of cues utilized	9.86 (2.32)	8.27 (2.18)	9.82 (2.31)	9.73 (4.25)

Table 6.3 Number of hypotheses: repeated-measures analysis of variance.

Source of variation	df	Adj. df[a]	MS	F
Group	1	—	0.01	0.00
Subjects: group	20	—	80.81	
Problems	3	2	94.31	7.69[b]
Problems x groups	3	2	1.73	0.14
Problems x subjects: group	60	47	12.26	

[a] Adjusted degrees of freedom for reference distribution test (Greenhouse and Geiser estimate).
[b] $p < .01$.

Table 6.4 Number of serious hypotheses: repeated-measures analysis of variance.

Source of variation	df	Adj. df[a]	MS	F
Group	1	—	14.58	1.51
Subjects: group	20	—	9.63	
Problems	3	2	67.38	17.94[b]
Problems x groups	3	2	0.74	0.20
Problems x subjects : group	60	49	3.76	

[a] Adjusted degrees of freedom for reference distribution test (Greenhouse and Geiser estimate).
[b] $p < .01$.

Table 6.5 Maximum cues associated: repeated-measures analysis of variance.

Source of variation	df	Adj. df[a]	MS	F
Group	1	—	3.83	0.63
Subjects: group	20	—	6.05	
Problems	3	1	19.17	7.17[b]
Problems x groups	3	1	5.68	2.12
Problems x subjects: group	60	31	2.67	

[a] Adjusted degrees of freedom for reference distribution test (Greenhouse and Geiser estimate).
[b] $p < .03$.

Table 6.6 Mean cues associated: repeated-measures analysis of variance.

Source of variation	df	Adj. df [a]	MS	F
Group	1	—	0.65	1.71
Subjects: group	20	—	0.38	
Problems	3	2	4.53	10.69[b]
Problems x groups	3	2	0.18	0.43
Problems x subjects: group	60	43	0.42	

[a] Adjusted degrees of freedom for reference distribution test (Greenhouse and Geiser estimate).
[b] $p < .01$.

Table 6.7 Number of early hypotheses: repeated-measures analysis of variance.

Source of variation	df	Adj. df [a]	MS	F
Group	1	—	1.77	0.12
Subjects: group	20	—	14.95	
Problems	3	2	9.77	1.98
Problems x groups	3	2	1.41	0.29
Problems x subjects: group	60	45	4.94	

[a] Adjusted degrees of freedom for reference distribution test (Greenhouse and Geiser estimate).

Table 6.8 Number of cues utilized: repeated-measures analysis of variance.

Source of variation	df	Adj. df [a]	MS	F
Group	1	—	23.61	1.28
Subjects: group	20	—	18.40	
Problems	3	1	12.95	2.57
Problems x groups	3	1	4.97	0.99
Problems x subjects: group	60	34	5.03	

[a] Adjusted degrees of freedom for reference distribution test (Greenhouse and Geiser estimate).

Table 6.9 Scheffé post hoc comparisons on several variables.

Variable	Comparison	Contrast tested
Number of hypotheses	Diagnostic specificity[a]	0.89
	Cue consistency[b]	2.34[c]
Number of serious hypotheses	Diagnostic specificity[a]	0.44
	Cue consistency[b]	1.94[d]
Maximum cues associated	Diagnostic specificity[a]	0.46
	Cue consistency[b]	1.32
	Pairwise comparisons:	
	Problem 1 - problem 2	2.14[c]
	Problem 1 - problem 3	0.86
	Problem 1 - problem 4	0.36
	Problem 2 - problem 3	-1.28
	Problem 2 - problem 4	-1.78[c]
	Problem 3 - problem 4	-0.50
Mean cues associated	Diagnostic specificity[a]	-0.14
	Cue consistency[b]	-0.35
	Pairwise comparisons:	
	Problem 1 - problem 2	0.34
	Problem 1 - problem 3	-0.21
	Problem 1 - problem 4	0.83[d]
	Problem 2 - problem 3	-0.55
	Problem 2 - problem 4	0.49
	Problem 3 - problem 4	1.04[d]

[a] $\hat{\psi} = (\bar{X}_3 + \bar{X}_4 - \bar{X}_1 - \bar{X}_2)/2$.
[b] $\hat{\psi} = (\bar{X}_1 + \bar{X}_4 - \bar{X}_2 - \bar{X}_3)/2$.
[c] $p < .05$.
[d] $p < .01$.

As a general summary statement of results, it may be said that whenever significant differences are found, they are attributable to the problems and their structure and *not* to the physician variable. In this section we shall analyze first the absence of a physician effect on the results and then the effects of the problems (the repeated measures) and their underlying structural dimensions. A more extensive consideration of the results in the light of a cognitive theory of medical inquiry is reserved for the discussion. The reader should bear in mind that these results were obtained with a small sample of physicians and a small set of possible problems;

conclusions must therefore be tentative until replication studies are conducted.

Differences between criterial and noncriterial physicians were uniformly nonsignificant, sometimes dramatically so. In three of the six analyses F ratios of less than 1.00 were obtained. The differences between the groups were so minute that the almost inevitable conclusion is that we are dealing here with only one group of physicians. Therefore, the means and standard deviations in Table 6.2 are presented by problem only.

Let us now consider the effects of the repeated measures (the problems) on the dependent variables.

Significant differences ($p < .01$) were found for number of hypotheses and number of serious hypotheses (Tables 6.3 and 6.4). Post hoc comparisons (Table 6.9) showed that more hypotheses and more serious hypotheses were produced in response to problems with high-consistency cues than when low-consistency cues were presented. There was no effect for the diagnosis dimension.

Similar results were obtained for maximum cues associated (Table 6.5) except that the overall significance level was $p < .025$. Post hoc comparisons showed that, as had been expected, the maximum number of cues associated with a hypothesis was greater with highly consistent data than with low-consistency cues. As before, there was no effect on the diagnosis dimension.

Results on the variable, mean cues associated, are a bit more difficult to interpret. Here a clear difference ($p < .01$) over all four problems was found (Table 6.6), but it was not attributable to the cue-consistency dimension. The comparisons presented in Table 6.9 show that only problem 4 (high cue consistency, one diagnosis) had a lower mean cues associated score than either problems 1 or 3, where one dimension or the other was more complex. These are the only results that suggest an interaction among cognitive dimensions. Some speculations on this issue will be offered in the discussion.

Finally, no significant differences were found on number of early hypotheses and number of cues utilized (Tables 6.7 and 6.8).

To summarize the results: no significant differences in behavior were found between the criterial and noncriterial groups of physicians. Significant differences were found on four of the six dependent variables, once at $p < .025$ and three times at $p < .01$. In three of these four variables, post hoc comparisons showed that the overall significant difference was mainly a result of the cue-consistency dimension.

Discussion

Criterial and Noncriterial Physicians

The finding that the groups of criterial and noncriterial physicians could not be discriminated by these fixed-order problems duplicates results reported in Chapters 4 and 5. It is evident that the procedures used to construct these two groups did not allow us to differentiate between them. These procedures may, in retrospect, be criticized; here it is sufficient to point out that inability to differentiate between the groups of criterial and noncriterial physicians is not a unique property of fixed-order, low-fidelity simulations and does not therefore reflect adversely on their validity. On the contrary, this property is shared by the other types of simulations used in our study.

Consequently, fixed-order problems should not be dismissed as a research tool on grounds of low face validity and lack of discriminant validity, since instruments with higher face validity also failed to discriminate between groups. Fixed-order problems may be attractive research and/or evaluation instruments because they are fairly easy to design, they can be administered more cheaply and quickly to more subjects than higher-fidelity situations, and their very brevity permits a broad sampling of both medical content and structural features within a fixed time span. Since there is little evidence in our studies to support a unidimensional concept of clinical competence, broad sampling of the domain of medicine will be needed to adequately assess a physician's capabilities.

Effects of Problem Structure on Dependent Variables

In three of the four variables where significant differences were found (number of hypotheses, number of serious hypotheses, and maximum cues associated), the findings are attributable to the effect of the cue-consistency dimension upon physician performance. Let us first discuss the results concerning number of hypotheses and number of serious hypotheses and their implications for a cognitive theory of medical diagnosis.

Subjects tended to generate more hypotheses, total and serious, when all of the cues were consistent with a single diagnosis than when a portion of the data were inconsistent. In other words, low-consistency data did not lead to increased hypothesis generation. This is a striking finding, not at all intuitively obvious, for it suggests that inconsistencies in the data were ignored instead of serving as stimuli to consider additional possibilities. The physicians tended to treat each problem as if it were a fairly typical case that would fit textbook descriptions of disease. Given this orientation, departures from textbook descriptions were treated as irrelevant noise rather than a signal.

Of course, this finding may not generalize beyond these simulations. On the other hand, it is possible that scattered, inconsistent, nonclustering cues are ignored more generally, on the grounds that real diseases commonly produce more than one cue from which to infer their existence. Accordingly, a generally safe and useful medical heuristic would be to ignore isolated cues and trace only the causes of clusters of cues. This heuristic assumes an ability to discriminate clusters, and to know what cues can and do cluster, but this is part of medical knowledge. Like other heuristics, it does not invariably produce diagnostic solutions. There surely exist some cases where a patient presents a number of cues that cannot be conveniently clustered because he has multiple, previously undetected ailments or because the effect of one unknown ailment is to alter the usual clinical picture of another unknown ailment. Our data imply that the strategy of working to cluster cues may be a disservice to the patient in these instances, since the tactic leads to reduced generation of serious hypotheses. But in many cases, the heuristic would lead to satisfactory formulation of the problem.

Figure 6.2 presents two possible models for generating hypotheses with consistent cues. Model 1 shows later cues leading to elaboration and refinement of early hypotheses with increasing specificity but with no new problem subspaces generated. Model 2 retains this mechanism, but adds another when a problem is reformulated: later cues are clustered with early cues to generate new hypotheses in new problem subspaces. The models suggest two heuristics for generating later hypotheses, either (a) that new hypotheses should be more elaborate, specific versions of earlier hypotheses, or (b) that cues should be clustered to generate warranted, justified hypotheses. In the second model it may be that the later a cue is presented the stronger is the tendency to try to cluster it with some of its predecessors and to ignore it if it cannot be clustered, but this is surely a theory for subsequent investigation. While it is not yet known which of these two models is more nearly correct, either can operate only on high-consistency cues and tends to ignore low-consistency data. Only consistent cues can be clustered properly with their predecessors and only they can lead to greater specificity of early hypotheses.

Figure 6.2 Models for generating hypotheses with consistent cues.

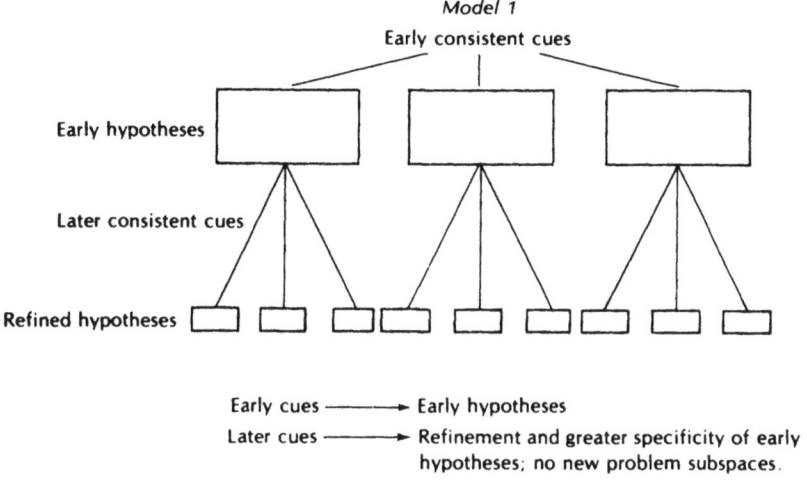

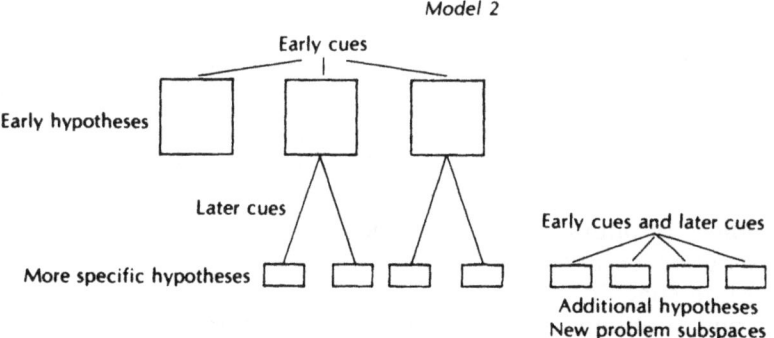

The strategy of clustering cues to generate diagnostic hypotheses and of ignoring inconsistent cues suggests how dependent diagnostic thinking is on finding a match between the case at hand and patterns or lists retrieved from memory. Cue clustering is used to find matches between recalled patterns and possible organizations of the data presented. Similarly, increasing the specificity of hypotheses can be accomplished only if guided by the aim of reorganizing the data to better match patterns or lists retrieved from long-term memory. Finally, inconsistent cues would not be ignored if hypothesis generation were not so linked to memory organization. More hypotheses are generated with consistent cues because these cues better match packets or descriptions already in memory. Of course, these descriptions are in textbooks and are learned by physicians because they are the typical, frequent manifestations of disease. Hence trying to match particular cases to these memory patterns will generally be rational and appropriate.

Since these heuristic principles are most adapted to consistent cue clusters, it follows that they will be less well adapted to inconsistent cues that do not cluster. For instance, if the heuristic followed with inconsistent data were "generate multiple competing hypotheses and disregard clustering of cues where necessary," then inconsistent data would generate as many or more hypotheses than consistent data. The results suggest that this is a difficult heuristic to follow. In so many problems, heeding it will lead to needless proliferation of exotic possibilities and will delay diagnosis unnecessarily. The principles that new hypotheses should be more specific versions of earlier ones, and that new hypotheses and problem subspaces should be generated by clustering early and late cues, are ordinarily justified and will facilitate diagnosis because most medical problems have the coherence upon which these principles depend for rational justification. Behavior along these lines is generally adaptive and so is frequently reinforced. Physicians become conditioned to anticipate coherence and to work by clustering cues. The trick is to know when to disregard these heuristics and to adopt others more appropriate for inconsistent data. Since there is no evidence in our studies that recognized expert diagnosticians are better than other physicians at changing strategies, it may be helpful to consider whether modern aids to data organization and interpretation, notably computers and flow diagrams, could solve this problem.

CUE-ASSOCIATION VARIABLES. Maximum cues associated with

a hypothesis should be greater in instances where the cues can reasonably be clustered with a hypothesis. Physicians as a group did respond to this property of consistency, though not as strongly as might be anticipated; the overall effect for maximum cues associated is significant at the .025 level. It is more intriguing to observe that the mean scores on the variable are essentially identical for both consistent problems and that there is no observable effect for the diagnosis dimension. Since all cues on problem 4 are consistent with one diagnosis, while the cues for problem 1 could properly be clustered with two diagnoses, it might have been anticipated that maximum cues associated scores would be greater on problem 4.

However, the findings on mean cues associated cannot be attributed to cue consistency. Pairwise comparisons disclosed differences between problems, to be sure, but what is at issue is not entirely clear. Tables 6.2 and 6.9 show that mean cues associated for problem 4 is significantly lower than for problems 1 and 3. Does this mean that a simple problem, high on both diagnostic specificity and cue consistency, calls forth less effort to justify a hypothesis than problems that lack one of these attributes? If so, why is this effect not duplicated on maximum cues associated? Or are we dealing here with an artifact of the particular medical content of four cases, unrelated to their psychological structure? Further inquiry is certainly needed.

EARLY HYPOTHESES. The role of early hypotheses was partially discussed earlier, in the section dealing with models for hypothesis generation. Here it is worth noting that the mean values for the early hypotheses plus their standard deviations, are just about in the range (between 5 and 7) that has been reported by Mandler (1967), Wortman (1970), and others as the value for the number of items retained in each chunk in short-term memory. Early hypotheses may be thought of as representing the initial subspaces used to define each problem space. Similar values for this parameter are reported by Allal in her study of early hypothesis generation, summarized in Chapters 7 and 8. (The values reported in Chapter 4 for number of hypotheses active one-quarter of the way through a workup are lower, but these values surely reflect a considerable reduction of hypotheses. By that point there were generally many more data available to cluster than in the early stages of the fixed-order problems, and fewer hypotheses fit. Besides, the rules for defining hypotheses in Chapter 4 were more stringent.)

An upper limit of about 5 to 7 on number of early hypotheses seems to be a regular feature of human information processing, invariant across a fairly broad selection of problems. While specific problem conditions frequently lower this value, as noted in Chapter 5, it is rarely exceeded. This further confirms the notion of an upper limit to capacity.

Conclusion

Four medical problems were administered to twenty-two physicians. In each problem the data were presented in the same order. Two cognitive dimensions, diagnostic specificity and cue consistency, were varied on two levels (high and low) to create the structural matrix for the four problems. The effects of physician type (criterial versus noncriterial) and problem structure of six dependent variables were assessed by performing a repeated-measures analysis of variance on each dependent variable. Each analysis included group (criterial versus noncriterial physicians) as an independent variable and problem as the repeated-measures dimension.

Differences between criterial and noncriterial physicians were uniformly nonsignificant. Significant differences were found on four of the six dependent variables: number of hypotheses, number of serious hypotheses, maximum cues associated with any hypothesis, and mean cues associated with a hypothesis. Post hoc comparisons showed that the differences resulted mainly from the cue-consistency dimension. No significant differences were found on two dependent variables, number of early hypotheses and cues utilized to generate hypotheses.

The phenomenon of early generation of diagnostic hypotheses replicates a finding of Chapters 4 and 5. This consistency implies that early hypothesis generation is a widespread, if not ubiquitous, feature of medical problem solving. When the size of the data base used to generate hypotheses is controlled, as in this study, the estimate of the magnitude of this parameter closely accords with measures of "chunking" obtained in other studies of short-term memory. This suggests once again that hypotheses function as memory organizers.

Two related heuristics may be proposed as a strategy for hypothesis generation: (a) cues are clustered to generate hypotheses, and inconsistent cues tend to be ignored; and (b) later diagnostic hypotheses are generally elaborations or refinements of earlier ones. Using these principles would lead to a decline in hypothesis generation when inconsistent cues are presented, and this has been observed. These heuristics also suggest that later hypotheses would only infrequently be new structures in the problem spaces. This question could be studied fruitfully by comparing tree structures of different problems and groups of physicians.

For future research, fixed-order problems (easily designed simulations of fairly low fidelity) can be used effectively to study certain aspects of medical reasoning. Many of the phenomena observed in higher-fidelity simulations of greater face validity are observed also with fixed-order problems. They have the further advantages of easy administration and greater possibility for experimental manipulation of selected variables, while preserving the sequential-data-presentation characteristic of medical problem solving.

7 / Generation of Initial Problem Formulations: Performance of Experienced Physicians[1]

A major finding of the research described in Chapter 4 is that nearly all experienced physicians began to generate diagnostic hypotheses, or problem formulations, within the earliest minutes of a clinical encounter.[2] Chapters 7 and 8 describe an investigation designed to focus on this initial hypothesis-generation phase of medical inquiry.

The primary purpose of this study was to develop and test experimentally a procedure for training medical students in the task of generating diagnostic problem formulations based on cues obtained during the first four to six minutes of a clinical workup. The training procedure that was developed included two major components: having the student practice the task under conditions that simulate the early part of the clinical encounter, and providing the student with feedback on the performance of this task by experienced physicians. Color films that present a "physician's-eye view" of the initial doctor-patient encounter were used to simulate the conditions of the early part of the workup. The feedback materials were developed on the basis of data—pertaining to initial problem-formulation outcomes and processes—that were collected from a sample of eight experienced physicians.

The present chapter will briefly describe the production of the films and the method used to collect data from the physicians. It will then present a fairly detailed descriptive analysis of the physician data. Chapter 8 will describe the design of the training exper-

---

[1] Chapters 7 and 8 are based on the Ph.D. dissertation of Linda K. Allal, "Training of Medical Students in a Problem-Solving Skill: The Generation of Diagnostic Problem Formulations" (Michigan State University, 1973).
[2] Analysis of the data in Chapter 4 indicated that the percentage of physicians who began generating hypotheses within the first five minutes of the workup was 95.2, 81.8, and 100 for simulations 1, 2, and 3, respectively.

iment with second-year medical students and will report and discuss the experimental results. In both chapters the term *problem formulation* (rather than *hypothesis*) has been employed to refer to the diagnostic labels generated on the basis of cues obtained from the workup. This term was selected because it was one with which the medical-student population participating in the experiment was familiar. For consistency's sake its use was continued in the two chapters related to this experiment. Conceptually, however, its meaning is the same as that of the term *hypothesis*, employed elsewhere in this book.

Method

The Films

Eight 16-millimeter films in color and with sound were produced. Each film presents the first four to six minutes in a physician's encounter with a new patient. The setting of the interview is a doctor's office; the patient is ambulatory, and his problem is of a nonemergency nature. Since the purpose of the films is to provide the viewer with a realistic simulation of participation in a clinical encounter, they were produced from the standpoint of the physician. Throughout the film the camera remains on the patient. The physician's voice is heard, but he is never seen. By focusing on the patient, the films attempt to facilitate the viewer's task of adopting the role of physician vis-à-vis the filmed patient.

The cases for the eight films were selected to represent a cross-section of problems in internal medicine, as well as a variety of patient demographic characteristics (age, sex, occupation).[3]

Table 7.1 lists the eight films, titled according to the demographic characteristics of the patient and numbered in the order they were presented during the training experiment. The table also indicates the presenting complaint(s) of the patient in each film.

Production of each film involved the following steps:
A case outline was prepared.
An experienced amateur actor was selected to play the role of the patient.

---

[3] Films 1 and 5 were based on the same case materials as two of the simulations (numbers 1 and 2, respectively) described in Chapter 3. Films 4 and 7 were based on the case materials developed for two of the fixed-order problems (numbers 1 and 3, respectively) described in Chapter 6. The cases for the other four films were developed specifically for this study.

Table 7.1 The eight training films used in generating diagnostic problem formulations.

Film no.	Title	Presenting complaint
1	A 21-year-old college senior	Fatigue and weakness
2	A 43-year-old landlady of a boarding house	Substernal chest pain
3	A 30-year-old taxi driver	Urinary distress
4	A 40-year-old carpenter	Left chest pain
5	A 19-year-old college sophomore	Headache and sleepiness
6	A 29-year-old lawyer	Low back pain
7	A 57-year-old executive	Cough and fever
8	A 19-year-old student nurse	Abdominal pain and vomiting

After the actor had familiarized himself with the case outline, a warm-up session was held in which the actor was coached with respect to his role—both the verbal presentation of his complaints and the nonverbal aspects of his role (gait, posture, gestures, facial expressions, and so forth).

A trial run of the interview was videotaped, with immediate replay to permit discussion and critique.

The interview was filmed.

Four physicians assisted with preparation of the case outlines and coaching of the patient-actors. Two of them played the role of the physician in the films (four films each). Given the constraint that each of the major topics in the case outline be covered, the physician-actor was free to conduct the interview in accordance with his usual practice. He was, however, instructed to use a relatively standard, unobtrusive questioning technique and in particular to avoid any questions that would obviously imply a particular problem formulation. During the warm-up session, a general sequence of events was worked out, but in order to preserve naturalness of dialogue any tendency to establish a fixed script was avoided.

Each film presents the viewer with both verbal and nonverbal information. Information presented in the verbal mode (that is, the dialogue between the doctor and the patient) consists primarily in a brief review of each of the patient's current complaints (history of present illness), but includes a few items of personal, past medical, or family medical history that have particular relevance to the present illness. The types of nonverbal information presented include: physical appearance of the patient (posture, build, dress); psychological state of the patient (gestures, manner of speech, facial expression); and nonverbal cues of particular relevance to the patient's current medical problem (cough, photophobia, clutching of abdomen).

The Physician Sample

In selection of the physician sample the objective was to obtain a group of subjects whose academic backgrounds and clinical experience would be representative of the population of physicians who would generally deal with the type of medical cases presented in the films—that is, office visits pertaining to problems in internal medicine. It was therefore decided to select a sample of eight physicians that included four specialists in internal medicine (with M.D. degrees) and four family-medicine physicians (two with M.D. degrees, two with D.O. degrees). The eight subjects were selected from among the physicians associated with the Michigan State University Colleges of Human and Osteopathic Medicine. Table 7.2 summarizes the characteristics of the sample.

Given the lengthy data-collection procedure for each film and the limited amount of time some of the subjects could make available, it was not possible to obtain data for all films on the performance of all eight subjects. For each film data were obtained from a minimum of three (out of the four) internists and three (out of the four) family-medicine physicians. For one film (number 6) data were obtained from a total of seven subjects. In all, a total of forty-nine sets of responses were obtained.

Table 7.2   Characteristics of the physician sample.

| | | | Average no. years experience ||
| | | | As practicing clinician | As medical educator |
n	Degree	Specialization		
4	M.D.	Internal medicine	11.0	11.7
2	M.D.	Family practice	8.0	2.5
2	D.O.	Family practice	8.5	1.5

Materials

Two types of materials were used in collecting the physician data: response sheets and a process checklist.

The response sheets were used by the subject to record the problem formulations he had generated while viewing a film. The sheets had a very simple format: a line across the top of the sheet for a problem-formulation title, and space underneath for listing the cues of relevance to that title.

A review of the protocols of the simulations described in Chapter 3 revealed that some subjects had difficulty in providing an introspective description of the mental processes by which they generated problem formulations. It was therefore decided that in addition to tape recording his introspective reconstruction of his thinking process while viewing the film, the physician would be given a checklist to fill out after the viewing. Details of this checklist are given below.

Procedure

The physician data were collected in individual sessions lasting about three hours, during which three or four films were viewed. The session began with the administration of a set of general instructions. For each film, two types of data were collected: (a) data on the *outcomes* of the physician's information processing as he viewed the film (principally, the set of problem formulations he generated and the cues associated with each), and (b) data on the *processes* by which the physician generated his set of problem formulations.

The following were the steps in collecting outcome data.

(a) The subject was first shown the initial brief segment of the film in which the patient walks into the doctor's office and sits down to await the arrival of the physician. The film was stopped at this point, and the subject was asked to comment on his impression of the patient and on any ideas that came to mind about what problems the patient might have. These comments were tape-recorded.

(b) The subject was given a written "nurse's sheet," which listed the patient's major demographic characteristics (age, sex, occupation) and his temperature. His comments were again tape-recorded.

(c) The subject was then shown the rest of the film. At the end of the film, he was asked to fill out a response sheet for each problem formulation that he had generated while viewing the film.

(d) The subject was asked to provide his tentative assessment of the case. He was asked to indicate how well substantiated he considered each of his problem formulations to be on the basis of the data obtained; whether he anticipated that the patient had a single illness or multiple disorders; whether he considered there to be any functional relationship among his problem formulations (for example, some formulation that could be considered secondary to, superimposed on, or contributing to some other formulations). All comments were tape-recorded.

The following were the steps in collection of process data.

(a) The subject was asked to attempt "to reconstruct your thinking while viewing this film," and to include such things as the point in the film when each problem formulation came to mind, the cues that were significant in generating each problem formulation, and any revision of initial formulations as the interview progressed. These comments were tape-recorded. The physician was offered the opportunity to view the film again as he reconstructed his thinking, but only occasionally did a subject elect to do so.

(b) The process checklist was administered. The experimenter used the items checked by the subject as a basis for asking additional questions pertaining to processes of problem formulation. The subject's responses were tape-recorded.

Although the checklist was used after each film, it is believed that the length of the list (twenty-five items) and the number of activities intervening between each application of the list were sufficient to minimize any effect that exposure to it might have had on subsequent problem-formulation activity.

Results

The remainder of this chapter will present an analysis and discussion of the data that were collected from the sample of eight physicians. This presentation will be organized in terms of three sections, each dealing with one of the following questions:

(a) How early in the clinical workup does the physician begin to generate problem formulations?

(b) What is the structure of a set of initial problem formulations?

(c) What cognitive processes are involved in the generation of initial problem formulations?

Given the small size of the physician sample, the findings reported in this chapter must be regarded as highly tentative. Nevertheless, because the procedure used in this study permitted appraisal of initial problem-formulation outcomes and processes in greater detail than have previous investigations, the findings may be of value in suggesting hypotheses to be explored in future research.

Generation of the First Problem Formulation

As indicated earlier, the physician was asked to report what thoughts had come to mind after the initial thirty-second view of the patient, and again after having read the nurse's sheet. When problem formulations were not reported at either of these points, the physician was asked at the end of the film to attempt to recall the point in the interview at which he first generated a problem formulation.

On the basis of a frequency distribution of these data over the forty-nine responses, the following were ascertained:

(a) In seventeen instances (35 percent) the physician generated his first problem formulation after the initial thirty-second view of the patient. The formulations generated at his point were of two types: formulations of "psychological problem," based on the patient's general appearance and manner; and formulations pertaining to organic disorders (such as "respiratory problem"), based on specific nonverbal cues (for example, "the patient's cough").

(b) In four instances (8 percent) the physician generated his first problem formulation after reading the nurse's sheet. In all four instances a formulation of "infection" was generated on the basis of the cue of elevated temperature.

(c) In twenty-six instances (53 percent) the physician generated his first problem formulation on the basis of the patient's presenting complaint. These formulations varied across cases depending on the nature of the complaint, but there was a high degree of consistency within each case with respect to the type of formulation generated.

(d) In two instances (4 percent) the physician generated his first problem formulation after the patient had presented several complaints. Both of these instances occurred with film 1, in which the patient's presenting complaint (fatigue and weakness) was highly general. It was not until the patient mentioned that he also had abdominal pain that, in these two instances, a problem formulation was generated.

Two factors must be borne in mind in attempting to generalize on the basis of these data. First, the demand characteristics of the experimental task, as well as the fact that the subject did not have to devote part of his attention to the task of data elicitation (that is, he obtained data by viewing a film rather than by actively engaging in an interview), may have led the physicians to generate problem formulations somewhat earlier than they would do in actual practice. Second, except in the instances where problem formulations were reported after the initial view of the patient or after the presentation of the nurse's sheet, some degree of retrospective distortion may have affected the physician's report of the point at which he first generated a problem formulation. The findings probably overestimate the earliness with which problem formulation typically occurs in clinical practice. Nevertheless, the fact that in 96 percent of the responses a first problem formulation was generated no later than one minute into the interview provides evidence that physicians are able to generate problem formulations very early, on the basis of minimal data; in actual practice most probably do generate problem formulations relatively early, at least within the first five minutes of the workup.

The Structure of a Set of Initial Problem Formulations

Newell and Simon's (1972) information-processing theory of problem solving includes two fundamental propositions: (a) that the task environment is represented internally as a "problem space," and (b) that the structure of the problem space determines the "programs" (that is, the information-processing activities) to be used in the search for a solution. In clinical medicine, as in other domains of problem solving, the potential size of the problem space is enormous: there are a vast number of elements (states of knowledge about the patient) that could be obtained, and an exceedingly large number of potential operators (interview questions, physical-examination maneuvers, laboratory tests) for obtaining them. The early generation of diagnostic problem formulations would appear to be a major strategy that is used by physicians to determine the regions of the potential problem space that are most likely to yield a solution. In sum, we may propose that a set of problem formulations defines the dimensions of the *functional* problem space in which a physician's search for a diagnosis is conducted.

The purpose of this section is to describe the way in which a set of initial problem formulations is structured. Thus, in terms of the theoretical perspective presented in the preceding paragraph, the analysis pertains to the functional problem space within which the physician is operating during the early part of the workup. In the analysis of a set of initial problem formulations, two topics were dealt with: its characteristic features and its size and organization.

STRUCTURAL FEATURES. An examination of the physician data indicated that the result of the physician's information-processing activity during the early part of the workup is not a unidimensional list of problem formulations. Rather it is a *structured set* of formulations that may be described in terms of four features: hierarchical organization, competing formulations, multiple subspaces, and functional relationships.

(a) Hierarchical organization. A set of problem formulations may include formulations organized into a general-to-specific hierarchy that pertains to a single diagnostic category (an organ system or a disease mechanism, for instance). A physician may generate a problem formulation such as gastrointestinal (GI) disorder and, as subcategories under this formulation, one or several more specific formulations such as inflammatory bowel disease and/or intestinal malignancy.

(b) Competing formulations. A set of problem formulations may include some that provide alternative explanations for some group of symptoms. For example, a physician may generate inflammatory bowel disease and intestinal malignancy as competing problem formulations.

(c) Multiple subspaces. A set of problem formulations may include subsets of formulations that pertain to different types of diagnostic categories (such as different organ systems, and/or different disease mechanisms). Each of these categories may be considered to designate a subspace within the functional problem space in which the physician is operating. For example, a physician may generate a set of formulations that consists in four subspaces: GI disorder, diabetes mellitus, anemia, cardiovascular problem.

(d) Functional relationships. A set of initial problem formulations may include functional relationships that the physician hypothesizes to exist between certain problem formulations. For example, a physician may consider anemia to be secondary to GI disorder.

In order to illustrate the way in which the four features characterize the structure of a set of initial problem formulations, a structural diagram of the composite set of problem formulations generated by the physician sample for one film has been prepared (Figure 7.1). Although the diagram pictures a more extensive set of problem formulations than would normally be generated by any single individual, it may serve as a useful illustration for the following commentary on the four features. The number of subspaces indicates the scope (or range) of diagnostic categories included in the problem space. It is the superordinate horizontal dimension of a set of formulations. Subspaces may be competitors (GI disorder versus diabetes mellitus); they may be compatible but unrelated (diabetes and anemia); or they may be functionally related (anemia, secondary to GI disorder). Some subspaces may consist in a hierarchy of formulations (GI disorder hierarchy), while others may consist in a single formulation that is highly general (cardiovascular problem) or very specific (diabetes mellitus). Hierarchical organization of formulations indicates the degree to which the problem space is elaborated on a vertical dimension. Competing formulations may exist within subspaces (inflammatory bowel disease versus intestinal malignancy), or between subspaces (anemia versus cardiovascular problem). Functional relationships may be hypothesized at the level of subspaces (anemia, secondary to GI disorder), but may also by hypothesized at the lower levels of subspace hierarchies (blood loss anemia, secondary to ulcerative colitis).

The set of problem formulations generated by each physician for each film was coded in terms of the features it exhibited. The results of this analysis are summarized in Table 7.3, by film

Figure 7.1 Structural diagram of the composite set of problem formulations generated by the physician sample for film 1.

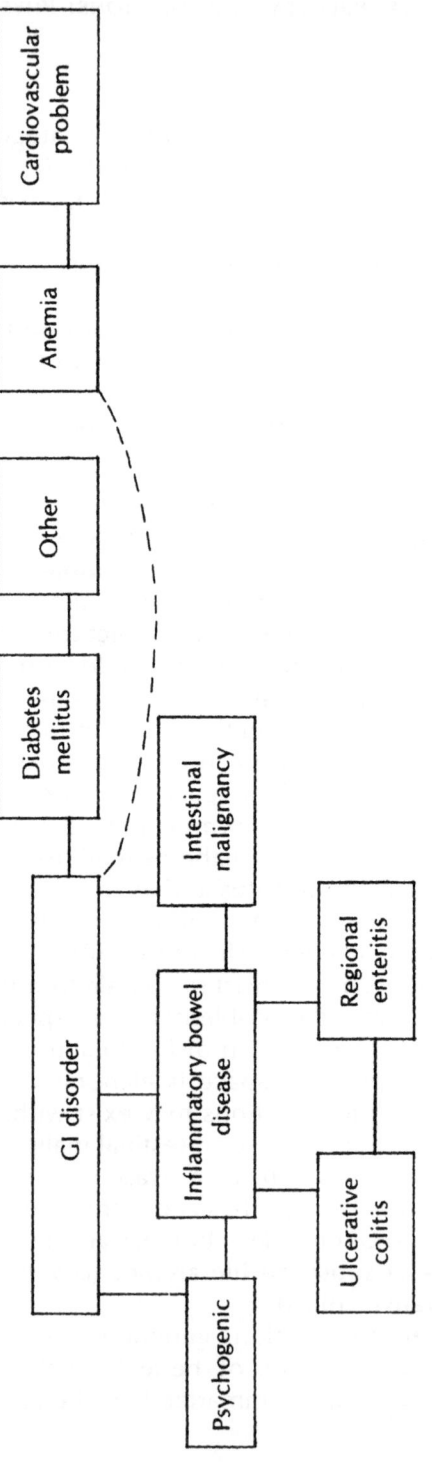

Key:

Hierarchical organization: indicated by vertical lines joining boxes.
Competing formulations: indicated by horizontal lines joining boxes.
Subspaces: GI disorder, diabetes mellitus, anemia, cardiovascular problem, other.
Functional relationships: indicated by dashed lines joining boxes.

Table 7.3 Features characteristic of individual sets of problem formulations, by film and by subject.

Variable	Hierarchical organization	Competing formulations	Multiple subspaces	Functional relationships
Film [a]:				
1	67	100	83	67
2	100	100	100	100
3	100	100	33	0
4	67	100	100	100
5	83	100	67	33
6	57	100	100	0
7	33	100	100	100
8	83	100	100	50
Subject [b]:				
A	38	100	75	38
B	57	100	100	71
C	75	100	100	100
D	75	100	75	50
E	86	100	71	43
F	100	100	71	43
G	75	100	100	63
H	100	100	100	50

[a] Figures are percent of subjects whose sets of formulations exhibited each feature.
[b] Figures are percent of films for which a subject's set of formulations exhibited each feature.

(percent of subjects whose sets of formulations exhibited each feature) and by subject (percent of films for which a subject's set of formulations exhibited each feature).

Of the four features, *competing formulations* is the only one that is consistently characteristic of all physicians' sets of formulations for all eight films. Thus, the present data suggest competing formulations as an essential feature of any experienced physician's set of initial problem formulations. It is not surprising that this feature stands out as the most salient characteristic of a set of initial problem formulations. Numerous scientists and philosophers of science have argued that the entertaining of multiple competing hypotheses is a primary means by which the scientific thinker seeks to avoid the pitfall of becoming prematurely wedded to a favored, but possibly incorrect, hypothesis (Chamberlin, 1890; Kessel, 1969).

The feature *hierarchical organization* is present a high proportion of the time for most films and for most subjects. But it also shows a good deal of variability across subjects and across films. In contrast to competing formulations, the occurrence of this feature appears to be influenced by both task environment and individual differences.

Comments in several of the physicians' recall protocols indicated that, having generated a hierarchy of problem formulations, they would evaluate data subsequently collected with respect to formulations at each level in the hierarchy. It may be hypothesized that a hierarchy of formulations serves a dual purpose. On the one hand, the early generation of specific formulations helps guarantee that those cues of particular relevance to the establishment of a differential diagnosis are elicited and interpreted. On the other hand, by continuing to entertain a more general problem-formulation category (that subsumes the specific formulations), the physician is more likely to avoid the "blind-alley" pitfall that could result if data collection and interpretation were narrowly focused on specific diagnostic hypotheses and these hypotheses were disconfirmed.

A further rationale for the feature of hierarchical organization is suggested by the research literature on the role of organization in memory (for example, Mandler, 1967; Collins and Quillian, 1969). A hierarchy of problem formulations permits more parsimonious storage of cues. Consider this example:

—A physician obtains eight cues of relevance to X_0 (where X_0 is a relatively general problem formulation, such as GI disorder). Of the eight cues, three (2, 3, 7) are of particular relevance to X_1, two (2, 6) to X_2, and two (2, 8) to X_3 (where X_1, X_2, and X_3 are more specific problem formulations, such as ulcerative colitis, intestinal malignancy, and psychogenic diarrhea).

—If the physician generates a two-level hierarchy of problem formulations, the cues may be stored as follows:

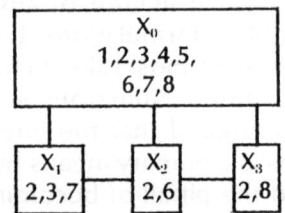

—If on the other hand, if the physician generates a single-level list of specific formulations, the cues must be stored as follows:

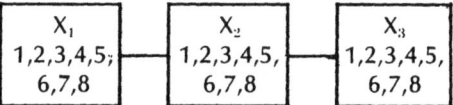

As the above example illustrates, hierarchical organization increases the number of categories to be stored (from three to four), but greatly reduces the amount of information to be stored within categories (from a total of twenty-four units to fifteen).

The feature *multiple subspaces* is present a high proportion of the time. With respect to subjects, this feature shows a relatively restricted range of variability (that is, it is present for at least 70 percent of the films viewed by each subject). Individual difference variables appear to have less of an effect on the occurrence of this feature than on the occurrence of hierarchical organization. With respect to films, the range of variability is fairly broad, but the distribution is highly skewed (for five films all subjects generated formulations in more than one subspace). This would appear to suggest that for many medical cases (such as films 2, 4, 6, 7, 8) task-environment variables are of primary importance (and thus consistently elicit this feature), while for other medical cases (films 1, 3, 5) task-environment variables are less powerful and individual difference variables may play a greater part. There are two task-related factors that probably contribute to the high frequency with which this feature typically occurs. One is the fact that a patient may often have more than one medical disorder. Resolution of such cases would require that multiple disease mechanisms and/or disorders in multiple organ systems be considered. A second factor is the ambiguity of the cues obtained during the early part of the workup: many cues are inherently nonspecific (for example, weakness and fatigue), and even relatively specific cues (such as substernal pain) may be compatible with multiple disease mechanisms and/or multiple organ-system involvements.

The feature *functional relationships* is more likely to be absent from a set of initial problem formulations than any of the other three features. It displays a considerable degree of variability across subjects, with some subjects showing a much greater tendency to hypothesize functional relationships than others. With respect to films, the data appear to suggest that for many cases (films 2, 3, 4, 6, 7) task-environment variables are powerful enough to elicit consistent outcomes across all physicians (in other words, either all subjects hypothesized functional relationships or none did), while for other cases (films 1, 5, 8) the occurrence of this feature is likely to vary and may be largely a function of individual difference factors. One task-environment variable that appears to influence the occurrence of this feature is age of the patient: several physicians noted when the patient is older than forty (films 2, 4, 7) he is more likely to have multiple disorders that are functionally related.

SIZE AND ORGANIZATION. The size of a set of initial problem formulations may be measured in terms of two variables: the number of problem formulations and the number of subspaces. Table 7.4 presents the mean and range on these variables, by film (across subjects) and by subject (across films). For films, the average number of problem formulations ranged from 3.5 to 8.8,

Table 7.4 Number of problem formulations and number of subspaces: average and range, by film and by subject.

Variable	Number of problem formulations		Number of subspaces	
	Average	Range	Average	Range
Film:				
1	4.8	3-7	3.2	1-5
2	8.2	5-14	5.0	3-6
3	3.5	3-6	1.3	1-3
4	5.0	3-7	3.7	3-6
5	4.3	3-7	2.0	1-3
6	6.9	4-12	3.4	2-3
7	4.7	3-7	3.8	3-5
8	8.8	4-11	4.3	3-5
Subject:				
A	3.6	3-5	2.6	1-4
B	6.0	4-11	4.3	2-6
C	6.5	3-9	3.8	3-5
D	5.3	3-7	2.8	1-4
E	5.3	3-7	2.6	1-5
F	5.7	3-11	2.9	1-5
G	7.8	3-14	4.3	2-6
H	7.0	3-10	3.5	1-6

and the average number of subspaces from 1.3 to 5.0. For subjects, the average number of problem formulations ranged from 3.6 to 7.8, and the average number of subspaces from 2.6 to 4.3.

The two measures of the size of a set of problem formulations are highly correlated: the product-moment coefficient is .70 with film as the unit, and .78 with subject as the unit. These correlations indicate that the two measures have a very sizable proportion of variance in common. Thus, the question arises of the rationale for considering that the two measures pertain to distinct psychological entities, a rationale that derives from an evaluation of the data in Table 7.4 in terms of the research literature on the role of organization in memory.

Studies by Mandler (1967) have indicated that material in working memory is ordinarily organized and stored in 5 ± 2 categories. Moreover, there is some evidence (Wortman, 1972; Wortman and Kleinmuntz, 1972) that this value also applies to the information-processing behavior of physicians. An examination of Table 7.4 reveals that the number of initial problem formulations a physician generates may in some instances considerably exceed the storage capacity of working memory (for example, films 2, 6, 8; subjects B, F, G, H). However, the number of subspaces generated for a given case, or by a given subject, never exceeds six. Thus it would appear that however many problem formulations a physician generates, the maximum number of subspaces into which these formulations are grouped is consistent with the upper bound of the parameter that has been determined to govern the storage of information in working memory. This finding would seem to attest to the psychological reality of the subspace as the superordinate unit in a set of problem formulations.

The number of subspaces a physician generates (within the limit imposed by memory capacity) is probably a function of both individual-difference variables (for example, the physician's knowledge of relevant medical content) and task-environment variables (the complexity of the case). It was possible to identify one task-environment variable that appears to have influenced the performance of this physician sample: namely, the number of different organ systems to which the patient's complaints pertained. When this variable is correlated with the minimum number of subspaces generated for each film, a product-moment coefficient of .72 is obtained. It would appear that while memory capacity imposes a limit on the maximum number of subspaces a physician generates, the number of organ systems to which the patient's complaints pertain is one task-environment variable that governs the minimum number of subspaces generated.

Let us now consider the way in which problem formulations are organized into subspaces. Examination of the physician data reveals that problem formulations are never evenly distributed across subspaces. In the typical case (a problem space containing two to five subspaces) there are usually several subspaces that contain only one problem formulation, and several other subspaces that contain from two to at most four problem formulations at the same level of specificity. The subspaces that are hierarchically elaborated typically include only two (or at most three) levels of specificity. Thus the number of units included in a subspace never exceeds, but in many instances falls considerably below, the value proposed by Mandler. There are several factors that may account for this finding: (a) in some instances the subspace category may be at a level of specificity that does not admit further hierarchical elaboration of diagnostic relevance (an example is the subspace "diabetes mellitus" in Figure 7.1); (b) in other instances it would be possible to generate a hierarchy of subordinate formulations, but the current data base is so limited with respect to that subspace that further hierarchical elaboration would be fruitless (for instance, the subspace "cardiovascular problem" in Figure 7.1).

CONCLUSIONS. On the basis of the preceding analyses, several tentative conclusions may be proposed regarding the structure of a set of initial problem formulations:

(a) The subspace is the superordinate unit in a set of problem formulations. Generally there are two to five such units.

(b) In the typical case some subspaces contain two to four hierarchically organized formulations, while others contain only a single formulation.

(c) In virtually every case there are competing formulations at the level of subspace categories and/or at the level of specific formulations within subspaces.

(d) In some cases there may also be functional relationships that link subspaces and/or specific problem formulations.

Processes Involved in Generating Initial Problem Formulations

Two types of data relevant to problem-formulation processes were collected: retrospective-recall data and process-checklist data. This section will present findings that were derived from an analysis of both types of information.

For each film the subjects' recall protocols were collated by means of a process summary sheet. This sheet summarized in outline form the time sequence of mental events reported by the physicians, including a notation of the number of subjects who reported each event.

A review of the process summary sheets for all eight films yielded several observations regarding the processes underlying the generation of initial problem formulations. The discussion of these observations will relate the problem-formulation processes to each of the structural features described in the first section of this chapter.

GENERATION OF A HIERARCHY OF PROBLEM FORMULATIONS. Kleinmuntz (1968; Wortman and Kleinmuntz, 1972) has proposed that the diagnostic process is characterized by hierarchical search, which proceeds from general problem-formulation categories to increasingly specific diagnostic formulations. The data from the present study indicate that a physician's initial problem formulations cannot be characterized as either highly general or highly specific. In fact, a set of initial problem formulations typically includes hierarchies of formulations at various levels of specificity. Moreover, the data from the physicians' recall protocols indicate that the elaboration of a problem-formulation hierarchy may proceed in three ways: (1) from general to specific, (2) from specific to general, or (3) generation of general and specific formulations almost simultaneously. Each of these processes may be illustrated by examples from the recall protocols.

Example of process 1:
In viewing film 1, nearly all physicians generated the general formulation of GI disorder on the basis of the patient's complaint of abdominal pain. Subsequently, when the patient mentioned having diarrhea (with blood and mucus in his stools), they generated the more specific formulations of ulcerative colitis and/or regional enteritis.

Example of process 2:
In viewing film 6, nearly all physicians generated the specific formulations of rheumatoid arthritis and/or ankylosing spondylitis relatively early, on the basis of certain cues (stiff back in the morning, but loosens up during the day; back pain plus dyspnea). Subsequently, when it was learned that the patient also had knee and ankle inflammation, they generated the more general formulation of polyarthritis.

Example of process 3:
In viewing film 5, nearly all physicians generated the general formulation of acute infectious illness very early, on the basis of the cues fever, headache, and sleepiness of three days' duration. They noted that almost simultaneously they thought of several specific types of infectious illnesses (viral flu, infectious mononucleosis, infectious hepatitis) that are highly prevalent in a college student population.

To summarize: it is necessary to distinguish between the processes involved in generating a problem-formulation hierarchy and the product of these processes. While the product may be represented as a general-to-specific hierarchy of formulations, the process of generating the hierarchy may take one of three forms. For a given case, however, there was a substantial degree of consistency (across subjects) in the process reported. It would appear that task variables, rather than individual-difference variables, were the major determinants of which process was employed.

GENERATION OF COMPETING FORMULATIONS. The recall protocols provided evidence of two types of processes underlying the generation of competing formulations: (1) generation of competitors at a single point in time on the basis of the same set of cues; and (2) generation of competitors at several points in time on the basis of different cues. Examples from the recall protocols will serve to illustrate each of these processes.

Example of process 1:
In viewing film 1, nearly all physicians generated a list of competing formulations (ulcerative colitis, regional enteritis, intestinal malignancy) at almost the same point in time, on the basis of the patient's report of diarrhea with blood and mucus.

Example of process 2:
In viewing film 8, all physicians generated the formulation of GI disorder early in the interview, on the basis of the cues abdominal pain and vomiting. Much later, they generated the formulation of diabetes as a competitor to GI disorder, on the basis of the patient's report of increased appetite, thirst, and urination.

It is probable that the associative mechanisms underlying the above processes are quite different. In the case of the first process, we may hypothesize two types of underlying associative mechanisms: association from cue(s) to a list of competing formulations; and association from cue(s) to one formulation, from this formulation to another competing formulation, and so on. In the case of the second process we may hypothesize an associative mechanism of the following sort: association from one set of cue(s) to a formulation; association from another set of cue(s) to another formulation; and associative linkup of the two formulations as competitors. As was the case for hierarchical problem formulations, diverse associative processes may result in the same product—that is, a set of competing formulations to be stored in memory.

GENERATION OF MULTIPLE SUBSPACES. Evidence from the recall protocols indicated that there are two types of processes underlying the generation of multiple subspaces: (1) generation of multiple subspaces at a single point in time on the basis of the same set of cues, and (2) generation of multiple subspaces at several points in time on the basis of different cues. Examination of the recall data revealed that there are several task variables that appear to govern the generation of multiple subspaces. The first process listed above generally occurred under two circumstances: (a) when the patient's complaint was of a general or multisystem nature, and (b) when the location of a specific complaint indicated that several organ systems could be involved. The second process listed above generally occurred when complaints, reported at different points in the interview, pertained to different organ systems or implied different disease mechanisms. These generalizations may be illustrated by the following examples.

Example of process 1a:
In film 1, the patient's presenting complaint of fatigue and weakness is highly general and could be compatible with diverse organ-system involvements and/or disease processes. Thus some physicians generated formulations that belong to two distinct subspaces: anemia and cardiovascular problem.

Example of process 1b:
In film 2, the patient indicates a substernal location of chest pain. On the basis of this cue, all physicians generated formulations that belong to two subspaces: cardiac problem and upper GI problem.

Example of process 2:
In film 7, the patient's presenting complaints of two days' duration led all physicans to generate formulations belonging to the subspace, acute respiratory infection. Subsequently, when the patient reported symptoms of several years' duration, they generated formulations in two additional subspaces: chronic respiratory problem and cancer.

When multiple subspaces were generated by processes 1a and 1b they were usually competitors, whereas multiple subspaces generated by process 2 most often pertained to disorders that were not mutually exclusive (that is, some sort of functional relationship between subspaces was hypothesized, or the subspaces pertained to concomitant but unrelated disorders).

GENERATION OF FUNCTIONAL RELATIONSHIPS. The data from the recall protocols indicate that, as each new problem formulation is generated, the physician usually considers how it might be related functionally to the formulations he has previously generated. Functional relationships between problem formulations therefore are usually not hypothesized until the physican has generated at least two noncompeting formulations. However, this is not always the case. In viewing film 2, for example, several physicians noted that because of their initial impression of the patient (a middle-aged, obese woman who appeared to be anxious) they expected from the outset that she might have multiple, interrelated problems of both organic and psychological nature.

Having presented and discussed the findings from the analysis of the recall-protocol data, let us now consider the findings from the analysis of the process-checklist data.

The process checklist devised for this study comprised a series of twenty-five statements that pertain to four aspects of the act of generating problem formulations: modes of mental representation; strategies of problem formulation, including initial routines and general strategies; associative processes of problem formulation; and cue utilization.

The classification of checklist items according to the above categories, and a brief description of each item, appear in Table 7.5. Instructions to the subject were to check the items that "characterize your thinking while viewing this film."

Construction of the checklist was based primarily on a review of the protocols obtained from the studies of reasoning in the high-fidelity simulations. Statements pertaining to problem-formulation processes were selected from the physicians' "think-aloud" and recall protocols and, with some modification of wording, included in the checklist. In addition, some items were devised to describe processes that were not explicitly stated by the physicians, but that could be inferred from the protocols of their workups.

The analysis of the checklist data was designed to determine, for each item: (a) its overall importance as a characteristic of the

Table 7.5 Analysis of the relative frequency with which each process checklist item was checked.

Category	Item no. and description	Relative frequency (percent)
Modes of mental representation	1. Mental list	84
	7. Mental image—general	49
	21. Mental image—anatomical	45
	23. Mental image—previous patient	29
Strategies of problem formulation:		
Initial routines	16. Organic vs psychogenic	22
	10. Assume organic	63
	18. Acute vs chronic	47
	11. Localize organ system	59
General strategies	12. Incidence	73
	19. Incidence, plus complaints	71
	2. Seriousness	45
	4. Pathophysiological processes	35
	17. Convergence	24
	9. Divergence—(1)	35
	24. Divergence—(2)	69
	3. Quick "rule-outs"	43
Associative processes of problem formulation	8. Association—salient cue	84
	15. Association—combination of cues	82
Cue utilization	25. Focus on verbal cues	61
	20. Focus on nonverbal cues	39
	6. Impression of patient	71
	13. Presenting complaint—more weight	43
	14. Selective focus on cues	24
	22. Interrelate cues progressively	88
	5. Store cues, interrelate later	65

act of generating initial problem formulations, (b) its stability with respect to subjects (across tasks), and (c) its stability with respect to tasks (across subjects).

The first step in the analysis was to construct a subject x task (film) data matrix for each item. In the forty-nine matrix cells for which data were available, a "1" was entered to indicate that the nth subject checked the item on the tth task.

The overall importance of an item as a characteristic of the act of generating problem formulations was measured by the relative frequency with which it was checked. The results of these calculations are presented in Table 7.5.

The subject stability and task stability of each item was measured in terms of the following criteria:

(a) *Subject stability.* An item was considered to be a stable characteristic of a subject's performance if the item was checked for all but one of the films he viewed.

(b) *Task stability.* An item was considered to be a stable characteristic of performance on a given task if the item was checked by all but one of the subjects who had viewed the film.

A "1" was entered in the margin(s) of the item matrix for each subject or task that met the stability criteria defined above.

In order to determine the proportion of cell entries that could be accounted for by using the stability criteria defined above, the following formula was employed:

$$(N_t - N_e)/N_t,$$

where N_t = the total number of cells in the item matrix (49)

and N_e = the number of cells in the item matrix whose entries deviated from those that would be predicted on the basis of the entries in either matrix margin (that is, a cell entry of 1 but no entry in either the subject or task margin; or, conversely, no cell entry but a 1 in either the subject or task margin).

The coefficients for each item calculated according to this formula ranged from 65.3 percent to 89.8 percent, with an average of 81.8 percent across all twenty-five items. In general, the criteria adopted for measuring subject and task stability accounted for a very large percentage of the observed responses.

In order to summarize the data on item stability with respect to subject and tasks, each item was classified along two crossed dimensions: degree of subject stability—that is, the number of subjects for whom the item was a stable characteristic of performance across tasks, and degree of task stability—that is, the number of tasks for which the item was a stable characteristic of performance across subjects. Table 7.6 presents the results of this classification.

The results of the analysis of the checklist data, presented in Tables 7.5 and 7.6, will now be discussed with respect to each of the

Table 7.6   Classification of checklist items in order of increasing stability along two dimensions: degree of subject stability and degree of task stability. Entries in cells are the item numbers as given in Table 7.5.

		Degree of task stability[a]								
		8	7	6	5	4	3	2	1	0
Degree of subject stability[b]	8		8							
	7		1		15					
	6		22							
	5					6				
	4				10	12, 19, 24		5		
	3							11, 25		
	2								2, 13	3, 7, 9, 18
	1								21	14, 20, 23
	0									4, 16, 17

[a] Number of tasks on which the item was a stable characteristic of performance across subjects.
[b] Number of subjects for whom the item was a stable characteristic of performance across tasks.

major areas involved in the generation of problem formulations.

MODES OF MENTAL REPRESENTATION.   This topic was concerned with two modes of mental representation, the verbal and the figural. Four checklist items (1, 7, 21, and 23) were of relevance to this topic.

Generation of verbal lists of problem formulations (item 1) occurred a very high proportion of the time (84 percent) and was found to be a stable characteristic of nearly every subject's performance on nearly every task. The generation of figural images occurred considerably less frequently (49, 45, and 29 percent, for items 7, 21, and 23, respectively). Moreover, the occurrence of mental images showed a very low degree of stability with respect to subjects or tasks: there were only two subjects who consistently reported mental images, and only one task for which mental images were consistently reported. Examination of the relative frequency scores for the three mental-image items revealed that when images are generated, they usually pertain to the anatomical location of the patient's problem (item 21) and, less frequently, may consist of an evocation of a previous patient (item 23). In sum, we may conclude that the generation of problem formulations is typically carried out in a verbal mode of mental representation, but that for a few individuals—or occasionally for all individuals on certain tasks—mental imagery accompanies the predominantly verbal train of thought.

STRATEGIES OF PROBLEM FORMULATION: INITIAL ROUTINES. This topic concerns what may be termed *initial routine strategies* for the generation of problem formulations. The items relevant to the subject were designed to determine whether one of the physician's first steps in the problem-formulation process was to consider the patient's complaint(s) in terms of an organic versus psychogenic distinction (items 10 and 16); to consider the patient's complaint(s) in terms of an acute versus chronic distinction (item 18); or to localize the patient's complaint(s) in terms of an organ system (item 11). All three of these strategies pertain to highly general principles of problem formulation. Thus this topic is also concerned with whether the physician begins the process of generating problem formulations at a high level of generality. The data in Tables 7.5 and 7.6 suggest the following conclusions regarding initial routine strategies.

Examination of the relative frequency scores reveals that the physician does not generally begin by trying to make an organic versus psychogenic distinction (item 16, 22 percent); most often he tends to assume that the patient's problem is organic (item 10, 63 percent). Item 16 was not a stable characteristic of any subject's performance on any task. On the other hand, item 10 was consistently checked by four subjects (across tasks) and on five tasks (across subjects). The relative frequency scores of items 18 (47 percent) and 11 (59 percent) indicate that these two routines occurred with more frequency than the first routine (item 16), but like the first routine they showed little or no subject or task stability. We may conclude that initial routines that involve highly generalized distinctions are not typically the first step(s) in the process of generating problem formulations. Only a few individuals consistently follow such routines, and there are few tasks that consistently prompt their use.

GENERAL STRATEGIES OF PROBLEM FORMULATION. In contrast to the previous discussion, which was concerned with the physician's initial strategies, this topic analyzes the strategies that the physician may use throughout the entire four- to six-minute encounter. Four items included under this topic sought to determine whether the physician follows a strategy based upon consideration of disease incidence (items 12 and 19); consideration of disease seriousness, that is, its life-threatening implications (item 2); or consideration of pathophysiological mechanisms (item 4). Three of the items sought to determine whether the physician follows a convergent strategy, that is, attempts to come up with one problem formulation that will account for all the data (item 17), and/or either of two divergent strategies: a brainstorming strategy of attempting to think of as many formulations as possible that fit the cues (item 9), or a more modest divergent strategy of attempting, as each formulation is generated, to think of other possible formulations (item 24). There was also one item (number 3) designed to determine whether the physician had already, within the initial interview, performed some quick rule-outs of certain problem formulations. The following conclusions are suggested.

Consideration of disease incidence is relatively more important than consideration of disease seriousness in determining the type of problem formulations a physician generates (relative frequency scores of 71 percent and 73 percent for the incidence items versus 45 percent for the seriousness item). Consideration of incidence was consistently checked by four physicians, and on four tasks, while consideration of seriousness was consistently checked by two physicians, and on only one task. We conclude that although the physician may not give consideration to either of these factors, he is relatively more likely to direct his search toward diseases of high incidence (which are usually not very serious) than toward diseases of great seriousness (which usually have low incidence).

The item pertaining to consideration of pathophysiological processes (17) was checked a relatively small proportion of the time (35 percent). Since knowledge of pathophysiological processes is considered to be one of the foundations of clinical medicine, this result is somewhat surprising. It may be that for the experienced physician the utilization of such knowledge is so well established (routinized) that he is no longer consciously aware of its use in generating problem formulations. On the other hand, it is also possible that the generation of problem formulations is essentially a cue-to-disease associative mechanism that does not require consideration of the pathophysiology underlying disease processes. This second hypothesis receives some support from data to be discussed under the topic "associative processes of problem formulation."

Examination of the data for the items on convergent versus divergent strategies of problem formulation reveals that the convergent item was checked rather infrequently (item 17, 24 percent), while one divergent item was checked relatively frequently (item 24, 69 percent) and the other was not (item 9, 35 percent). The convergent item was not consistently checked by any subjects, or on any task. The data for the divergent items indicate that item 24 was consistently checked by four subjects, and on four tasks, while item 9 was checked consistently by only two subjects, and on none of the tasks. It is not surprising that experienced physicians rarely follow a convergent strategy of problem formulation during the initial minutes of the workup. To do so would entail the risk of premature closure—acceptance of a formulation that may be intellectually appealing (because it can account so parsimoniously for the available data), but possibly incorrect. Divergent strategies of problem formulation would of course help to counteract any tendency toward premature closure. Of the two divergent strategies that were considered, one (the strategy of attempting, each time a formulation is generated, to think of other formulations) was consistently employed by a sizable number of physicians, and on a sizable number of tasks, while the other (a brainstorming strategy of attempting to think of as many causes of the patient's symptoms as possible) was not. The less frequent use of the second divergent strategy may be a result of the risks brainstorming could entail (such as information overload taxing the capacity of working memory or insufficient data collection to test numerous potential but implausible hypotheses).

The item on quick rule-outs was checked with a relative frequency of 43 percent. However, it was checked consistently by only two subjects, and not consistently for any tasks. We may conclude that while a few physicians consistently rule out some problem formulations generated during the first four to six minutes of a workup, most physicians retain all formulations they generate as components of their initial problem space.

ASSOCIATIVE PROCESSES OF PROBLEM FORMULATION. The items under the two previous topics were designed to determine whether the physician attempts to follow various strategies of problem formulation. The items under the present topic were designed to determine whether the act of generating problem formulations entails associative processes, that is, rapid cue-to-problem formulation retrieval, essentially outside the realm of conscious search. There were two items of relevance to this topic. They sought to determine whether problem formulations were immediately brought to mind by some particularly salient cue (item 8), and/or by a combination of cues (item 15). Both of these items were checked a very high proportion of the time (84 and 82 percent, respectively). Item 8 was checked consistently by all eight subjects, and on seven of the tasks; this was the highest degree of subject and task stability of any item on the checklist. Item 15 was checked consistently by seven subjects, and on five tasks; it was among the top four items with respect to degree of subject and task stability.

When the data for these items are compared with the data on problem-formulation strategies, we are led to conclude that the generation of problem formulations is largely an associative process. Search strategies are employed, more or less frequently depending on the individual and the case, but appear to be adjuncts to the primary process of associative retrieval. Moreover, the finding that generation of problem formulations is based more consistently on single salient cues than on combinations of cues would appear to indicate that the physician's long-term storage of potential problem-formulation categories (disease processes) may be indexed in terms of a very small number of pathognomonic cues for each category, rather than in terms of a complex system of multiple-entry, cross-referenced cues. In sum, the checklist data tend to support the notion that the generation of diagnostic problem formulations is composed primarily of rapid cue-to-problem category associative retrieval. As Barrows and Bennett (1972) noted in their study of neurologists, hypotheses seem to literally pop into the head of the clinician.

CUE UTILIZATION. The items under this topic were designed to measure several aspects of the physician's behavior with respect to detecting, interpreting, and utilizing cues: whether he focuses on verbal cues (item 25) or nonverbal cues (item 20); whether he gives more weight to the patient's presenting complaint then to subsequent cues (item 13); what role his initial impression of the patient plays in interpretation of the reliability of cues (item 6); whether he focuses his attention on certain cues and pays less attention to others (item 14); whether he attempts to look for relationships among cues progressively as each cue is presented (item 22), or stores cues and attempts to interrelate them after obtaining data on each major complaint (item 5). The data for these items suggest the following conclusions regarding cue utilization.

Although in many instances the physician does not selectively focus on either verbal or nonverbal cues, there is a greater tendency to focus on verbal than on nonverbal cues (relative frequency scores of 61 and 39 percent, respectively). Focusing on nonverbal cues (item 20) was a stable characteristic of only one subject (and no tasks), while focusing on verbal cues (item 25) was a stable characteristic of three subjects (and two tasks). However, the data for item 6 indicated that physicians generally do make use of nonverbal data to form an early impression of the patient (his personality, intelligence, background, and the like), which is then used as the basis for judging the accuracy and objectivity of the symptoms the patient reports. This item had a relative frequency score of 71 percent and was consistently checked by five subjects, and on three tasks. It appears that some physicians make greater use of their initial impression of the patient than others; and some patients provide more of a basis for doing so (for instance, they have more salient nonverbal characteristics) than others.

The items that deal with giving more weight to the patient's presenting complaint than to other cues (item 13), and with giving more attention to certain cues than to others (item 14) had moderate to low relative frequency scores (43 and 24 percent, respectively) and were consistently checked by only one or two subjects, and on only one (or none) of the tasks. The comments of several physicians in their recall protocols suggest a reason why the physician does not typically give more weight to the patient's presenting complaint: they noted that with some patients there may be a "hidden agenda" of medical problems, which must be uncovered by careful questioning and which may prove to be more important than the presenting complaint.

The two items pertaining to the manner in which the physician attempts to interrelate cues were both checked relatively often (item 22, 88 percent; item 5, 65 percent). In constructing the checklist, we considered that these two items described contrasting strategies for dealing with cues. However, four subjects consistently checked both of them. Several subjects' comments in discussing the checklist items with the experimenter provided an indication of why this occurred. They noted that although they do not consciously adhere to either of the strategies described by the two items, both refer to aspects of their processing of cues and were therefore checked. They noted that it is not a matter, as the items imply, of "trying" (or "not trying") to relate each new cue to previous cues; rather, they suggested, relationships among cues simply "come to mind," usually as each new cue is obtained, but sometimes later.

Conclusions

Several tentative conclusions may be drawn from the analysis of the recall protocol and checklist data regarding the processes involved in the act of generating initial problem formulations.

(a) The mode of mental representation involved in the generation of problem formulations is, for all physicians, predominantly verbal. For most individuals mental imagery occasionally occurs, and for a few individuals such imagery consistently occurs. But for all individuals mental imagery appears to be an adjunct to the primary verbal mode of representation.

(b) Although physicians show some tendency to focus on verbal cues, they do make use of nonverbal cues. One major use of such cues, consistently reported by over half of the physicians, is to form a general impression of the patient that will aid in judging the accuracy and objectivity of the cues reported verbally by the patient.

(c) The generation of problem formulations appears to be primarily a process of direct associative retrieval, rather than one of strategy-guided search. The checklist data indicated that only two strategies were consistently employed by at least half of the physicians: focusing on diseases of high incidence for the patient's demographic group, and attempting to think of alternatives (or competitors) to each formulation generated. On the basis of the recall protocol data, it was possible to identify various processes underlying the generation of each of the four structural features of a set of initial formulations. In general, these processes appeared to be governed by the effect of various task variables on associative retrieval, rather than by consistent use of strategies on the part of the subject. In particular, it may be noted, the data failed to support Kleinmuntz's (1968) notion that the physician follows a "general-to-specific" strategy, at least so far as the generation of initial problem formulations is concerned. To summarize: both the recall protocol and checklist data suggest that the physician's information-processing activity during the early part of the workup consists primarily in associative retrieval of problem-formulation labels on the basis of cues, and that this process is mediated to only a limited extent by search strategies.

8 / Generation of Initial Problem Formulations: Training of Medical Students[1]

This chapter describes an experiment that was conducted to test the effectiveness of a model for training medical students to generate initial problem formulations based on cues obtained during the early minutes of a clinical encounter.

The rationale for training medical students in this task rests on two arguments:

(a) A major conclusion drawn from much of the psychological literature on problem solving and inquiry (Dewey, 1938; Shulman, Loupe, and Piper, 1968; Newell and Simon, 1972) is that, when confronted with any complex problematic situation, the human information processor inevitably generates some sort of conceptual framework as an early step in his search for a solution. The research described in Chapter 4 provides evidence that this conclusion applies to medical problem solving. Thus, training medical students in the early generation of diagnostic problem formulations is consistent with what is known about the cognitive processes of human problem solvers in general and of experienced physicians in particular.

(b) Since experienced physicians, despite their training in the traditional "reserve judgment" approach to diagnosis, are found to generate problem formulations very early in the workup, it is anticipated that clinical experience alone would lead the medical student to do likewise. We believe, however, that by providing the medical student with training that focuses explicitly on this process, it may be possible to improve his ability to generate *ap-*

---

[1] Chapters 7 and 8 are based on the Ph.D. dissertation of Linda K. Allal, "Training of Medical Students in a Problem-Solving Skill: The Generation of Diagnostic Problem Formulations" (Michigan State University, 1973).

propriate initial problem formulations and thereby aid him in making the transition from classroom studies to clinical practice.

The Training Model

The training model developed and tested in the present experiment included two major components: having the student practice the task of generating initial problem formulations under conditions that *simulate* the early part of the clinical encounter, and providing the student with *feedback* based on the performance of this task by experienced physicians.

The first component in the model, the use of simulation exercises, is based on the educational principle that problem-solving skills can be taught best by providing the student with opportunities to encounter and attempt to solve a range of problems that closely approximate, in breadth and complexity, the problems he will encounter in the real world (Dewey, 1963; Bruner, 1966; Gagné, 1971). In the present case the student's encounter with a series of patients having various medical complaints and diverse demographic characteristics was simulated by color films that give a physician's-eye view of the first four to six minutes of a clinical workup (see Chapter 7). Simulations, by definition, are designed to contain the parts of reality essential to the learning task, while ignoring the aspects of reality that are to some degree unnecessary to the learning task (Twelker, 1971). The use of films to simulate the student's encounter with patients relieves the student from carrying out some of the activities in which the physician must normally engage, such as formulating and asking questions, and establishing rapport and handling interpersonal relations. Viewing the film does, however, provide the student with the opportunity to carry out the two types of information-processing activities that are of concern in the present study: the detection and encoding of cues from naturalistic observation of what a patient says and does, and the use of these cues in generating diagnostic problem formulations.

The second component in the training model, the provision of feedback by experienced physicians on the performance of the task, was designed to enable the student to evaluate his own performance on a given exercise and, across the full set of exercises, to increase his skill in attaining problem-formulation outcomes similar to those of the experienced physician. Two types of feedback were employed in the experiment: feedback on the *out-*

comes of physicians' problem-formulation activity during the earliest part of the workup, and feedback on the *processes* by which physicians arrive at these outcomes. Both types were based on the data obtained from the sample of experienced physicians described in Chapter 7.

The first type of feedback consisted in written materials that presented the problem formulations generated by the physicians and the cues associated with each formulation. The materials were designed to indicate both the commonalities and the range of diversity found in the physician outcomes. The second type of feedback included a special version of each of the training films in which think-aloud recordings were interposed at various points in the dialogue. The purpose of these films was to provide for the student a simulated portrayal of the problem-formulation processes typically going on inside the physician's head as he observes and interviews the patient. In addition, written materials were used to summarize the similarities and differences among physicians with respect to processes of generating a set of initial problem formulations.

The feedback employed in this study has special features that distinguish it from most traditional types: first, the notion of using feedback to provide the learner with "process models" is obviously quite foreign to the behaviorist tradition of feedback; and second, the type of outcome feedback provided in this study is closer to what has been termed "cognitive" feedback (Hammond and Summers, 1972) than to the classical types of outcome feedback used in learning experiments or programmed instruction. A major feature is that it does not provide the student with a single "correct" model of either outcomes or processes. Rather, it indicates both the convergent and the divergent aspects of the performance of experienced physicians—that is, the common and differing characteristics of nearly all physicians with respect to the generation of a set of initial problem formulations. Thus in using the feedback to evaluate his own performance, the student must engage in a series of relatively complex cognitive activities. He must examine, synthesize, and draw inferences from a sample of the performances of experienced practitioners in his field.

Hypotheses

The training model, therefore, comprised problem-solving exercises in which films were used to simulate the conditions of the early part of the clinical workup and feedback based on data from a sample of experienced physicians. The experiment was designed to test two hypotheses: first, that the training model will significantly improve second-year medical students' skill in generating an initial set of diagnostic problem formulations; and second, that the training model will be significantly more effective when it provides outcome and process feedback than when it provides outcome feedback only.

Method

Subjects

A sample of forty-eight students in the third term of their second year of medical school participated in the experiment. The decision to sample second-year students was based on consideration of several criteria. First of all, it was believed that training in the generation of problem formulations using filmed case presentations would be most appropriate prior to the student's participation in clinical clerkships (in other words, before summer term of his second year). Then, for the training to be effective it was necessary that the student have acquired sufficient medical science background to be able to deal with the range of cases in internal medicine presented by the films. It was also necessary that the student have not already attained a level of skill in the experimental task that would preclude improvement in this skill via participation in the training experiment. Pilot testing indicated that, of two potential populations that met the first criterion (first-year and second-year students at the College of Human Medicine, Michigan State University), the second-year population most adequately met the other two criteria.

Out of a target population of seventy-seven students, a total of sixty-eight persons were randomly selected to obtain forty-eight willing to participate in the experiment. Thus, the acceptance rate was 70.6 percent. To determine whether those who refused to participate (or who could not be contacted) differed systematically from the sample of participants, it was possible to examine the students' final examination scores for the Focal Problems course in which they were enrolled the term preceding the experiment. Inspection of these data revealed that the four students with exam scores considerably lower than all other students (that is, scores in the 40s, whereas the range of all other students' scores was 61 to 87) were among the refusals. In this way the weakest students in the population may have eliminated themselves systematically from participation in the experiment. With these four students excluded, the mean exam scores for the participant and refusal/no-contact groups were virtually identical (72.06 and 72.67, respectively). This finding lends support to the argument that, with the exception of the students in the bottom 6 percent of the class, the results of the experiment may be generalized to the target population of second-year medical students.

The target population of real interest, however, extends beyond the students actually sampled. One would wish, using the arguments of Cornfield and Tukey (1956), to generalize the experimental results to a hypothetical target population of all second-year students similar to those actually sampled. The characteristics of this hypothetical population may be inferred from the description of the characteristics of the sample—at both the individual and the institutional level—that is provided in Allal (1973).

Experimental Procedure

The experiment employed a posttest-only, control-group design, with subjects assigned at random to one of three experimental conditions:

Treatment 1: training with outcome feedback; posttest.

Treatment 2: training with outcome and process feedback; posttest.

Control: posttest only.

Since both treatment conditions were based on the general training model described in Chapter 7, they had a number of features in common.

(a) Both conditions comprised three training sessions (with two films presented at each session) and a posttest session (at which two films were presented). The general format of each session was the same under both conditions.

(b) Under both conditions the subject carried out the same basic task with respect to each of the films: having viewed the film, he filled out a set of response sheets that indicated the problem formulations he had generated, and he wrote a brief tentative assessment.

(c) Under both conditions the subject was provided with feedback materials based on the physician performance data.

The two training conditions differed, however, with respect to the type of feedback provided. Under one condition (treatment 1), the feedback materials provided the student with "outcome models"—examples of the problem formulations and tentative assessments generated by the physicians for each of the training films. Under the other condition (treatment 2), the feedback materials provided the subject with outcome models *and* "process models"—materials that portrayed the processes by which the physicians arrived at their problem formulations. The outcome feedback furnished under both treatments was presented in written booklet form. The process feedback furnished under treatment 2 included written material and audio supplements to each of the training films.

Training was conducted in three weekly sessions, with the posttest administered at a fourth session. All experimental manipulations were administered by means of individual booklets in self-instructional format. At the beginning of the first training session, this booklet provided the subject with a set of orientation materials designed to acquaint him with the problem-formulation task. At the beginning of the next three sessions the subject was given review materials. The instructional sequence (or posttest task) for each of two films was then administered by means of the self-instructional booklet. The role of the experimenter was limited to a small number of preliminary verbal instructions.

A single session for the subject under the control condition was considered undesirable for two reasons.

(a) Because a single control-group session would require administration of the orientation materials prior to presentation of the two posttest films, it would be longer than the treatment-group posttest session and of course not fully equivalent in content.

(b) On a subject's first exposure to the task his performance possibly might be depressed, or affected in some other unknown way, by the novelty of viewing a filmed interview and then having to fill out a set of relatively unfamiliar response sheets. It was believed that any "novelty effect" would be eliminated after a subject's first exposure to one of the films and to the task of filling out the response sheets. To make the posttest session conditions as similar as possible across all three groups and to control for the possibility of a novelty effect, it was decided to conduct two sessions for control-group subjects. During the first session the subject was given orientation materials (similar to those administered at the first session under the treatment condition), and he carried out a task designed to control for a possible novelty effect during

Table 8.1 The experimental procedure for training medical students in the generation of initial problem formulations.

Week	Experimental conditions	
	Treatments 1 and 2	Control
1	Training session 1 Orientation Film 1 Film 2	
2	Training session 2 Review Film 3 Film 4	
3	Training session 3 Review Film 5 Film 6	Orientation session Orientation Film 6
4	Posttest session Review Film 7 Film 8	Posttest session Review Film 7 Film 8

the subsequent posttest session: namely, the sixth training film was presented, and the subject recorded his problem formulations and tentative assessment. (Feedback, of course, was not provided.) The second control-group session involved the same procedure as the treatment-group posttest sessions: review of the orientation materials, followed by presentation of the two posttest films. The format of the experimental procedure is outlined in Table 8.1.

Instructional Sequence

The same instructional sequence was followed under both treatment conditions for each of the six filmed training cases. This sequence involved five steps, which are summarized below.

Step 1: The subject read the "nurse's sheet" for the patient in the film.

Step 2: The subject viewed the film of the four- to six-minute interview with the patient. He was given the following instructions in advance: While viewing the film, you should generate a set of initial problem formulations that you would want to investigate more thoroughly if you were to continue the workup beyond the first four to six minutes presented in the film.

Step 3: The subject recorded the problem formulations he had generated and the list of cues relevant to each formulation. He then wrote a brief paragraph giving his tentative assessment of the case, after instruction that his assessment should indicate:

—how well-substantiated he considered each of his problem formulations to be on the basis of the data obtained thus far;

—whether he anticipated that a single illness or multiple disorders accounted for the patient's various problems;

—whether he considered there to be any relationships among his problem formulations. For example, he might consider one problem formulation to be secondary to, superimposed on, or contributing to some other problem formulation.

Step 4: The subject was provided with feedback on the performance of the experienced physicians.
(a) Feedback sheet 1 was presented.
(b) Treatment 1: The film of the interview was presented a second time.
Treatment 2: The process-feedback version of the film was presented.
(c) Feedback sheet 2 was presented.

Step 5: The subject filled out a self-evaluation checklist.

The first three steps in the sequence constituted the basic experimental task. Step 4, which embodied the experimental manipulation of feedback, was the only step in the instructional sequence that differed for the two treatment conditions.

The feedback was presented to the subjects in three parts. The first part (feedback sheet 1, "Major Problem Formulations") was designed to provide the subject with feedback on the problem-formulation outcomes that were common to the responses of all, or nearly all, of the physicians. This sheet enabled the subject to determine whether he had generated those formulations which the physician data indicated were of major importance for the case under consideration.

The second part of the feedback was a film presentation: in the case of treatment 1, a second presentation of the standard film of the interview; in the case of treatment 2, a presentation of the process-feedback version of the film. Under both treatment conditions a second exposure to the interview provided the subject with implicit feedback on the adequacy of his detection and recall of cues. The conditions differed, however, with respect to the provision of process feedback. The film presented under the treatment 2 condition provided explicit feedback, via the physician's think-aloud comments, on the processes by which the physician sample generated each of the problem formulations listed on feedback sheet 1. Under the treatment 1 condition, on the other hand, the second presentation of the standard film provided the student with the opportunity to attempt to reconstruct, on his own, the processes by which the problem formulations on feedback sheet 1 were generated.

The third part of the feedback (feedback sheet 2) contained one section that was the same for subjects under both conditions. This section ("Additional Problem Formulations") was designed to provide the subject with feedback on the range of diversity in the physicians' problem-formulation outcomes.

The second section of feedback sheet 2 ("Summary") differed for the two treatment groups. Under treatment 1, it summarized the comments included in the physicians' tentative assessments. Under treatment 2, it consisted in a reconstruction of the physicians' reasoning about the case and included a description of the processes by which the problem formulations listed on both feedback sheets were generated and a summary of the comments in the physicians' tentative assessments. Feedback sheet 2 pointed out both the commonalities and the range of diversity that were characteristic of the physicians' problem formulation processes and their tentative assessments. Table 8.2 outlines the properties of the feedback presented under the two treatment conditions.

The fifth and final step in the instructional sequence consisted in filling out a self-evaluation checklist, designed to serve two functions: to ensure that the subject carried out the process of comparing his own performance to that of the experienced physicians, and to provide the subject with a sense of closure at the completion of the instructional sequence for a case. The first part of the checklist listed the titles of the problem formulations generated by the physicians. The second part listed the statements regarding functional relationships between problem formulations that were found in the physicians' tentative assessments. The subject was instructed to check each item in the list that corresponded to one of his own responses.

Table 8.2 Properties of the feedback presented to medical students under the two treatment conditions. PF = problem formulation; TA = tentative assessment; C = feedback indicating commonalities found in the performance of all or nearly all physicians; and D = feedback indicating the range of diversity found in physician performance.

Feedback material	Treatment 1	Treatment 2
A. Feedback Sheet 1	PF outcomes (C)	PF outcomes (C)
B. Film Presentation	Standard film	Supplemented film: PF processes (C)
C. Feedback Sheet 2:		
Section 1	PF outcomes (D)	PF outcomes (D)
Section 2	TA outcomes (C, D)	PF processes (D) and TA outcomes (C, D)

Materials

Each subject received two booklets: an instructional booklet that contained directions and the written feedback materials; and a response booklet that contained the response sheets and self-evaluation checklists.

OUTCOME FEEDBACK. Each problem formulation presented on a feedback sheet had two components: a problem-formulation title, and a list of cues of relevance to that title. Problem formulations were organized on the feedback sheets to indicate hierarchical relationships (if any) among subsets of formulations. Cues of relevance to all formulations in a hierarchy were listed under the problem-formulation title at the head of the hierarchy; only those cues of particular relevance to each more specific formulation in the hierarchy were listed under the subordinate title(s) in the hierarchy (see Figure 8.1).

PROCESS FEEDBACK FILMS. Each of these films included three or four think-aloud segments interposed at appropriate points in the standard film of the interview. After each segment the dialogue between the doctor and patient stopped, an image of the patient was frozen on the screen, and the physician was heard thinking aloud about such matters as:

—the problem formulations he had generated up to that point;
—the cues that had led to the generation of these formulations;

Figure 8.1 **Sample of outcome feedback for film 1.**
GI disorder:
Ulcerative colitis, or regional enteritis/ileitis

GI disorder
   pain in right lower quadrant of abdomen, for 4 months
      occurs in evening, lasting several hours
      not relieved by aspirin or Darvon
      not related to foods
   diarrhea: increase in number of stools, from 1 to 4-5/day,
      over 3-month period
   mucus in stools
   blood in stools
   pieces of food in stools
   weight loss, 25 lbs in 1-2 months
   good appetite, eating more than usual
   extreme fatigue and weakness, for 2 months
   no vomiting

Ulcerative colitis, or regional enteritis/ileitis
   diarrhea
   blood and mucus in stools
   weight loss of 25 lbs, with good appetite
   age 21
   college senior: under academic stress, concerned about
      keeping up with studies

—alternative interpretations being considered for certain ambiguous cues;
—any strategies that were guiding his thinking;
—his impressions of the patient;
—his revisions of previous formulations in the light of new data.

In sum, the thinking-aloud segments attempted to provide the viewer with simulated access to the processes going on in the physician's head as he conducted the interview.

Posttest Tasks

THE BASIC POSTTEST TASK.   At the posttest session the subject carried out the basic experimental task (steps 1 to 3 described earlier in the chapter) with respect to each of two films. Selection of the films was based on two considerations. First, to obtain as broad a sample as possible of the content domain (that is, internal medicine), films that presented dissimilar cases, with respect to type of medical complaints and patient demographic characteristics, were selected. Second, to avoid a possible ceiling effect, the films were selected from among those found, upon examination of the physician data, to provide the basis for generation of a relatively large number of problem formulations.

ADDITIONAL POSTTEST TASK.   After the subject had completed the basic posttest tasks, he was given two additional tasks pertaining to the second posttest film. Their purpose was to determine the extent to which perceptual and memory factors (factors in the processes of detecting, encoding, and retrieving cues rather than in generating problem formulations per se) may have affected the subject's performance on the basic posttest task. Since the results of the experiment indicated that performance on these additional tasks was *uniformly* high (that is, there was no evidence that performance of the basic task was inhibited by perceptual or memory factors), a description of these tasks, and of the data pertaining to them, will not be presented here (see Allal, 1973, for details).

QUESTIONNAIRE.   At the end of the posttest session a questionnaire was administered to subjects in the two treatment conditions. The primary purpose was to elicit the subject's opinion of, or attitude toward, various aspects of the training procedure.

The Covariate: Controlling for Differences in Entry Skills

Since earlier Medical Inquiry Project studies had found a high degree of variability on most medical problem-solving variables, it was considered important that an appropriate covariable be obtained to increase the precision of the statistical analysis. That is, if the participants differed from one another significantly in their initial problem-solving capabilities, the precise magnitude of the training could be masked.

Probably the best measure would have been a pretest in which the subject carried out the same task as on the posttest. However, this possibility was rejected for several reasons. First, it was believed that to obtain reliable pretest measures on the dependent variables at least two filmed cases would have to be employed. This would have reduced the number of films available for training from six to four. It was believed that insufficient training was more likely than lack of precision to result in a nonsignificant treatment effect. Moreover, a nonsignificant outcome caused by failure to carry out an adequate test of the treatment would be a more serious experimental failure than the occurrence of a Type 2 error caused by lack of precision. It was, therefore, decided to attempt to obtain covariate measures from some source other than a pretest.

The source decided on was the final examination in the Focal Problems course, in which all second-year medical students had been enrolled the term prior to administration of the experiment. This measure was selected for several reasons. Since it comprised a hundred multiple-choice and true-false questions, it could be expected to provide relatively reliable and objective data. Furthermore, it could be expected to correlate better with the dependent variables in the present analysis than any other available measure. Although the majority of items in the test were designed to measure the student's knowledge of the medical science content covered in the course, a substantial number of items attempted to assess his ability to use data about a patient to make a differential diagnosis or to select diagnostic or therapeutic options. It was therefore anticipated that use of this exam as a covariate would be effective in reducing intragroup variability on the dimension "pre-experimental knowledge of medical science content" and, secondarily, on the dimension "pre-experimental ability in solving medical problems."

Dependent Variables

A subject's performance on the basic posttest tasks was evaluated in terms of four dependent variables: a cue-utilization score, a problem-formulation score, a score that reflected the classification of cues with respect to problem formulations, and a relationships-among-problem-formulations score.

The first three variables were based on the information recorded by the subject on his problem-formulation response sheets. Each of these variables was designed to measure one component of the interrelated cognitive outcomes that resulted from the subject's simulated encounter with a patient. The cue-utilization score pertained to the functional data base (set of cues) that the subject extracted from the film and used to generate problem formulations; the problem-formulation score pertained to the set of problem formulations he generated; the cue-classification score pertained to the way in which he classified the cues obtained with respect to the problem formulations he generated. The fourth dependent variable, the score reflecting relationships among problem formulations, was based on information the subject recorded in his tentative assessment and pertained to functional relationships which he hypothesized to exist among the problem formulations he had generated.

For each variable the adequacy of the subject's performance was measured by means of a scoring key derived from the physician performance data. The subject's score on each variable was calculated separately for each of the two posttest tasks, but for purposes of statistical analysis his scores were summed across tasks, so that there were four dependent measures per subject.

Each scoring key was designed to measure the degree to which the student's performance on a given variable approximated that of the experienced physicians. Each key contained a list of various potential responses, with points assigned to each. The number of points assigned to a response was weighted to reflect the relative frequency with which the response occurred in the experienced physician data. Certain additions to the keys and validation of several key components were carried out by means of independent consultations with two physicians who were not part of the sample of eight. A detailed description of the construction and properties of the scoring keys may be found in Allal (1973).

To aid in interpreting the experimental outcomes of primary interest (namely, intergroup differences in the four variables), a number of other measures were calculated. These will be described subsequently in the section entitled "Supplemental Analyses."

Results

Tests of Experimental Hypotheses

RELIABILITY. For each of the four dependent variables, two types of reliability estimates were calculated by means of the intraclass correlation coefficient (Ebel, 1951). The coefficients were calculated on the basis of a random sample of six subjects' posttest responses, scored independently by the experimenter and a second person. As shown in Table 8.3, the coefficients for cue utilization, problem formulation, and cue classification are nearly 1.0. Inspection of the data revealed that the very low coefficient for relationships among problem formulations was the result of a high degree of restriction in range on this variable, rather than a substantial degree of divergence between scorers. Since the operations involved in obtaining a subject's score on relationships among problem formulations were similar to those in-

Table 8.3 Interscorer reliability and generalizability coefficients on the variables cue utilization, problem formulation, cue classification, and relationships among problem formulations.

Variable	Interscorer reliability	Generalizability coefficient[a]
Cue utilization	.97	.73
Problem formulation	.99	.66
Cue classification	.97	.55
Relationships among problem formulations	.09[b]	.48

[a] Generalizability coefficient modified to exclude between-group variation: $r = (MS_{S:G} - MS_{T:G})/MS_{S:G}$, where $MS_{S:G}$ = mean square for subjects within groups and $MS_{T:G}$ = mean square for treatment effects within groups.
[b] Index of interscorer agreement = .83 (see text for discussion).

volved in conducting a content analysis, a content analysis formula (Holsti, 1969, p. 140) for estimating percent of interscorer agreement was calculated for this variable. The coefficient obtained was .83. It was concluded that on all four dependent variables, scorer variation would not constitute a source of unreliability in the data.

To determine the degree to which it would be possible to generalize from subjects' performance on the two posttest tasks to a hypothetical population of randomly equivalent tasks in the domain of internal medicine, *generalizability coefficients* were calculated for each dependent variable on the basis of all subjects' posttest scores. These coefficients were calculated by means of Hoyt's (1941) analysis of variance technique, which is equivalent to Cronbach's (1951) coefficient alpha. So that estimation of the generalizability of the instrument would not be contaminated by treatment effect, the formula was modified to exclude intergroup variation. As shown in Table 8.3, the generalizability coefficients ranged from .48 to .73. Given that the posttest included only two tasks and that the tasks were selected to represent very different cases (with respect to type of medical complaints and patient demographic characteristics), the magnitude of the generalizability coefficients is quite substantial. In fact, compared to coefficients obtained by other investigators (Lewy and McGuire, 1966) and in other Medical Inquiry Project studies (see Chapters 4 and 10), the coefficients are very high.

Results of Hypothesis Tests

The experimental hypotheses were tested in the following manner.

(a) A multivariate analysis of covariance was conducted to determine whether the training procedures had enhanced the problem-formulation performances of the participants, as measured by the set of four dependent variables (Table 8.4).

(b) To identify the specific dependent variable(s) responsible for any significant treatment effect, a stepdown analysis was conducted. Since the four dependent measures are interrelated, this analysis requires that the investigator specify a logical order for examining these scores. Univariate analyses were also conducted on these measures (Tables 8.5 and 8.6).

(c) For each variable having a significant univariate F ratio, the Scheffé post hoc confidence-interval procedure was used to test for significant differences between each pair of experimental conditions. Thus, given a significant treatment effect, was it attributable to *both* treatments, one but not the other, or differences between the treatments? A one-way fixed-effects model was used for both the multivariate and univariate analyses.

The decision to order the dependent variables for the stepdown F tests (Table 8.5) was based on the following considerations.

(a) Since performance on cue utilization is a prerequisite for the generation of problem-formulation titles, the variable cue utilization was ordered first and problem formulation second. Thus, for cue utilization the stepdown F test was the same as a

Table 8.4   Adjusted means on the dependent variables, by experimental condition.

Variable	Experimental condition		
	Treatment 1	Treatment 2	Control
Cue utilization	79.52	76.45	72.66
Problem formulation	59.46	50.58	40.09
Cue classification	83.49	75.27	58.12
Relationships among problem formulations	9.10	6.32	7.33

Table 8.5 Multivariate analysis of covariance on cue utilization, problem formulation, cue classification, and relationships among problem formulations.

F tests	df	F	p
Multivariate F test	8, 82	3.01	.0052
Stepdown F tests:			
On cue utilization	2, 44	1.94	.16
On problem formulation	2, 44	8.27	.001
On cue classification	2, 44	0.43	.66
On relationships among problem formulations	2, 44	1.83	.17

Table 8.6 Univariate analyses of covariance on problem formulation, cue classification, and relationships among problem formulations.

Variable	df	F	p
Problem formulation	2, 44	11.01	.001
Cue classification	2, 44	7.20	.002
Relationships among problem formulations	2, 44	2.27	.12

univariate F test, while for problem formulation the stepdown F provided a test of treatment effect on the generation of problem-formulation titles with intergroup differences on cue utilization partialed out.

(b) Since the classification of cues with respect to problem-formulation titles is a function of both cues obtained and problem-formulation titles generated, cue classification was ordered third. The stepdown F ratio for cue classification thereby provided a test of treatment effect on this variable with intergroup differences on both cue utilization and problem formulation partialed out.

(c) Since statements of functional relationships among problem formulations are dependent on the subject's prior processing of cues and generation of problem formulations, this variable was ordered last. The fourth stepdown F ratio therefore tests for treatment effect on relationships among problem formulations with intergroup differences on the other three variables partialed out.

To aid in interpretation of the stepdown F tests, univariate F tests were calculated on problem formulation, cue classification, and relationships among problem formulations (Table 8.6).

The results of the above analyses indicate the following conclusions.

(a) The multivariate F test indicates that for the *set* of dependent variables taken together there was a significant main effect for treatment ($p < .0052$).

(b) For the variables cue utilization and relationships among problem formulations, differences among adjusted group means were nonsignificant.

(c) For problem formulation, a significant treatment effect was found on both the stepdown and univariate tests ($p < .001$ and $p < .0002$, respectively).

(d) For cue classification, differences among adjusted group means were significant, as tested by a univariate F ratio ($p < .002$). However, when cue classification was conditioned on cue utilization and problem formulation (via a stepdown F ratio), differences among groups were not significant. Since significant intergroup differences were found on problem formulation but not on cue utilization, and since the intragroup correlation of problem formulation and cue classification was .75, the nonsignificant stepdown F for the latter variable could be attributed to the partialing out of intergroup differences on problem formulation.

Once a significant univariate treatment effect on problem formulation and cue classification had been determined, the Scheffé post hoc confidence-interval procedure was used to test for significant differences on these variables between each pair of experimental conditions.[2] The results of this procedure are presented in Table 8.7.

Similar results were found for both dependent variables: the difference between the two treatment groups is nonsignificant; the difference between treatment 1 and the control group is significant at the .001 or .005 level; and the difference between treatment 2 and the control group is significant at the .05 level.

The average correlations (within treatment groups) between earlier problem-solving performance (the covariate) and the de-

---

[2] The more powerful Tukey post hoc procedure is not considered applicable after analysis of *covariance*, because the estimates of the regression intercepts do not in general meet the requirement of equal variances and covariances (Scheffé, 1959).

Table 8.7 Scheffé post hoc comparisons on problem formulation and cue classification. Comparisons are made on adjusted group means. T1 = treatment 1; T2 = treatment 2; and C = control.

Variable	Comparison	Confidence interval	Degree of confidence (percent)
Problem formulation	T1-T2 8.88	±10.32	95
	T1-C 19.37[a]	±16.66	99
	T2-C 10.49[a]	±10.32	95
Cue classification	T1-T2 8.21	±17.06	95
	T1-C 25.37[a]	±23.66	99
	T2-C 17.16	±17.06	95

[a] Significant group differences at the .05 level or better.

pendent variables were .15 for cue utilization, .26 for problem formulation, .22 for cue classification, and .36 for relationships among problem formulations. Given the low magnitude of the four coefficients, we may conclude that the covariate was not effective in increasing the precision of the analysis. Problem-solving performance measured in a course prior to the experiment did not correlate with performance after training. While some of the statistical tests were found to be significant despite the ineffectiveness of the covariate, it is possible that others would have proved significant if a more powerful covariate had been available.

CONCLUSIONS. The results of the preceding analysis supported hypothesis 1 (treatment versus control difference) with respect to problem formulation and cue classification, but not with respect to the other two variables.

If the means on cue utilization are expressed as a percentage of the maximum possible score on this variable, it is found that the average performance under all three conditions was high (77 percent for treatment 1, 74 percent for treatment 2, 71 percent for the control group). This would suggest that the subjects already had attained, prior to the experiment, a high level of cue-acquiring skill.

On problem formulation, the treatment groups both differed significantly from the control group. Since the treatment and control subjects did not differ in cue utilization, the significant differences in problem formulation cannot be attributed to a failure of the control subjects to acquire sufficient cues to generate problem formulations. We conclude that the effect of the training was to improve the subject's skill in using the cues he obtained to generate a thorough and appropriate set of initial problem formulations.

On cue classification, the treatment group means both differed significantly from the control group mean. Thus the training was also effective in improving subjects' performance on the task of classifying cues with respect to the problem-formulation categories of major importance for the case. However, the results of the stepdown F test on cue classification indicate that intergroup differences on this variable can be attributed to the intergroup differences in problem formulation. We may conclude that although training significantly improved the subjects' performance on cue classification, this effect was a function of improvement in the thoroughness and appropriateness of the problem formulations they generated.

The second hypothesis, that outcome plus process feedback (treatment 2) would be superior to outcome feedback alone (treatment 1), was not supported with respect to any of the dependent variables. Moreover, the direction of observed differences indicated a trend in the direction opposite to that hypothesized: the means for the "outcome feedback only" condition were consistently higher than the means for the "outcome plus process feedback" condition. Except for cue utilization, the treatment 1 group means did not closely approach the maximum possible score on each variable (the problem formulation mean was 51 percent of the maximum, the cue classification mean 40 percent, and the mean for relationships among problem formulations 38 percent). Thus, the lack of significant differences between treatment groups cannot be attributed to a ceiling effect. As indicated in Table 8.4, differences between the treatment conditions were sizable on problem formulation and cue classification. It is possible that these differences would have proved significant if the covariate had been more powerful. While neither treatment was found to be more effective than the other, the results suggest a possible superiority of treatment 1 over treatment 2.

Supplemental Analyses

TREATMENT-CONTROL DIFFERENCES.   To evaluate more precisely the nature of the treatment-control differences on problem formulation, several supplemental analyses were undertaken.

The first analysis consisted in an evaluation of the structural properties of the sets of problem formulations generated by subjects under each experimental condition. The variables were the same as those employed in the analysis of the physician outcome data reported in Chapter 7, namely, four structural features that may characterize a set of problem formulations (hierarchical organization, competing formulations, multiple subspaces, functional relationships), and two measures of the size of a set of problem formulations (number of problem formulations, number of subspaces).

With respect to the structural features of a set of problem formulations, the most salient finding was that under treatment 1 virtually all subjects generated competing formulations for each posttest film (16 subjects—film 7; 15 subjects—film 8), while under the control condition 50 to 70 percent did so (11 subjects—film 7; 8 subjects—film 8). One effect of the training, at least under the "outcome feedback only" condition, apparently was to increase the number of subjects who generated competing formulations. Competing formulations, it will be recalled from Chapter 7, constituted the one feature found to be *uniformly* characteristic of experienced physician performance (across subjects and across films).

For the two measures of the size of a set of problem formulations, the method of analysis was the same as that employed in testing the experimental hypothesis (that is, multivariate analysis of covariance, followed by Scheffé post hoc comparisons). Table 8.8 reports the means on each variable by experimental condition. The statistical analysis revealed: (a) a significant multivariate main effect ($F = 5.03$, $p < .001$); (b) a significant main effect on number of subspaces (univariate $F = 6.24$, $p < .004$); (c) a significant main effect on number of problem formulations conditioned on number of subspaces (stepdown $F = 4.01$, $p < .025$); (d) a sig-

Table 8.8   Means and ranges on two measures of the size of a set of formulations, by experimental condition.

	Treatment 1	Treatment 2	Control
Film 7:			
Number of problem formulations	6.9 (4-11)	5.5 (3-7)	4.2 (1-8)
Number of subspaces	4.0 (3-6)	3.7 (3-5)	3.1 (1-5)
Film 8:			
Number of problem formulations	8.4 (5-13)	6.8 (3-10)	5.1 (3-9)
Number of subspaces	4.4 (3-5)	4.2 (3-5)	3.3 (2-5)

nificant treatment 1—control difference on both number of problem formulations and number of subspaces ($p < .001$ and $p < .05$, respectively); and (e) no significant difference between treatment 2 and the control group or between the treatment groups on either variable.

The larger number of subspaces generated by the treatment 1 subjects indicates that one effect of the outcome-feedback training was to increase the scope (or horizontal dimension) of the problem space in which the student was operating. Moreover, the significant stepdown F ratio for number of problem formulations conditioned on number of subspaces (which indicated that the intergroup difference in number of problem formulations could not be accounted for by the intergroup difference in number of subspaces) suggests that the outcome-feedback training also led to an increase of problem-space size on the vertical dimension of hierarchical elaboration within subspaces.

It is also interesting to note that the range of subspaces (per film) generated under both treatment conditions coincides very closely with Mandler's (1967) proposition that human information processors typically organize and store items in terms of (5 ± 2) categories. Under the control condition the number of subspaces generated never exceeded the upper limit of Mandler's parameter, but in the case of five subjects on each task it did fall below the lower limit.

The data on number of subspaces provide a quantitative measure of the scope of subjects' problem spaces, but do not indicate whether the (5 ± 2) subspaces typically generated were the most appropriate ones for the case. To address this question, a second type of analysis was undertaken. The subjects' problem-formulation responses were evaluated in terms of the major problem-subspace categories that were found to characterize the performance of all the experienced physicians on the two posttest films. For film 7 there were three major categories in which every physician generated at least one problem formulation; for film 8 there were five such categories. Tabulation of the student data revealed that for film 7 the number of subjects who generated at least one problem formulation in each of the three categories was fifteen under treatment 1, twelve under treatment 2, and six under the control condition. For film 8 the number of subjects generating at least one problem formulation in four (or five) of the five categories was fifteen under treatment 1, twelve under treatment 2, and seven under the control condition. Examination of the data indicated that failure to generate formulations in each of the major categories could generally be attributed to insufficient consideration of competing explanations for various subsets of symptoms, rather than to insufficient consideration of multiple concurrent or functionally related disorders.

In sum, the results of the supplemental analyses would appear to support two conclusions. The first is that the performance of the trained subjects (especially under treatment 1) was superior not only on a quantitative dimension (number of problem formulations and subspaces generated), but also on a qualitative dimension (number of subspaces of major importance in which at least one formulation was generated). The second conclusion is that skill in generating competing formulations was a major factor contributing to treatment–control differences in performance.

COMPARISON OF THE TREATMENT CONDITIONS. Although treatment group differences were found to be nonsignificant on the posttest tasks, it was noted that on every variable examined, the direction of the differences was in favor of treatment 1 (outcome feedback only). This section will present the results of several supplemental analyses regarding the treatment groups and address the question of why the process feedback proved so ineffective.

Univariate F tests on the subjects' problem-formulation scores for each of the six training films indicated a significant intergroup difference in favor of treatment 1 on the sixth film ($F = 7.11$, $p < .01$). Although there was not a well-established trend across the training tasks, it is possible that with a longer period of training the cumulative effects of the treatments would have led to a significant contrast between groups on the posttest and thus have provided clear evidence of the superiority of treatment 1 for problem formulation.

A second supplemental analysis was based on the responses to the questionnaire administered at the end of the posttest session. The subjects' responses to each item in the questionnaire were scored on a five-point scale: +2 = strongly agree; +1 = agree; 0 = no opinion; −1 = disagree; −2 = strongly disagree. Scores on three summary variables were then calculated in the following way.

Film evaluation: The subject's evaluation of the six filmed interviews was calculated from the mean of his responses to items 3 to 9, with the sign reversed for item 5.

Feedback evaluation: The subject's evaluation of the feedback materials was calculated from the mean of his responses to items 10 to 13, with the sign reversed for item 11.

General evaluation: The subject's evaluation of the overall effectiveness of the training materials and procedures was calculated from the mean of his responses to items 12, 17, and 20.[3]

The group means and standard deviations on these variables and the results of the one-way fixed-effects analysis of variance performed on each variable are reported in Tables 8.9 and 8.10.

First, it may be noted that, with one exception, both groups evaluated the films, feedback materials, and training procedure in a positive manner (as indicated by mean scores close to 1.0 on each variable in Table 8.9). The one exception was the treatment 2 mean on feedback evaluation, which was halfway between the positive and neutral points on the scale.

There were, however, some differences between the groups with respect to their opinions. As indicated in Table 8.10, the treatment 1 mean on feedback evaluation was significantly higher than the treatment 2 mean ($p < .003$). Thus, on type of feedback, the factor that differentiated the two groups, the opinion of treatment 1 group was more favorable than that of treatment 2 group.

---

[3] In the present chapter consideration of the questionnaire data will be limited to these three summary variables. For information on responses to items not included in these variables, see Allal (1973).

Table 8.9 Means and standard deviations of treatment group scores[a] on questionnaire.

Variable	Treatment	
	1	2
Film evaluation	1.16 (0.40)	0.88 (0.43)
Feedback evaluation	1.03 (0.35)	0.56 (0.45)
General evaluation	1.10 (0.36)	0.83 (0.63)

[a] Range of scale is from + 2 (highly positive) to - 2 (highly negative).

Table 8.10 Analyses of variance on questionnaire scores for film evaluation, feedback evaluation, and general evaluation.

Score	Sources of variation	df	F	p
Film evaluation	Between groups	1	3.60	.07
	Within groups	30		
	Total	31		
Feedback evaluation	Between groups	1	10.71	.01
	Within groups	30		
	Total	31		
General evaluation	Between groups	1	2.22	.15
	Within groups	30		
	Total	31		

Although the groups did not differ significantly on the other two variables (film evaluation and general evaluation), it should be noted that treatment 1 had slightly higher means and slightly lower standard deviations on these variables than treatment 2. At the level of the individual subject, then, more persons reported relatively unfavorable opinions under treatment 2.

In sum, analysis of the questionnaire data yielded results that closely paralleled those obtained from analysis of the posttest data. While differences between treatment groups were largely nonsignificant, there was some evidence to suggest that the "outcome feedback only" training elicited more favorable student opinions.

We shall now address the question of why providing the subject with process feedback, in addition to outcome feedback, clearly did not have a positive effect on the development of his problem-formulation skills and may even have had a negative effect. Although several potential explanations were considered, it is believed that the most plausible explanation is offered by two hypotheses. First, having been given the outcome feedback, the treatment 1 subjects had no difficulty in inferring what the physicians' reasoning process must have been to generate the formulations listed on the outcome-feedback sheets. They were able to provide themselves with self-generated process feedback and thereby received, in essence, the same "treatment" as the other group. This factor could explain equivalence of posttest performance by the two groups. However, a second hypothesis is needed to account for the evidence suggesting a possible superiority of outcome feedback alone. It would appear that the treatment 2 condition may have provided the subject with *too much* feedback and thereby led to a diminishing of interest in the task. Two observations support this hypothesis. First, the experimenter noted that during presentation of the process-feedback films some of the treatment 2 subjects did not appear to be overly attentive. Second, the questionnaire item on which the largest difference was found between the groups was number 11, on which the majority of the treatment 2 subjects agreed that "the feedback materials were sometimes overly redundant," while the majority of the treatment 1 subjects disagreed. In response to another item (14), the majority of treatment 2 subjects indicated that the supplemented films did convey "an understanding of the process by which experienced physicians generate initial problem formulations." However, the real issue seems to be whether the films were necessary to this effect or whether *self-generated* process feedback, as apparently occurred under the treatment 1 condition, is not more effective from both a cognitive and a motivational standpoint.

Conclusions and Implications

Conclusions

The results of the training experiment support two major conclusions:

(a) That a training model composed of the following is an effective means of improving the second-year medical student's skill in generating a set of initial problem formulations: (1) problem-solving exercises in which films are used to simulate the conditions of the early part of the clinical workup; and (2) feedback based on data from a sample of experienced physicians.

(b) That the training model is just as effective, if not more effective, for second-year students when it provides outcome feedback only, rather than outcome and process feedback.

Implications for Future Research

Given the effectiveness of the "simulation exercises plus feedback" model as a means of training medical students in the generation of initial problem formulations, one line of future research would be to consider ways of applying the model to other problem-solving skills involved in the remainder of a clinical workup: namely, the testing of initial problem formulations by further data collection; the revision of initial formulations and the generation of new formulations in light of additional data obtained as the workup progresses; and, ultimately, the making of diagnostic decisions at the close of the workup. Since an essential feature of the physician's activity after the earliest part of the workup is the *selection* of clinical procedures that will provide data to test his problem formulations, it would be necessary to use some medium other than films to simulate the conditions of the remainder of the workup. Booklets with "rub-out" answer sheets, of the type employed in the patient-management problems developed by McGuire and Solomon (1971), provide an effective yet relatively low-cost means of simulating sequential decision making regarding the selection of clinical procedures. Modification of the McGuire format to provide feedback, based on physician performance data, at various key decision points in the workup (for example, between history and physical or between physical and lab) would be one means to test the effectiveness of the training model with respect to skills other than the generation of initial problem formulations.

A second line of research would be to determine if there are not less expensive means of simulating the early part of the workup than motion pictures of the type used in this experiment. It seems probable, in retrospect, that a set of color slides of a patient, plus a tape recording of the doctor-patient dialogue would be as effective as a film and much less costly. A slide-tape combination would maintain the realism of the audio aspect of the simulated encounter with the patient, but would of course reduce the realism of the visual aspect. The question, therefore, is how much does a moving picture of the patient, as compared to a series of still images, contribute to the development of the student's skill in generating problem formulations. Certain types of visual cues—such as the patient's gait as he enters, the way he sits down, his shifts of position in the chair, the movements of his head and arms, his changes of expression—could not be adequately conveyed by slides. However, examination of both the physicians' and the students' responses reveals that no cues of this type were used to generate problem formulations. The visual cues that the physicians and students did use to generate problem formulations were either essentially static in nature (the patient's physical build or his dress) and could be easily conveyed by means of slides, or were movements and gestures whose cue properties could be fairly effectively captured in slides (for instance, the patient points to the location of his pain, clutches his abdomen, or splints his chest wall with his arm; the patient rests his head on his hand, squints his eyes, or exhibits an expression of pain). Slides would simplify the learner's task by providing still images of the visual cues of relevance to the generation of problem formulations, whereas a film requires the student to detect such cues from the ongoing flow of images of the patient. However, the results of the experiment indicate that, at least in the case of second-year medical students, the ability to detect relevant cues on the basis of naturalistic observation of the patient in motion was *already* well established; films were not needed to develop the students' skill in this domain. For first-year medical students, on the other hand, a motion picture might provide needed practice in cue detection and therefore contribute substantially to the training's effectiveness.

A third line of future research that may be proposed pertains to the feedback component of the training model. It would be of interest to determine the degree to which feedback contributes to the effectiveness of the model by comparing students' performance under two experimental conditions: simulation exercises with feedback, and simulated exercises without feedback. A second question of interest is whether there may be an interaction between the type of feedback provided (outcome versus outcome and process) and the level of medical knowledge and skill of the student. Although provision of process feedback, in addition to outcome feedback, clearly had no positive effect in the case of second-year students, it is possible that it *would* be effective with students at an earlier point in the medical school curriculum. Unlike the second-year student, the first-year student may not have acquired a sufficient level of medical knowledge and skill to be able to reconstruct for himself the processes by which the experienced physician arrives at a given set of problem-formulation outcomes. In this way, process feedback materials could be effective in enabling him to understand and assimilate the outcome feedback materials.

Instructional Applications

In conclusion, it may be suggested that even without further research and development the materials produced and tested in this study may have a number of useful applications within the current medical school curriculum.

(a) Self-instruction. Each of the simulation exercises could be easily packaged as a self-contained unit (film cassette plus instructional and response booklets), and the set of such units made available to students for use on an individual basis. The students' responses to the questionnaire indicated that if a library of such units were available, most students would use it.

(b) Group instruction. The materials could also be used in group settings, such as a Focal Problems class. In such a setting it would probably be effective to have a group discussion (in which the students compare and criticize the various outcomes at which they arrive) prior to presentation of feedback on the physician outcomes. In responding to the questionnaire, many students indicated a preference for using the materials in a group discussion setting, rather than on an individual, self-instructional basis.

(c) Evaluation. The films produced in this study could be used in designing more effective evaluation instruments for clinically oriented coursework or clerkships. Although the films provide a simulation of only the early part of the workup, they could be combined with booklets of additional clinical findings (further history plus physical and lab data) to evaluate a wide range of clinical competencies.

9 / Effects of Hypothesis Generation and Thinking Aloud[1]

Medical care has many facets, one of which is diagnosis, the "investigation or analysis of the cause or nature of a condition . . . or problem" (Webster's New Collegiate Dictionary, 1977). One approach to diagnostic problem solving (Weed, 1971) emphasizes acquiring a comprehensive data base and fosters comparative conservatism of judgment. Another approach (Morgan and Engel, 1969) advocates the use of incoming information to guide subsequent data acquisition and tends to foster more speculation in judgment. Although both approaches yield the same outcome (differential diagnosis and management plan), the route to that outcome is quite different. While one important element, the generation of diagnostic hypotheses, is shared, a major difference seems to lie in the reasoning process recommended. The problem-oriented approach, utilizing an extensive data base, encourages reasoning from accumulated facts to the generation of hypotheses and discourages speculation. The process described by Morgan and Engel, and apparently used frequently by physicians, encourages proceeding from hypothesis generation to the acquisition of data relevant to those hypotheses, as well as vice versa, and permits more speculation on the part of the problem solver.

Physicians' accounts of medical thinking abound with instances of hypothetico-deductive reasoning. Price and Vlahcevic (1971) asserted that diagnostic decisions are arrived at by eliminating erroneous hypotheses while confirming accurate ones. Similarly, Dudley (1971) sees data as being gathered and incorporated into Boolean-type nets, in such a way that the physician's search be-

---

[1] This chapter is based on the Ph.D. dissertation of Sarah A. Sprafka, "The Effect of Hypothesis Generation and Verbalization on Certain Aspects of Medical Problem Solving" (Michigan State University, 1973).

comes more and more specific and converges on a solution to the problem.

Early hypothesis generation is a central feature of the theory of medical inquiry developed in this book. The findings of Chapters 4, 5, and 7 point to the ubiquity as well as the occasional riskiness of early hypothesis generation. This research has shown that physicians uniformly tend to generate early diagnostic hypotheses and are usually able to interpret diagnostic information relevant to these hypotheses and arrive at an accurate solution. This research has also demonstrated that a diagnostic hypothesis can be a strong determinant of data acquisition and interpretation. If hypotheses are generated early and are not revised, the problem solver may be led to an erroneous solution.

These considerations formed the basis for an investigation of the effect of hypothesis generation on problem solving and the effect of instructions on hypothesis generation. The following questions were formulated:

(a) Do instructions to use early as opposed to late hypotheses have any effect on the diagnostician's approach to a diagnostic problem?

(b) Do instructions to use one or the other of these approaches have any effect on the quality of diagnosis?

(c) Independent of instructions, is there any relation between the number of hypotheses, the time of their generation, and the quality of a diagnostic workup?

The second major concern of this chapter is the use of thinking aloud or verbalization as a method in research on medical problem solving. Thinking aloud was used early in this century by Claparède (1934) and has been used extensively since that time in the information processing approach to cognition (de Groot, 1965; Newell, 1966; Newell and Simon, 1972), and in another psychological paradigm by Gagné and Smith (1962). Claparède considered it a credible procedure since it involved neither retrospection nor introspection, but he noted certain drawbacks. First, it required training, and second, some subjects did not talk during the most interesting and active moments of problem solving. Neisser (1968) criticized the procedure on the grounds that speech is perforce sequential, and the use of speech to report the problem-solving process may make it sound or even become sequential, when actually it may be operating on many levels at one time. Similarly, McGuire (personal communication, 1972) expressed concern that thinking aloud may make problem solving seem (or even be) more orderly than it is. Gagné and Smith (1962) reported that students who verbalized in their experiment were more likely to solve a problem accurately than those who did not.

Since several of our studies depend upon the problem solver's verbalizations as a fundamental source of data, it was advisable to formulate some questions about the effect of this research method on the data obtained:

(d) Do instructions to verbalize during problem solving have any effect on the diagnostician's approach to the problem?

(e) Do instructions to verbalize have any effect on the quality of diagnosis?

Research Design

Subjects

Thirty students entering their fourth year of medical school served as subjects. Fifteen were from the Michigan State University College of Human Medicine; fifteen were from the University of Michigan Medical School. Subjects were contacted individually by telephone and asked to participate. Each participant was paid twenty dollars.

The sample was chosen because the task was deemed to be at a level of difficulty appropriate for them, they were accessible, they had similar backgrounds, and they would be interested in the materials and format of presentation, since it closely resembled part III of the National Board Examination that they would be taking within a year.

Procedures

Subjects were given a modified version of three patient-management problems developed by the Interdepartmental Appraisal Committee of the University of Illinois College of Medicine (McGuire and Solomon, 1971). The experimenter administered each problem individually to each subject. After the students had read and checked the common instructions as well as instructions specific to each experimental group, each was asked to request information from the available data pool. This was provided by a cue sheet containing numbered items. As subjects requested information, they recorded the number identifying each item. The experimenter then handed over that information, printed on a file card. All subjects were requested to record a differential diagnosis at the end of each problem. The order of the three problems was the same for all subjects.

The independent variables manipulated were instructions concerning hypothesis generation and verbalization. Each subject was assigned to one of six groups:

(a) Group E-V (instructions to generate hypotheses early and verbalize).Subjects in this group were instructed to generate diagnostic hypotheses as early in the problem as possible and, if they wished, to use these hypotheses to guide data gathering. They were also stopped periodically during the problem and asked to write down any diagnostic hypotheses they had at that point, as well as describe how and when those hypotheses were generated.

(b) Group E-NV (instructions to generate hypotheses early without verbalization). Subjects in this group were instructed to generate diagnostic hypotheses as early in the problem as possible, and, if they wished, to use them to guide data gathering. At the end of each problem, the subject was asked to review the problem orally with the experimenter and indicate what hypotheses were generated and at what point in the problem generation occurred.

(c) Group L-V (instructions to generate hypotheses only after all the data were in and to verbalize). Subjects in this group were admonished to withhold judgment about diagnostic hypotheses until most or all of the data had been collected. They were stopped periodically during the problem and asked how they were coming along and what their thoughts were about the data they had gathered up to that point.

(d) Group L-NV (late generation, no verbalization). Subjects in this group were similarly admonished to reserve judgment about diagnostic hypotheses until the end of the problem. They were then asked to review the problem orally and comment on what their thoughts had been about the progress of the problem at certain points.

(e) Group C-V (control: no hypothesis generation instructions and verbalize). Subjects in this group were given no instructions concerning hypothesis generation but periodically were asked to think aloud. They were stopped occasionally and asked if they had any idea where the problem was going or any other comments on the problem up to that point.

(f) Group C-NV (control: no hypothesis generation instructions and no verbalization). As in group C-V above, subjects were given no instructions about hypothesis generation. At the end of each problem, subjects were asked to review the problem orally with the experimenter. Review questions emphasized where the subject thought that problem was going at certain points.

The instructions read to the E-V group are given in Appendix B.

The hypotheses tested concerned the effect of verbalization (thinking aloud) on problem solving and the effect of instructions and approach on solution. The following specific hypotheses were tested:

Effect of instructions on efficiency, thoroughness, and accuracy.

Subjects instructed to generate hypotheses early or given no instructions about hypothesis generation will give a more efficient, less thorough, and more accurate performance than those instructed to withhold judgment.

Subjects reminded to verbalize will reach a more accurate solution than those not so instructed, but these instructions will have no effect on the efficiency or thoroughness of performance.

Effect of instructions on earliness of hypothesis generation.

Subjects instructed to generate hypotheses early or given no instructions to generate hypotheses will generate hypotheses earlier than those instructed to withhold judgment.

Instructions to verbalize will have no effect on how early hypotheses are generated.

Effect of instructions on number of hypotheses generated.

Subjects instructed to generate hypotheses early or given no instructions about hypothesis generation will generate more hypotheses than those instructed to withhold judgment.

Instructions to verbalize will have no effect on the number of hypotheses generated.

Effect of hypothesis generation on efficiency, thoroughness, and accuracy.

Subjects who generate hypotheses early will give more efficient, less thorough, and more accurate performance than those who generate hypotheses later.

Subjects who generate comparatively many hypotheses will give a more efficient, less thorough, and more accurate performance than those who generate comparatively few hypotheses.

Earliness of hypothesis generation and number of hypotheses generated will be statistically independent.

Modifications of Patient-Management Problems

The materials for this study were taken from a series of patient-management problems (PMPs) developed over a number of years by the Interdepartmental Appraisal Committee of the University of Illinois College of Medicine. All problems deal with a patient who has some kind of ailment that requires a physician's care; none are of the insurance physical or healthy recruit variety. The problems were modifications of the PMPs discussed in Chapter 5: problem 1, PMP 2; problem 2, PMP 1; and problem 3, PMP 4. Each problem begins with a brief introduction that presents some information about a patient, including chief complaint. Having obtained the initial information, the examinee (problem solver) is to gather more information and make certain decisions in an attempt to diagnose and manage the patient's problem. Information is given in verbal form (printed answers to the examinee's questions) as well as nonverbally (chest roentgenograms, photos of lesions, reproductions of electrocardiogram tracings).

This study used PMPs more as an instrument for observation than for evaluation. Subjects were not scored relative to any criterion and judgment was not passed on the quality of a workup, only on the accuracy of diagnosis. This use justified certain changes in the format as well as in the scoring of the problem. For comparison, a summary of the usual rules for scoring PMPs, developed at the University of Illinois College of Medicine, is provided in Appendix C.

Format Modifications

The PMP ordinarily presents available information in booklet format. The booklet also includes instructions for progressing through the problem, that is, about what section of the problem the subject should attempt next. In the interest of observing the sequence a subject would naturally choose in this situation, the booklet was changed to a set of cue sheets and printed instructions were omitted.

The usual PMP format makes information available by having the subject rub out an opaque overlay or use a chemical pen to reveal the "answer." This format enables the subject to obtain more than one item of information at a time and denies the experimenter the opportunity to keep track of the order in which information is requested within each section. In this study information was presented one item at a time on printed cards. This procedure assured that the subject would receive no more information than requested, and it facilitated recording the order of presentation of items.

Scoring Modifications

The PMP proficiency (or selective thoroughness) score is a calculation of the percentage of positive points (or total weights of positive items) chosen by the subject. This formula rewards subjects as much for choosing a larger number of items with low weights as for selecting a few heavily weighted ones.

For purposes of this experiment a more straightforward non–criterion-related thoroughness score was deemed appropriate. Thus, thoroughness for this experiment was the percent of positively and zero-weighted items chosen by a subject (see formula below). This method of calculating thoroughness yields a score having the same metric as the efficiency score, which is the percentage of all positively weighted items chosen.

Errors of omission or of commission were not calculated. Furthermore, no separate efficiency and thoroughness scores for diagnosis and management were computed, nor was an overall competency score determined.

Accuracy, which is not ordinarily calculated for the PMP, was computed on a five-point scale (0 to 4). The accuracy of each subject's definitive diagnosis was determined by comparing his diagnostic formulation with a set of often-entertained diagnostic hypotheses that had been weighted for their appropriateness by the developers of the PMP.

In summary, problem scores calculated were the following:

$$\text{efficiency} = \frac{\text{number of positively weighted items selected}}{\text{total number of items chosen by subject}},$$

$$\text{thoroughness} = \frac{\text{number of positively and zero-weighted items selected}}{\text{total number of positive and zero items in problem}},$$

and diagnostic accuracy = 0, 1, 2, 3, or 4.

Validity of the Modified Problems

To make judgments about content and concurrent validity of the modified problems, performance on two of these problems by the subjects in the present study was compared to performance of physicians on the same two problems in the original PMP form, as well as to the performance of those physicians on two similar problems presented as high-fidelity simulations. The original PMPs used for comparison are described in Chapter 5. The high-fidelity simulations used as criteria for judgments about concurrent validity were two of the cases discussed in Chapter 4. These simulations were chosen because measures were available from them that could be compared to similar measures on the two types of PMP. Since the same subjects did not complete all three types of simulation (modified PMP, original PMP, and high-fidelity simulation), the comparisons are somewhat crude. Generally, it was hoped that students' thought processes as well as other aspects of their performance on the modified PMPs would closely resemble physicians' performance on the high-fidelity simulations. Regarding content validity, the intellectual processes used by students to solve the modified PMPs closely resembled those used by physicians on the high-fidelity simulations in at least three ways. First, in both types of simulations, subjects spontaneously generated diagnostic hypotheses early in the problem after having obtained very few cues. Second, problem solvers in both types of simulation used the cues they obtained to help evaluate these hypotheses. Third, there were instances where a cue was elicited specifically in the interest of testing a hypothesis.

Concurrent validity was evaluated by comparing means and standard deviations of thoroughness, efficiency, and accuracy scores on the three types of simulations. The relation of the modified PMP scores to high-fidelity simulation scores proved to be no stronger than the relation of original PMP and high-fidelity simulation scores. Any comparisons that favored the modified PMP might have been serendipitous. The data are taken from two different samples; the scores are obtained by different methods; and the content of the problems is not identical for all three types of simulations. Again, problems of case specificity make comparisons across formats difficult.

Table 9.1 Product-moment correlations r between process scores for modified patient-management problems 1 and 2, 1 and 3, and 2 and 3.

Variable	$r_{1,2}$	$r_{1,3}$	$r_{2,3}$
Thoroughness	.32	.77	.55
Efficiency	.09	.10	.32
Accuracy	.19	.09	-.15

Reliability of the Modified PMPs

In the interest of determining whether the three problems could be considered a three-item test that measured thoroughness, efficiency, and accuracy of diagnostic problem solving independent of experimental group assignments, the scores were intercorrelated. The results are shown in Table 9.1.

The variability in these correlations indicates that there is little consistency in thoroughness, efficiency, and accuracy across problems and that each problem therefore should be considered a separate test and analyzed individually.

The type of reliability estimates appropriate for these problems are those that reflect the consistency with which a test measures what it purports to measure. With this in mind, the internal consistency of each problem was calculated by one of the procedures described by Lewy and McGuire (1966). Each problem was divided into sections:

Problem 1—Credited introductory items
  Physical exam
  Laboratory
  Nonsurgical intervention
  Surgical intervention
Problem 2—Diagnosis, prognosis
Problem 3—Credited introductory items
  History
  Physical exam
  Laboratory
  Therapy.

A subproblem was then constructed from each problem by picking every third item, beginning with the first item in each section. Scores on the whole problem and the subproblem were calculated for ten randomly selected subjects. The score was the sum of weights of the items chosen in the total and the subproblem. The weights were those assigned the items by the University of Illinois criterion group. These scores served as the basis for estimation of the reliability (internal consistency) of each problem.

Internal consistency was calculated from the formula derived by Angoff (1953) and his correction for spuriousness (1956). The resulting internal consistencies were problem 1, .80; problem 2, .34; and problem 3, .87.

These coefficients indicate that problems 1 and 3 were internally consistent. Internal consistency is interpreted here as meaning that the set of items chosen for the subtest was a representative sample of the items used in the whole test. This apparently was not the case for problem 2. The items that made up the subtest were not a representative sample of the frequency distribution for subjects' choices of items on the whole test. On the whole test the ratio of number of items chosen by more than half the subjects to number chosen by less than half the subjects was approximately two to one; on the subtest this ratio was closer to four to one.

These coefficients cannot be taken to reflect the generalizability of the results on this test to other tests that deal with the same type of patient and contain a similar factor structure. To attain generalizability, a set of parallel tests containing items selected from a pool representative of the universe of items appropriate for this type of patient would have to be constructed, and a test-retest reliability would have to be calculated.

Careful consideration should be given to interpreting any reliability coefficient for one of these tests that is based on a part-whole correlation. The choice of any one item may depend in one of two ways on the choice of another item. First, some items are redundant. If one of a pair is chosen in any problem, then the other member of the pair logically cannot be chosen. When the reliability of the test is calculated, one item cannot be automatically declared the redundant one and its weight dropped from the calculations. Thus all redundant items are included in the reliability estimate. It is sometimes possible to create a subtest that is equivalent in its redundancy to the whole test, but this cannot always be assured. Secondly, irrespective of redundancy, the items are interdependent from the point of view of the problem solver. What has been learned by a certain point in the problem should determine the choice of subsequent items. Most formulas for calculating reliability, especially single-administration procedures such as the split-half coefficient or the Angoff formula used here, depend heavily on the assumption that the test items are independent of one another. That assumption is violated in these problems.

Results

Hypothesis Generation and Verbalization

The test of hypotheses was begun with establishment of the statistical independence of earliness of hypothesis generation and number of hypotheses generated. The hypothesis of independence should be rejected at the 5-percent level if $x^2 > 3.84$. A statistic of $x^2 = 1.87$ was obtained, which confirms the independence of the two variables.

The next hypotheses to be tested were those concerning the effect of instructions about hypothesis generation and verbalization upon number of hypotheses generated and upon thoroughness, efficiency, and accuracy of performance.

Table 9.2 presents the results of a multivariate analysis of variance relevant to those hypotheses. (This analysis was not done for problem 3 accuracy. All subjects arrived at a correct solution for this problem; thus it had no variance on the accuracy measure.) Instructions about hypothesis generation had no effect on the number of hypotheses generated or the thoroughness, efficiency, and accuracy of performance. On the other hand, instructions to verbalize did have an overall effect on the number of hypotheses generated, and on thoroughness, efficiency, and accuracy of performance. Inspection of the univariate F's shows that the effect is mainly on problem 3 (number of hypotheses): subjects instructed to verbalize produced more hypotheses for problem 3 than those not so instructed. There was an interaction between instructions about hypothesis generation and verbalization that affected the number of hypotheses generated for problem 3. This interaction is plotted in Figure 9.1.

The findings thus far suggest there is something different about problem 3 with respect to manipulations of variables that affect the number of hypotheses generated. To investigate further, the interactions between hypothesis generation instructions and verbalization as they affect number of hypotheses were plotted for the other two problems, and for average performance across problems. These interactions (though not significant) were similar in form to Figure 9.1, a finding that weakened speculation

Table 9.2 Effect of instructions on number of hypotheses, thoroughness, efficiency, and accuracy.

Problem:	Number of hypotheses			Thoroughness			Efficiency			Accuracy		
	1	2	3	1	2	3	1	2	3	1	2	3
Cell means												
Generate early												
Verbalization	8.6	9.0	13.6	46.0	51.6	57.6	61.0	63.0	88.4	2.5	1.0	4.0
No verbalization	10.6	6.8	6.0	40.5	49.4	48.8	63.0	65.8	83.8	3.0	1.8	4.0
Generate late												
Verbalization	11.4	6.0	8.6	35.8	45.2	45.6	66.8	68.4	84.4	3.1	2.4	4.0
No verbalization	11.6	9.4	10.8	42.0	48.0	54.8	63.0	63.0	84.8	3.0	1.8	4.0
Control												
Verbalization	11.6	9.8	12.0	42.0	53.6	52.4	63.0	68.4	89.4	2.6	2.8	4.0
No verbalization	9.6	9.0	7.8	48.2	49.2	55.8	59.0	58.0	89.6	3.4	1.0	4.0

Multivariate analysis of variance
Effect of instructions on hypothesis generation ($F = 1.04$; $df = 22, 28$; $p < .45$)
Effect of verbalization instructions ($F = 2.42$; $df = 11, 14$; $p < .06$)
Interaction ($F = 2.35$; $df = 22, 28$; $p < .01$)
Univariate analysis of variance

F ($df = 1, 24$)	0.004	0.01	4.61	0.96	0.06	0.04	0.22	0.79	0.34	0.89	0.78	
p less than—	.95	.91	.04	.34	.81	.84	.65	.38	.56	.18	.39	

Univariate analysis of variance

F ($df = 2, 24$)	1.30	2.31	3.71	1.25	0.17	0.70	0.25	0.62	0.52	0.95	1.55	
p less than—	.29	.12	.04	.30	.84	.51	.78	.55	.60	.40	.23	

Figure 9.1 Interaction of instructions and verbalization for problem 3.

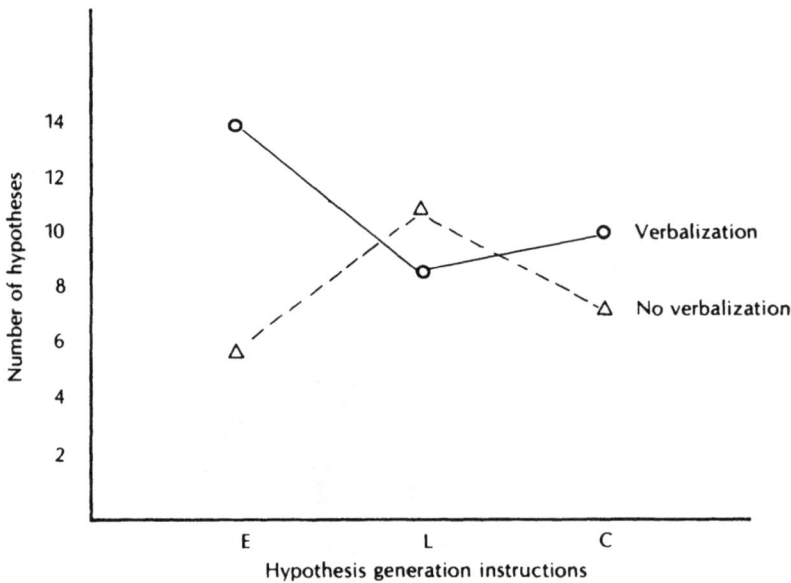

Key:

E = instructions to generate hypotheses early.
L = instructions to generate hypotheses late, after all data were collected.
C = control; no instructions concerning hypothesis generation.

about problem specificity, at least with respect to that dependent variable. The findings also suggest that the interaction of instructions and verbalization yields a reproducible pattern (that is, it was observed in two of the three problems, and in the average scores). A possible explanation for this may be in the similar structure of the problems. Both presented some ambiguity at the outset but became clearer toward the end. It is possible that subjects in the "early" and "control" groups who did not verbalize had changed their image of the problem by the end, and in retrospect may have suppressed some hypotheses generated but not expressed during the problem. Those in the "late" group may have shown an opposite trend, because the verbalizers were trying to follow instructions and thereby generated fewer hypotheses.

Attention was then turned to the topic of early hypothesis generation, defined as generation of the first hypothesis directly after reading the introduction to the problem. Table 9.3 shows that this

Table 9.3 Effect of instructions about verbalization and hypothesis generation on early hypothesis generation. Entries in cells are numbers of subjects.

Experimental condition	Problem	Early generation	Late generation
Verbalization:			
Generate hypotheses early	1	5	0
	2	5	0
	3	5	0
Generate hypotheses late	1	1	4
	2	5	0
	3	4	1
Control	1	3	2
	2	5	0
	3	4	1
No verbalization:			
Generate hypotheses early	1	3	2
	2	3	2
	3	5	0
Generate hypotheses late	1	5	0
	2	5	0
	3	5	0
Control	1	3	2
	2	5	0
	3	4	1

behavior occurred in seventy-five of ninety instances (85 percent of the time). Instructions about hypothesis generation or verbalization apparently had no effect on this behavior. It was noted that problem 1 produced the most late generation, a total of ten out of fifteen. A χ^2 test for homogeneity yielded a test statistic of 10.22, which confirmed the lack of homogeneity among the three problems on this dimension.

Although it was anticipated that there would be a tendency to generate hypotheses early, there was no idea that the outcome would be so dramatic. The medical students almost always generated hypotheses early, regardless of instructions. This finding has strong implications for medical school instruction and record-keeping systems that urge students to withhold judgment regarding diagnostic hypotheses. With respect to the clear difference in number of late hypothesis generations for problem 1, it is felt that some difficulty may have been encountered in establishing a problem space. The introduction to the problem is rather ambiguous and diffuse, with information that does not suggest a specific hypothesis or set of hypotheses on which to base further inquiry. For these reasons subjects may have felt a need to gather more data before generating the first hypothesis.

In summary, the only independent variables that produced any interesting results were instructions about hypothesis generation and verbalization. The interaction of these variables had an effect on the number of hypotheses generated for one problem. The general form of this effect was repeated for other problems.

The results that appear to have the strongest implications for medical education are incidental outcomes of this study. First, early generation of diagnostic hypotheses appears to be an inescapable fact. Despite exhortations to the contrary and regardless of the nature of the problem, subjects tend to generate the first diagnostic hypothesis based on a small number of data. Although early hypothesis generation does not seem to have any relationship to the other aspects of problem solving measured here, it would appear to be an inevitable component of the problem-solving process.

Secondly, it seems clear that the nature of a problem has a strong effect on how it is approached. The effects of manipulating different variables are not consistent across problems. The pattern of hypothesis generation varies from problem to problem. Problems vary in difficulty, too. Thus far the specific distinctive features of problems have not been identified.

Process Analysis

Following the statistical analysis of the performance variables, a process analysis was done on problems 1 and 2 to cast further light on why some subjects scored high and some scored low on accuracy of outcome. A number of new elements were found that seem to point up differences between high and low scorers. These elements deal with the acquisition and interpretation of cues relevant to the correct diagnostic hypothesis as well as the types of hypotheses generated.

ANALYSIS OF PROBLEM 1.   Table 9.4 shows the variables uti-

Table 9.4 Process analysis of problem 1.

	High scorers (n = 25)	Low scorers (n = 5)
Cue acquisition		
Thoroughness (mean %)	43.7	37.4
Efficiency (mean %)	61.1	66.4
Mean % of cues positive for correct hypothesis	41.8	40.1
Mean number of cues[a] per subject positive for correct hypothesis	24.7	20.5
Hypothesis generation		
Mean number of hypotheses	10.5	11.0
Mean number of cues[a] positive for correct hypothesis obtained:		
Before generation	16.8 (n = 10)	9.2
After generation	0.2 (n = 10)	7.6
Mean number of cues[a] positive for solution hypothesis obtained:		
Before generation		6.5 (n = 4)
After generation		12.5 (n = 4)
Early: late	7:3	4:1
Many: few	5:5	2:3
Cue utilization		
Mean % of cues misinterpreted	25	21

lized in this analysis and the mean values for high and low scorers. With respect to cue acquisition and hypothesis generation, very little difference can be observed. There is notable difference, however, in the "mean number of cues positive for correct hypothesis" for high scorers and the "mean number of cues positive for solution hypothesis" for low scorers. High scorers tended to collect more data before generating the correct solution, which was then retained. Furthermore, they gathered a relatively small number of cues positive for that hypothesis after generating it. On the other hand, low scorers tended to acquire a proportionally smaller number of cues that supported their favored hypothesis before generating it. Furthermore, they acquired a rather large number of cues relevant to that hypothesis *after* generating it. While high scorers tended to generate hypotheses early, generation of the accurate hypothesis came only after a large number of cues to support it had been gathered. Flexibility in reformulating the problem thus aids accurate outcome.

These observations suggest that all subjects, whether high or low scorers, had difficulty formulating the problem space. By gathering a large number of data, high scorers were able to develop an appropriate problem space. Low scorers apparently did not give as much consideration to the data they were gathering and may have jumped to an inaccurate conclusion too early. We also notice that after generating the hypothesis they used as a solution, the low scorers tended to pursue confirmation of that hypothesis, even though it was erroneous, by gathering substantial data to support it.

In summary, although the hypothetico-deductive approach involves early generation of hypotheses, and although most subjects used this approach, those who scored high on this problem tempered their approach by reserving judgment about the final problem solution until a substantial data base had been acquired and then reformulating the problem.

ANALYSIS OF PROBLEM 2. The variables used in the process analysis for this problem are shown in Table 9.5. The analysis again focuses on hypothesis generation and cue acquisition.

High scorers were generally more efficient in data gathering and particularly in gathering cues positive for a correct hypothesis. They did not, however, gather any more positive cues than did low scorers. High-scoring subjects presumably were better able to establish a problem space; this appears to hinge in part on their knowledge of what cues needed to be collected to solve the problem and what cues were not necessary for its solution. This knowledge helped them to focus their cue acquisition on those cues which were helpful in arriving at a correct solution.

The ability to use a focused problem-solving strategy is further borne out by a crude analysis of the types of alternative hypotheses generated by subjects in the various groups. These hypotheses are listed in Table 9.6, which also shows the frequency with which each hypothesis was entertained. Almost all subjects in all three groups entertained the hypothesis of sickle cell anemia,

Table 9.5   Process analysis of problem 2.

	High scorers (n = 10)	Low scorers (n = 16)	Low scorers who dropped correct hypothesis (n = 4)
Cue acquisition			
Thoroughness (mean %)	47.6	50.9	
Efficiency (mean %)	73.9	59.1	
Mean % of cues positive for correct hypothesis	41.9	29.0	
Mean number of cues per subject positive for correct hypothesis	6.4 (4-8)	6.1 (3-8)	
Hypothesis generation			
Mean number of hypotheses	6.7 (3-11)	9.2 (3-15)	
Mean % of workup complete when final hypothesis was generated	68.1	50.9	
Mean number of cues positive for correct hypothesis obtained:			
Before generation	4.3		0.8
After generation	2.2		5.0
Cue utilization			
Number of subjects who misinterpreted any cues	4	9	
Total number of cues misinterpreted for correct hypothesis	0		1

and a large number of these subjects entertained the hypothesis of G6PD deficiency. Both of these were strongly suggested by the introduction to the problem. Other hypotheses, considered by a smaller number of subjects, were hemolytic anemia, autoimmune anemia, leukemia, and iron deficiency anemia. These do not differentiate high scorers from low scorers. Low scorers do differ from high scorers in their generation of hypotheses such as hered-

Table 9.6 Representative hypotheses generated in the solution of problem 2, and the number of subjects who generated each.

		Low scorers	
Hypothesis	High scorers ($n = 10$)	Correct hypothesis generated ($n = 16$)	Correct hypothesis not generated ($n = 4$)
Sickle cell anemia	10	10	3
G6PD deficiency	8	6	4
Thallassemia	1	1	1
Hemolytic anemia	6	5	3
Autoimmune anemia	4	6	3
Blood loss anemia	1	4	0
Hereditary cell problem	0	5	0
Hypersplenism	0	2	3
Bone marrow repression	1	4	2
Leukemia	5	7	2
Lymphoma	1	1	1
Iron deficiency anemia	5	6	1
Vitamin B_{12} deficiency	3	4	0
Folic acid deficiency	2	3	1
Lead poisoning	1	7	3
Infection	1	1	1

itary cell problem, hypersplenism, and lead poisoning. Thus, although there was a good deal of overlap, there was also divergence. Furthermore, a greater number and a wider variety of hypotheses were considered by low than by high scorers, another indication that high scorers' thinking was more focused in this problem.

Table 9.5 shows that subjects who received high scores generated fewer hypotheses than low scorers. Furthermore, they generated their final hypothesis later and based it on more supportive cues. For this problem, as for problem 1, generation of the correct hypothesis should come rather late in the problem if one is going to obtain an accurate outcome.

Summary and Discussion of Process Analyses

The process analyses conducted on problems 1 and 2 identified aspects of diagnostic problem solving that differentiated between subjects who received high scores and those who received low scores. Some aspects are common to both problems, others are problem specific. Success on problem 1 is characterized by elements such as the ability to perceive and deal with a complex problem and to delay final decision about a solution until a comparatively large number of cues has been gathered. Elements that differentiate high scorers from low scorers on problem 2 are related to the ability to delineate a closely circumscribed problem space and to put off deciding on a solution until a large amount of information positive for that solution has been acquired.

The role played by knowledge and experience in solving these problems cannot be overlooked. Thus far it has been suggested that performance is a function of certain general, though ill-defined abilities. These apparent abilities may be the result of knowledge of a type of problem or a particular content area. Similarly, high scorers may have had more recent experience with the same sort of problem. Before firmer conclusions can be drawn, the relation of these abilities to knowledge and experience should be clarified.

Summary

Results of the Study

Fourth-year medical students completed three modified patient-management problems. Subjects were randomly assigned to six groups in a two-by-three design. On one dimension of the design, instructions concerning hypothesis generation were manipulated. Subjects were encouraged to generate diagnostic hypotheses early in the problem, to withhold judgment about diagnostic hypotheses, or were given no instructions about hypothesis generation. On the other dimension, subjects were either constrained to think aloud during problem solving or were asked to discuss the problem after they had solved it. Their performance on each problem was scored for thoroughness and efficiency of cue acquisition, as well as for accuracy of outcome and number of hypotheses generated.

Before results of the study were analyzed, efforts were made to estimate the internal consistency and concurrent validity of the modified PMPs. Two of the three problems turned out to be internally consistent and one was not. Furthermore, students' thoroughness and efficiency scores on one of the problems more closely resembled physicians' scores on the original PMP than those on a comparable high-fidelity simulation. Students' scores on the other problems showed the opposite trend; they more closely resembled physicians' scores on a comparable high-fidelity simulation than their scores on the original PMP.

After effect of instructions on number of hypotheses, thoroughness, efficiency, and accuracy had been determined, a process analysis that related certain aspects of performance to outcome was performed on two problems.

These are the major results:

Instructions to generate hypotheses early had no effect on thoroughness, efficiency, accuracy, or number of hypotheses generated.

For one problem, the constraint to verbalize prompted subjects to produce significantly ($p < .04$) more hypotheses than the absence of that constraint.

For the same problem, the interaction of instructions and constraint to verbalize had a significant effect on the number of hypotheses generated ($p < .04$).

Regardless of instructions, early hypothesis generation occurred 85 percent of the time.

One problem prompted significantly ($p < .05$) more late hypothesis generation than did the other two.

Obtaining a high score on problem 1 was associated with the ability to generate and retain the elements of a complex solution.

Obtaining a high score on problem 2 was associated with the ability to conduct a focused inquiry by gathering a small number of high-yield cues and generating a relatively small number of diagnostic hypotheses.

On both these problems, obtaining a high score was associated with postponing generation of the solution until a relatively large number of cues positive for it had been gathered.

Theoretical Considerations

Early hypothesis generation is an integral part of diagnostic problem solving. Moreover, how early in a problem hypotheses are generated is probably determined more by the problem and the way in which it is perceived by the problem solver than it is by training or exhortation from teachers. Although early hypothesis generation has no apparent relation to the ability to gather data about a case or to the ability to accurately solve a problem, it appears to be an integral part of clinical inquiry, a necessity in organization of the problem space.

One of the strongest influences on how a subject approaches a diagnostic problem is the nature of the problem itself. The amount of information presented at the outset, whether or not the situation is an emergency, and how complex the solution is, are only a few of the elements that combine to influence a subject's performance. There is great variability across the three problems used in this study. One presents a large amount of information at the outset and leaves the subject only a few options; the other two present less initial information and contain more options. One has a complex solution, the other two have simple solutions (that is, the patient has only one disease). Of the last two, one is apparently quite easy, since all subjects arrive at the correct solution; the other apparently is quite difficult, since the fewest subjects solve it. Lastly, different behaviors seem to characterize successful solvers of one problem than characterize successful solvers of another. Diagnostic problems are often differentiated based on organ system and clinical specialty area. These two factors are not sufficient to categorize problems. The other elements discussed above play an equal, if not more important, role in the characterization of clinical problems.

Although no conclusions can be drawn about the kinds of abilities that *lead to* success on patient-management problems, certain abilities were *associated with* success (arriving at an accurate solution) on two problems. In both cases, successful problem solvers did not generate the hypothesis they used as a solution until near the end of the problem, after a large number of cues had been acquired. This seems to imply that delay in arriving at a decision about a solution until a large number of cues are known, and being able to rule out other hypotheses generated early in the problem, may be helpful in reaching an accurate solution.

Methodology

Instructions can play a number of roles in a psychological experiment (Sutcliffe, 1972). Their usual role is to acquaint the subject with the task. The clearer the instructions, the more predictable the effect they will have on the outcome of the experiment. The instructions concerning hypothesis generation used in this study went beyond subject orientation to exhort the subject to approach a problem in a certain way. The results of the study indicate that the instructions about hypothesis generation had no measurable effect on any of the dependent variables. It can be concluded that an experimenter should never assume that a certain set of exhortations is going to have the desired effect on a group of subjects.

Verbalization during problem solving provides the experimenter with varied and reliable information about a subject's thought processes without apparently interfering with those processes. On the other hand, at least for certain problems, verbalization about thought processes *after the problem has been solved* may introduce retrospective distortion into the experiment.

Patient-Management Problems

Patient-management problems, particularly the more complex variety, are an attractive way of simulating the clinical setting. They involve sequential information gathering such as is practiced when working up a patient, and they give the problem solver the opportunity to use thought processes similar to those he would use in a real case. However, it has been demonstrated on a number of occasions that problem solvers perform differently on PMPs than they do on actual patients or even on higher-fidelity clinical simulations.

The two most recent estimates of the validity of PMPs are those of the present study and of Goran, Williamson, and Gonnella (1973). Our study found that physicians performed differently on the two PMPs analyzed than on two high-fidelity simulations with which they were compared. The Goran study also found that physicians and fourth-year medical students performed differently on a real patient (observed via chart audit) than they did on an analogous PMP. These differences may result partially from the lack of thoroughness of the charts audited. Studies to date of the validity of PMPs have demonstrated that the validity of these tests is difficult to ascertain and remains open to question.

The only types of reliability estimated for PMPs are the consistency of the scoring system and the internal consistency of the problems. The latter was estimated in the present study; although the problems sampled appear to be internally consistent, this measure of reliability is weak.

The reliability of a problem could be determined using a test-retest technique or by clearly establishing the universe of skills to which performance on a PMP can be generalized. The first approach is straightforward if done in the appropriate context. The two problems used must be essentially identical, since there are so many hidden variables that can cause apparently parallel problems to differ. Time lag between the administration of the two problems must be great enough so that performance on the one will minimally influence performance on the other. Further, the subjects used for the test should be at a stage in their career where a large amount of learning is no longer taking place. In this manner, the time lag between tests will not be accompanied by a noticeable change in the subject caused by new experiences and acquisition of large amounts of new knowledge. The establishment of a universe of generalizability is a more complex task and will not be pursued here.

10 / Use of Heuristics in Diagnostic Problem Solving[1]

Among the skills necessary for the practice of clinical medicine are the abilities to collect the pertinent facts about a case and to use these facts intelligently in order to arrive at an appropriate diagnosis. Medical educators have typically assumed that better diagnosis was to be achieved through the Baconian ideal of thorough and impartial gathering of facts, which are later objectively interpreted and evaluated in order to reach a single diagnosis or a few diagnostic possibilities that can best account for the assembled data. Systematic observation of competent practicing physicians, however, has led to the conclusion that the process of diagnosis is one in which hypotheses are continually advanced, tested, modified, ruled out, or presumptively confirmed. Physicians apparently collect medical case data as much for the purposes of generating hypotheses and aggregating evidence in their favor as for the sake of building a data base from which hypotheses are later generated. Cues are regularly reorganized and actively used by physicians at the earliest stages of a diagnostic interview.

Improved diagnostic problem solving may result from improvements in the ability to generate appropriate hypotheses and to test them adequately and efficiently. In this study subjects were trained to use a set of heuristics, or rules of thumb, that were intended to aid them in the application of their knowledge of medicine to the generation and testing of hypotheses.

There are obvious dangers in allowing hypotheses and conjec-

---

[1] This chapter is based on the Ph.D. dissertation of Michael J. Gordon, "Heuristic Training for Diagnostic Problem Solving among Advanced Medical Students," (Michigan State University, 1973). Thanks are extended to Dr. Robert Bridgham, also of Michigan State University, for his extensive analysis and assistance in interpretation of the data.

tures to influence data collection and interpretation at an early stage. These dangers include possibilities of premature closure, selective information gathering, and biased interpretation of information. Conversely, there is reason to believe that hypotheses may serve an indispensable function, even in the earliest stages of diagnostic interview. The formation of hypotheses appears to direct an economical search for information. Hypotheses also appear to function as an organizational structure for storage and recall of information in the physician's memory.

This study proceeds from the position that the dangers of hypothesis-guided diagnostic inquiry should not be countered by struggles to eliminate early hypotheses and their "biasing" effects, but instead by training in diagnostic heuristics that might help physicians to generate more adequate hypotheses and to test these hypotheses more effectively. A set of five experimental heuristics was derived from analysis of the reported and observed errors of diagnostic reasoning committed by medical students:

Planning heuristic. Each piece of information requested by the problem solver should be related to a plan of attack for solving the problem. There should be a plan and a well-defined purpose behind every question or set of questions asked.

Hypothesis-specificity heuristic. No diagnostic hypothesis should be more specific or more general than the evidence on hand justifies.

Competing-hypotheses heuristic. There should always be at least two or three competing hypotheses under consideration at a particular time. Each piece of information should be evaluated with respect to all hypotheses presently under consideration.

Reinterpretation heuristic. Whenever a new or revised hypothesis emerges, the information previously collected should be reviewed. The problem solver should attempt to categorize the previously elicited findings as either tending to confirm or tending to disconfirm his new hypothesis.

Negative-inference heuristic. When high-cost (expensive, uncomfortable, or risky) procedures are being considered to confirm a favored hypothesis, the problem solver should consider the possibility of lower-cost procedures that might instead rule out one or more diagnostic possibilities in order to make the high-cost procedure unnecessary or to increase the probability that the high-cost procedure will yield the definitive diagnosis.

Recent interest in heuristics stems principally from George Polya's popular book, *How to Solve It* (1957). Polya claimed that, at least in mathematics, knowledge of the process of problem solving is more important than knowledge of the content. This question of content versus process has been hotly debated in American medical schools, but it is safe to say that some knowledge of both is indispensable for medical practice.

Polya approaches the teaching of problem solving by asking students questions of a particular kind. The questions are not intended to be hints in the solution of a particular problem, nor do they fit the model of a Socratic dialogue. Instead, these heuristic questions have two required characteristics, common sense and generality: "As they proceed from plain common sense, they very often come naturally; they could have occurred to the student himself. As they are general, they help unobtrusively; they just indicate general direction and leave plenty for the student to do" (p. 4). Polya's expectation is that by repeatedly asking general, common-sense questions of a student, the student will become aware of fruitful problem-solving approaches and will begin to ask these questions of himself independently.

Research Design

In order to obtain evidence of the effects of heuristics on medical problem solving, thirty-two medical students were presented with a series of simulated medical cases. They were asked to diagnose each case by requesting any information they believed pertinent. Half of the subjects were trained to employ the experimental heuristics described above, and half were asked to generate and employ a set of personal or idiosyncratic heuristics that they had found to be helpful in past diagnostic problem solving. Within this division, half of the subjects were systematically prompted to use the heuristics and half were invited to use the heuristics at their own discretion. All subjects in the resulting four groups were asked to solve the diagnostic problems as efficiently and accurately as possible. Thus the design provided an opportunity to evaluate evidence with respect to four major questions:

(a) What are the relative effects of experimental versus idiosyncratic heuristics when used by advanced medical students?

(b) Do medical students who are prompted to use either the experimental or the idiosyncratic heuristics regularly and systematically perform differently from students who use either of these heuristics in a more casual and discretionary way?

(c) Are there any interactions between types of heuristics used and prompted use of the heuristics?

(d) Do medical students attending schools with different curricula perform differently?

The effects of heuristic usage were operationally defined in terms of four dependent measures:

(a) *Scope* of the early diagnostic formulations, reflecting the degree of generality or specificity of early hypotheses.

(b) Number of *critical* or highly diagnostic case *findings* elicited.

(c) *Cost* of the diagnostic workup defined as an additive function of financial expense, patient discomfort, and risk to patient health inherent in the diagnostic procedures ordered.

(d) *Accuracy* of the diagnosis.

The scope and critical findings measures were considered to be process measures, which might be related to diagnostic outcomes. The measures of cost and accuracy were considered to be diagnostic outcomes of paramount importance.

Subjects

Thirty-two medical students from two medical schools were divided into four treatment groups that encompassed all combinations of type of heuristics utilized (experimental versus idiosyncratic) and type of utilization (systematically prompted versus discretionary). While the kind of training and the instruction to students differed among the four treatment groups, the content of the task remained constant. Each student was individually presented with a short scenario that described a patient in the outpatient department of a community hospital. The task was to request any additional information that appeared to be pertinent in order to reach a diagnosis of the case. The experimenter supplied answers to each inquiry. All participants were presented with the cases in the same order, and the problem-solving sessions were recorded for later scoring.

Construction and Analysis of Dependent Measures

Four measures of performance were obtained from each subject on each diagnostic case presented. The first measure (scope) was intended to capture the range or scope of the subject's diagnostic formulations based on the data elicited in the early phases of a diagnostic workup. The scope of the early hypotheses is a concern of the hypothesis-guided approach because it sets limits on the kinds of information judged to be most useful in the subsequent search for data. Therefore, it is of interest to determine how the scope of early diagnostic formulations might vary among medical students trained in various modes of heuristic problem solving and how these variations might influence diagnostic outcomes.

The second measure (critical findings) was intended to determine whether different conditions of training and usage of heuristics would influence the number of important diagnostic findings elicited by a diagnostic problem solver. The hypothesis-guided method emphasizes efficiency rather than thoroughness, but it was not clear whether greater efficiency of information search would reduce the number of critical findings elicited, or whether a reduction in critical findings elicited would significantly influence the outcome of the problem-solving effort.

The third variable (cost) was considered to be an additive function of (a) the estimated financial expense of the diagnostic procedures, (b) the discomfort and inconvenience to the patient, and (c) the severity and probability of the risk to patient health inherent in the diagnostic procedures. With a variant of a method used by Rubel (1970), dollar equivalents for specific degrees of discomfort and risk were generated. Each diagnostic procedure could then be assigned a cost equivalent based on independently derived values for financial expense, discomfort, and risk.

Assessment of the fourth variable (accuracy) was made by asking subjects to complete a semistructured, short-answer diagnostic summary form at the completion of each case. Accuracy scores were computed with consideration taken of the number of diagnostic findings accurately identified, the relationships of the various diagnostic findings, and the specificity with which these findings were reported. Diagnostic accuracy was assessed as a scaled, rather than as a dichotomous (correct versus incorrect), variable.

Reliability of Dependent Variables

The reliability of the dependent measures was investigated in several ways. First, studies of agreement among experts were required in order to develop scoring keys on the critical findings and cost variables. Second, studies of the stability of subject scores over transformations in scoring rules were appropriate for the variables of cost and accuracy. Third, studies of interrater reliability on the scoring of subjects' performance were required for the scope and accuracy measures. Fourth, studies of consistency of subjects' performance across problems were appropriate for all four variables. The results of the reliability studies for each measure in turn are summarized in the following paragraphs.

The scoring format for scope was developed rationally and required no empirical judgments for the development of scoring keys. Substantial judgment by raters was required to score a subject's performance, and interrater reliability was high ($r = .90$). Internal consistency of subjects' performance across cases on the scope measure was $r = .68$ (Hoyt).

The critical findings variable required a key developed by a panel of three physicians. These physicians achieved reliabilities above $r = .90$ in their judgments of degree of importance, and an average of approximately 90-percent agreement on the designation of critical findings in the posttest cases. Once the key was developed for the critical findings variable, scoring was completely objective and no investigation of interrater reliability was necessary. Internal consistency of subjects' performance across cases for the critical findings measure was $r = .56$ (Hoyt).

The development of the cost measure required consistency of expert judgment for patient discomfort ($r = .88$) and risk ($r = .56$). Based on various relative weights applied to the components of expense, discomfort, and risk, differences in the aggregate cost scores were found to be negligible. Objective scoring procedures on this variable eliminated the need for interrater reliability studies. The internal consistency of subjects' performance across cases on the cost measure was $r = .47$ (Hoyt).

The accuracy measure did not require empirical keying, but the relative weights applied to subscores were arbitrary. Stability of the accuracy scores over transformations of subscore weights was extremely high ($r = .98$). The mean interrater reliability in the scoring of subjects' performance was also quite high ($r = .91$). Consistency of subjects' performance across cases on the accuracy measure was disappointing ($r = .25$, Hoyt).

Experimental Design

The hypotheses of this study were initially tested by means of four two-way analyses of covariance. The pretest score on each of the four dependent measures was used as the covariate in the analysis of posttest group differences.

Multivariate analyses of variance and covariance were subsequently performed to investigate differences among training groups that might be discernible when all four dependent measures were considered simultaneously. Exploratory product-moment correlation analyses were also performed on an expanded set of variables comprised of subcomponents of the dependent measures.

Results

Factorial Analysis of Dependent Measures

Univariate covariance analysis revealed no differences between the two schools on any measure. There were no significant differences among treatment groups in terms of the scope of early hypotheses, number of critical findings elicited, or cost of the diagnostic workups. Means and standard deviations for all four variables are reported in Table 10.1. Differences in accuracy of diagnosis among the treatment groups approached statistical significance ($p < .07$). The analysis of covariance for the accuracy measure is presented in Table 10.2.

Relation Between Diagnostic Cost and Accuracy

Figure 10.1 depicts the adjusted mean scores for each of the four heuristic treatment groups on the diagnostic cost and accuracy measures. While it suggests an inverse relationship between diagnostic cost and accuracy, this is misleading. Not only do the measures fail to reach statistical significance, but also inferences made would refer only to groups and not to individual subjects.

Correlations between diagnostic cost and accuracy on the pretest and posttest problems, with subjects as the units of analysis, were .13, .17, and −.05 respectively. These results support the conclusion that there is no significant linear relation between these two measures of diagnostic effectiveness.

Table 10.3 reveals an inconsistent pattern for most of the performance measures across cases. Measures 2 through 6, however, are significantly correlated across cases; all deal with what might be called the extensiveness of the search for data. Subjects exhibited characteristic styles of data collection in the history and physical-examination portions of their workups. Some preferred to be systematic and thorough; others preferred to obtain only a brief history and perform a selective physical examination. This difference in style is important to the questions of this study because it reflects the extent to which medical students are operating in either a stepwise approach or a hypothesis-guided

Table 10.1 Group means and standard deviations on four measures.

Measure	Group[a] (n = 8)	Mean	Adjusted mean	Standard deviation
Scope	1	68.25	68.54	27.05
	2	52.50	52.99	25.18
	3	60.00	59.74	30.37
	4	47.50	46.98	19.10
Critical findings	1	10.75	11.15	2.50
	2	10.25	11.02	1.30
	3	11.87	11.13	3.10
	4	10.75	10.32	3.37
Cost	1	185.87	205.35	75.94
	2	260.37	251.24	122.61
	3	370.75	371.13	342.19
	4	330.75	320.03	165.13
Accuracy	1	45.87	45.83	2.89
	2	41.00	41.03	8.28
	3	36.75	36.82	6.29
	4	40.00	39.94	6.58

[a] Group 1: Trained to employ experimental heuristics and prompted to use them.
Group 2: Trained to employ experimental heuristics and invited to use them at their own discretion.
Group 3: Asked to generate personal heuristics and prompted to use them.
Group 4: Asked to generate personal heuristics and invited to use them at their own discretion.

Table 10.2 Two-way analysis of covariance on accuracy of the definitive diagnosis.

Source of variation	df	MS	F	p
T (treatments)	3	144.78	2.69	.07
S (schools)	1	15.73	0.37	.55
T x S interaction	3	21.28	0.50	.69
Error	23	53.82		
Total	30			

Figure 10.1 Adjusted mean scores of treatment groups on cost and accuracy measures.

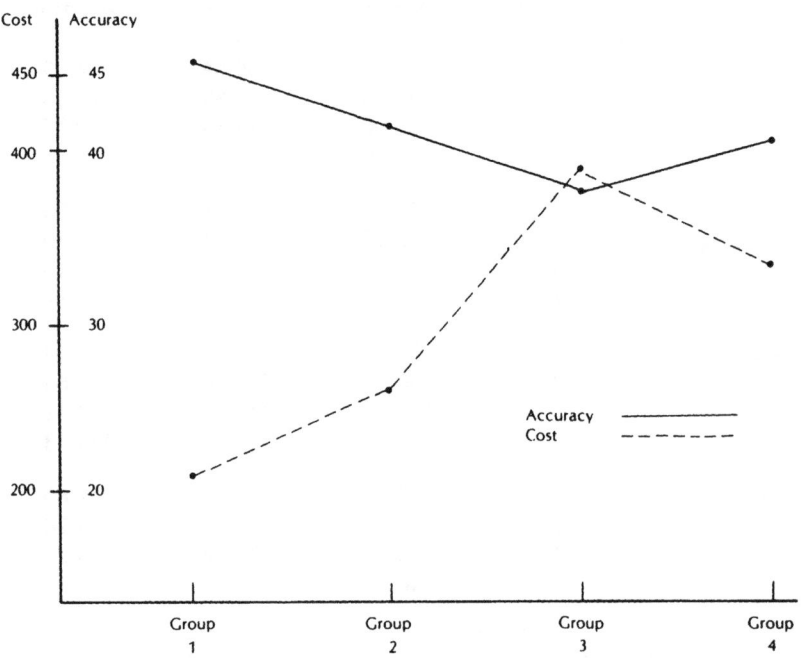

approach. The best indicator of this approach differential is probably a composite of the measures financial expense of history (a direct function of the number of historical inquiries made by the subject) and financial expense of the physical examination (a direct function of the estimated time to perform each segment of the physical exam). This composite will be labeled a "thoroughness" measure and will be included in subsequent discussions.

Results of Multivariate Analyses

The univariate analyses appeared to tell only a portion of the story. While the experiential heuristics produced no clear-cut differences on any of the four dependent variables, employment of the heuristics might have produced an orientation whose total effect would be observable when the entire ensemble of four de-

Table 10.3 Correlations on performance measures across cases. Case 1 was the pretest case, 3 and 4 comprised the posttest.

	Correlates ($n = 32$)		
Performance measure	$r_{3,4}$	$r_{1,3}$	$r_{1,4}$
1. Scope of early formulations	.45[a]	.06	.05
2. Critical findings elicited	.42[a]	.23	.39[c]
3. Moderately important findings elicited	.57[b]	.45[a]	.58[b]
4. Noncontributory findings elicited	.83[b]	.50[a]	.60[b]
5. Financial expense of history	.76[b]	.45[a]	.60[b]
6. Financial expense of physical exam	.61[b]	.32[c]	.34[c]
7. Financial expense of lab tests	.37[a]	-.03	.17
8. Discomfort of physical exam	.23	-.16	-.21
9. Discomfort of lab tests	.25	.03	.22
10. Risk of physical exam	1.00[b]	-.16	1.00[b]
11. Risk of lab tests	.15	.16	.21
12. Cost of workup	.35[c]	.02	.25
13. Accuracy of diagnosis	-.06	.03	-.19

[a] $p < .01$.
[b] $p < .001$.
[c] $p < .05$.

pendent variables was considered simultaneously. The data were therefore further studied by multivariate analysis of variance and covariance procedures. Multivariate analyses were used to investigate all three main effects (medical school, heuristics, and prompting) and their interactions. Multiple analyses of the same data must always be suspect, since each investigation adds to the probability of uncovering chance differences of spurious statistical significance. The present study is exploratory rather than definitive, however, and in this context the variables were manipulated further and new relationships were examined.

Multivariate Analyses of Variance

Analyses for the factor of medical school revealed no significant differences. In fact, F values for the main effect of schools and all interactions involving schools were less than 1.0. In subsequent analyses the design was collapsed across the variable of schools to create greater within-cell stability.

Multivariate analyses of variance were subsequently run to test for experimental effects of heuristics, prompting, and heuristics by prompting interaction. The only contrast that achieved or approached statistical significance was the main effect of heuristics ($F_{4,21} = 4.20$, $p < .012$). That is, considering all four dependent measures simultaneously, the vector of scores for subjects provided with the experimental heuristics differed significantly from the vector of scores achieved by subjects using their personal heuristics. The vector of scores achieved by those using the experimental heuristics, in comparison to subjects using their personal heuristics, was characterized by a pattern of more inclusive early hypotheses, slightly fewer critical findings elicited, lesser cost, and greater accuracy (see Table 10.1).

Multivariate Analyses of Variance with Transformations

An additional set of analyses was run to reduce the distributional problem of the cost and accuracy variables. A log transformation (transformed cost = $\log_{10}$ cost) was performed on the highly skewed cost data, which made the within-cell deviations approximately normal. A correction for strong ceiling effects suggested by Cox (1958, p. 16) was applied to the accuracy scores. The two normalizing transformations had no discernible effect upon univariate analyses of the individual variables, but did increase correlations between the dependent measures. Multivariate analysis of variance on the transformed variables produced slightly larger F ratios than the same analysis performed without the transformations. The contrasts achieving or approaching significance in the analysis of the transformed data were for the main effect of heuristics ($F_{4,21} = 4.63$, $p < .008$) and for the interaction of heuristics and prompting ($F_{4,21} = 2.29$, $p < .09$). This suggested the possibility that prompting had differential effects, depending upon which set of heuristics was being prompted.

Multivariate Analyses of Covariance with Transformations

In the univariate tests initially performed, pretest measures of the four dependent variables were not found to be effective covariates, since correlations between the covariates and dependent measures were low. The multivariate analyses on the transformed dependent measures were repeated, however, with the four pretest measures as covariates. Again, because of low correspondence between pretest and posttest performance, the effect of the covariates on the analyses was an overall reduction in F ratios. In this analysis the only contrast approaching statistical significance was for the main effect of heuristics ($F_{4,21} = 2.83$, $p = .0509$).

Discussion

Approximately 130 hours were spent by the experimenter in individual problem-solving sessions with the thirty-two subjects. This does not include time spent with medical students and physicians in the pilot-study phase of the project. Observations and anecdotes recorded during these encounters may aid in interpretation of the results. Collection of notes was fortuitous rather than systematic, however, so these interpretations should be viewed as speculative and tentative explanations of the results obtained.

The single most striking impression to emerge on completion of the data-collection phase of the study was the extreme variability in virtually every dimension of problem-solving behavior investigated. The theme of variability was manifested in great heterogeneity among subjects on all variables, large variability in performance by the same subject on different problems, and a noticeable lack of standardization in the approach to the same case by different subjects. The great variability in both processes and outcomes makes the use of terms such as *trends* and *tendencies* dangerous. Generalizations beyond narrow limits of experience are not warranted.

Discussion of Scope Results

Subjects trained in the experimental heuristics (groups 1 and 2) had been trained to employ the hypothesis-specificity heuristic among others. This heuristic was, in fact, a direct instruction to review each hypothesis generated and to alter the hypotheses to make them correspond more closely to the currently available data base. The difference between treatment-group means on the scope of hypotheses measure, therefore, can be said to be a direct reflection of the extent to which subjects understood and applied this particular heuristic in the posttest cases. In the training phase all subjects were quickly able to grasp the concept and rationale for keeping the scope of their diagnostic formulations consistent with the available supporting data. Subjects were able to generate examples of inappropriately narrow or broad hypotheses from their own experience. Despite uniform conceptual understanding, subjects varied greatly in their ability to apply this heuristic in the problem-solving posttest. This failure is seen as the primary reason for lack of significant differences among treatment groups on the scope score.

The different kinds of response to the hypothesis-specificity heuristic illustrate problems that may occur generally in the application of heuristic suggestions to problem solving. First, some subjects were either unwilling or unable to alter the statement of their hypotheses after review of the hypothesis-specificity heuristic. Under conditions where an unjustifiably specific hypothesis had been generated, these subjects indicated no recognition of the discrepancy between the specificity of the hypothesis and the deficiency of the supporting data base. Some appeared to be too involved to achieve a perspective on the problem. As one student remarked afterward, he "couldn't see the forest for the trees." It would seem that recognition of situations in which particular heuristics are applicable requires extensive training, even when the concept and rationale of the heuristic are well understood by the subject.

Other subjects who did not alter their hypotheses simply appeared reluctant to expend cognitive energy on refinements of hypotheses while they felt they were making good progress toward the solution. Voice intonations, impatient glances, and other nonverbal cues conveyed the message that alteration of hypotheses was considered to be an unwelcome distraction from some subjects' problem-solving train of thought. If such observations can be supported, it would seem that training for the use of heuristic suggestions must be made powerful enough to permit incorporation of the heuristic suggestions into the original formulation of plans, conceptions, and decisions, rather than in time-consuming or disruptive reformulation of these processes.

Another group of subjects did alter the verbal description of their hypotheses upon reviewing the heuristic prompts. It was discovered, however, that verbal reformulation of hypothesis statements does not always correspond to cognitive reformulation of the appropriate psychological problem space. For example, one subject initially interpreted the cough and shortness-of-breath symptoms of the case 4 patient as "pneumonia." On recognizing the overly specific character of this early formulation, she changed her hypothesis to "infectious process." However, instead of altering her data-collection plan to investigate the possibility of any infectious process (which would have been ruled out on the basis of several low-cost inquiries), she continued to request information specifically related to the hypothesis of pneumonia.

Finally, there was evidence that some subjects altered both the verbalization of the hypothesis and their conception of the problem through application of the hypothesis-specificity heuristic.

For example, in case 3 the symptom of left chest pain initiated a search by one subject for myocardial infarction or angina. On reviewing the hypotheses for undue specificity, the subject switched his questioning to general cardiovascular functioning, found no significant positive findings, and quickly turned his attention to more probable causes of the pain.

Because of the initial variability among subjects on the scope variable and the observation that only about 50 percent of subjects even minimally applied the hypothesis-specificity heuristic to their early formulations, significant treatment-group differences on the scope variable could not be demonstrated. For specific subjects, however, attention to the scope of hypotheses did appear to take place and to guide subsequent inquiry. It may be speculated that extensive practice in formulation and evaluation of hypotheses is necessary before the process can be integrated into diagnostic problem solving without interfering with the main line of diagnostic reasoning.

Discussion of Critical Findings Results

None of the five experimental heuristics was especially directed toward increasing or decreasing the number of critical findings elicited. Instead, each of the experimental heuristics was intended to bring about the more effective use of information as opposed to more thorough accumulation of information. It was not known whether increased effectiveness in the use of information would affect the number of critical findings elicited. Although the difference between group means was not statistically significant, the trends suggested the possibility that the effect of the heuristics may have been to reduce in number the critical findings elicited with no reduction in diagnostic accuracy. The correlations between accuracy of diagnosis and number of critical findings elicited, however, indicated a positive relationship between these two variables, which appears to be partially a function of the kind of data included among the critical findings. Critical findings, by definition, have high diagnosticity for the actual pathology of the patient. Prominent among them were the highly specialized tests used primarily as confirmations of presumptive diagnoses. Subjects who had already confirmed a correct diagnosis were able to inflate their critical findings score by reconfirming the diagnosis with additional exotic but unnecessary tests. Thus, greater accuracy might have resulted in eliciting more critical findings, rather than the reverse.

Correlational analysis indicated that the number of critical find-

Table 10.4 Proportion of critical findings to critical plus noncontributory findings, by treatment group.

Treatment group[a] (n = 8)	Proportion	Standard deviation of proportion
1	0.340	0.018
2	0.281	0.013
3	0.210	0.062
4	0.248	0.055

[a] Group 1: Trained to employ experimental heuristics and prompted to use them.

Group 2: Trained to employ experimental heuristics and invited to use them at their own discretion.

Group 3: Asked to generate personal heuristics and prompted to use them.

Group 4: Asked to generate personal heuristics and invited to use them at their own discretion.

ings appeared for most subjects to be a function of the thoroughness of their questions. The more thorough the collection of information, the more likely the subject was to elicit critical findings as well as moderately important and noncontributory findings. In order for the heuristics to produce greater efficiency, the "dross" rate should be reduced for those subjects exposed to the heuristics; that is, the ratio of critical findings to noncontributory findings would be greater for subjects trained and prompted to use the experimental heuristics (group 1) than for subjects trained and prompted to use their idiosyncratic heuristics (group 3). In fact, the ratio of critical findings to noncontributory findings for the four treatment groups suggests such a possibility. The proportion of critical findings to critical plus noncontributory findings is presented in Table 10.4 for each of the four treatment groups.

An analysis of variance failed to demonstrate statistically significant differences between treatment groups ($F_{3,23} = 1.49$, $p < .25$).

Discussion of Cost Results

As with differences on other variables, group means on the cost variable favored the use of the experimental heuristics. In terms of equivalent dollar values, the cost differential among the groups was quite large. The mean diagnostic cost of group 1 subjects, prompted to use the experimental heuristics, was approximately half of the mean diagnostic cost incurred by group 3 subjects, prompted to use their idiosyncratic heuristics. These large group differences were not statistically significant because of the extreme variability among subjects within groups. The standard deviation of the cost measure ($215) was much greater than anticipated, and positive skew was substantial.

Observation of subjects revealed at least three different reasons behind high costs. One might be called compulsiveness or inability to separate the important information from the unimportant. Subjects in this category typically elicited a complete history and physical examination, and noted any datum that might remotely resemble a clue. By and large, each of these marginal and perhaps unreliable findings was thoroughly followed up with additional costly procedures. For example, the patient in case 4, when asked about her history of previous surgery, reported that she had had a varicose vein stripped in her right leg at age fifteen. On further probing she explained that the surgery was done for cosmetic reasons and because she was told that it might give her problems later. This finding, in the light of other historical and physical evidence, appeared to most students to be what was commonly referred to as a "red herring." Yet some subjects, despite their frequent admission that the finding was probably noncontributory, felt compelled to follow up with expensive and risky procedures, including arteriography, in order to rule out the remote possibility of thromboembolic disease. On finding negative results of their costly procedures, subjects usually responded, "I thought so." This kind of student was fully aware of the high cost and low probability of payoff of his exotic procedures, but appeared to disregard these factors in his decision making. In postproblem interviews with these subjects, the explanation usually given was that good medicine demands that all possibilities be checked, even at some slight risk to the patient. Financial expenses were generally dismissed with references to third-party payment plans.

A second type of student incurred excessive costs because of what appeared to be either inefficient problem-solving skills or inadequate medical knowledge. In short, this kind of student may have had sufficient information on hand to make the diagnosis but failed to recognize the diagnostic significance of his data. Such students simply needed to collect additional information before eliciting evidence that they could correctly interpret in order to secure the diagnosis. Interviews with this kind of student revealed either that they simply did not know the diagnostic significance of an important finding or that they failed to put together the clues which in retrospect seemed obvious to them.

A third kind of performance was in some respects a combination of the previously mentioned two. In such cases the subjects both failed to interpret data correctly and disregarded diagnostic costs. This type of performance typically emerged when students became lost in the problem and exhausted reasonable hypotheses. Rather than admit to deficiencies of clinical skills, some students tacitly implied that they had deficiencies of data. Subsequent investigations often took the form of an unsystematic search for unlikely diagnoses through exotic procedures. Such students fortunately were represented by only three subjects in the present study, but their performance is worth mentioning because of the striking similarity among them, and because behavior patterns of this type would seem to warrant detection and remediation in the interest of future patient care. The three subjects all reached a point in the solution of at least one problem in which each of their seriously entertained hypotheses had been ruled out, either correctly or incorrectly. Other subjects, when they found themselves in a similar position, reviewed their data base, made a few more low-cost inquiries, and as the initial instructions suggested, they "referred" the case to a specialist. The three subjects in question were highly reluctant to refer. One of them subjected the patient in case 4, a young woman in extreme distress, to all of the following expensive, risky, or uncomfortable procedures: intravenous pyelogram, renal arteriogram, upper gastrointestinal series, cholecystogram, lung scan, bone marrow aspiration, retrograde pyelogram, lumbar puncture, renal biopsy, muscle biopsy, nasogastric tubing for analysis of stomach blood, and a barium enema!

The procedures, listed above in the order requested by the subject, attest to the undisciplined hunt for pathognomonic clues of unsupported hypotheses. While the performance cited above was the most bizarre example encountered, the other two subjects who resorted to this type of inquiry were notably similar in their attitude and approach to the patient. Remarks by the subjects indicated that they were unwilling to admit that the problem was beyond their competency ("I think I've got it now." "Now it's falling into place." "I think I should check out a few more things before referring.") and showed a callous disregard of the patient's condition ("This may kill her, but I'd like to have a renal biopsy.").

In summarizing the experimental performance on the cost variable, two particular points deserve mention. First, the variability in performance on the cost variable was so extreme that on this basis alone the factors of expense, discomfort, and risk in diagnostic settings may deserve the attention of those charged with clinical education. Second, the evaluation of diagnostic costs appears on a subjective level to be a promising indicator of diagnostic performance and of various kinds of problem-solving, medical content, and attitudinal deficiencies.

There was no clear explanation of why some subjects inflicted such a costly array of procedures on the simulated patients, but the approximately log-normal shape of the cost score distribution suggests one possibility. It may be that individuals tend to judge the costs of *contemplated* diagnostic expenditure by comparing them to costs already incurred. That is, a contemplated $100 test may seem to be a smaller matter if one has already accumulated expenses of $1,000 than if one has accumulated only $50 in previous expenses. If this kind of reasoning error is characteristic of human judgments in diagnostic decision making, the implications are great. By this reasoning, any clinician might occasionally find himself ordering "just one more test" because the patient had already endured so much.

Discussion of Accuracy Results

Cases were selected to be within the competence of most fourth-year medical students. Subjects were instructed to gather data about each case until they were satisfied with their identification of each patient's problem. Because of the open-ended nature of the task, most students eventually were able to reach a high level of diagnostic accuracy; the result was a substantial ceiling effect on the accuracy measure.

The pattern of means among the treatment groups on this measure suggests that subjects trained to use the experimental heuristics were more accurate in their diagnoses than subjects trained to use their idiosyncratic heuristics. The statistical significance level of $p < .07$ for differences among treatment-group means is encouraging, since ceiling effects tend to moderate differences between groups. On the other hand, it should be recalled that because each of the four dependent variables was analyzed independently, the probability of reaching statistical significance on the test of at least one variable was increased by four.

If we bear in mind that the null hypothesis was not rejected for the accuracy measure, it is possible to speculate on the pattern of group means obtained. The mean scores for groups 2 and 4, the unprompted groups, were very close to each other. It appears that although the list of experimental heuristics was available to the group 2 subjects, it was seldom used during the posttest problem-solving. Thus, for group 2 subjects, the effect of the heuristic training was probably residual—perhaps interpreted as a stronger admonition than that given in the initial instructions to all subjects to think carefully and avoid unnecessary procedures. Under these conditions it is not surprising that group 2 subjects performed more or less equally to the untrained, unprompted subjects in group 4.

Group 2 and group 4 subjects may be considered as a control group in the comparison of subjects trained and prompted to maximize use of either the experimental or the idiosyncratic heuristics. Viewed in this way, the experimental heuristics might facilitate diagnostic accuracy, while systematic use of the idiosyncratic heuristics might be detrimental in comparison to the unprompted controls. Why should this be so?

If the mean accuracy scores reflect treatment effects, the particular pattern of means is consistent with the hypothesis that the content of heuristic suggestions is crucial, and that systematic prompting to use heuristics will produce different results depending on the quality of the heuristics prompted.

One might ask which of the personal heuristics might have been detrimental to accuracy. This question is difficult to answer, since thirty-two different heuristics were generated and used by the eight group 3 subjects. It is interesting, however, that six of these subjects mentioned a heuristic that stressed thorough collection of data. Further, when asked periodically to select a heuristic that fit the present situation, subjects called upon this heuristic a disproportionate part of the time—almost to the exclusion of other heuristics. Compulsive thoroughness was virtually the only heuristic used by these six subjects. Those who employed the thoroughness heuristic repeatedly had a mean accuracy score 6.3 points lower than those not employing this heuristic and a mean thoroughness score 5.6 points greater than the mean of the remaining members of group 3. Standard deviations for the accuracy and thoroughness variables were 6.7 and 14.4, respectively.

Discussion of Multivariate Results

Multivariate results are difficult to interpret at best, and the meaning of a significant result is less clear when variables are transformed and adjusted for covariation. Nevertheless, the results of the three sets of multivariate analyses presented here are encouraging evidence that teaching of powerful heuristics may alter diagnostic problem-solving performance.

The findings of the multivariate tests suggest that while the experimental heuristics were unable to demonstrate clear influences on any of the four dependent measures considered separately, they may have altered the approach to the problem in such a way that their effects were discernible when all four variables were considered simultaneously.

The experimental heuristics embody an approach that deemphasizes thoroughness of data acquisition. They urge more careful selection of high-yield information and more intensive evaluation of the information elicited. The pattern of results among subjects exposed to the experimental heuristics (increased breadth of early hypotheses, slightly fewer critical findings, decreased cost, and increased accuracy) was consistent with expectations under the assumption that the experimental heuristics were effective.

The Relative Importance of Medical Knowledge and Problem-Solving Strategy

A central question of the present study is whether effective problem-solving skills can be taught, independent of specific medical knowledge. Obviously, the solving of medical problems requires an adequate understanding of specific disease processes and their manifestations.

In this study heuristic processes were often of secondary importance to the students' knowledge of the medical content required to solve the diagnostic cases. For example, in case 4 a finding of red-cell casts in the urine was almost invariably elicited, since it was reported to all subjects who requested a routine urinalysis. The significance of this finding, a nearly pathognomonic sign of glomerulonephritis, was missed by approximately 40 percent of all subjects. It was clear that regardless of the heuristic processes employed, failure to interpret this finding correctly had implications for both the cost and the accuracy of the workup.

Gaps in medical knowledge are easy to spot when they produce major obstacles to problem solving, and remedies are equally obvious. In contrast, failures to use efficient strategies are difficult to discern and even more difficult to remedy. It is no accident that medical schools traditionally have packed the curriculum with as much factual content as time and student capacities permitted, and have offered little or no formal guidance in problem-solving strategies.

Several recent curriculum experiments in medical education have specifically attempted to improve upon the problem-solving process. Subjects of the present study were drawn in equal numbers from a well-established, highly traditional medical school, and from a newly accredited medical school with a highly innovative curriculum stressing a problem-centered clinical approach. Yet comparison of performance between the two schools revealed no differences on any variable.

This finding invites a comparison between the two apparently dissimilar schools. The innovative curriculum has admitted new content and new teaching methods. It has also substantially reorganized subject matter so that the teaching of clinical medicine is more closely articulated with basic science underpinnings. Still, no fundamental changes have occurred with respect to rules for acquiring or utilizing information in order to solve problems.

In the present study an attempt has been made to alter the rules for acquiring and utilizing information and to make these rules more explicit. The results suggest that the ability to select and use information effectively in solving problems may be a teachable cognitive skill, independent of specific clinical knowledge.

Summary

The contribution of this study is twofold. First, a set of dependent measures for the quantification of important diagnostic outcomes has been defined and investigated. It has been demonstrated that diagnostic cost and accuracy performance can be evaluated objectively, although several cases are required to obtain acceptable coefficients of reliability. Second, the effects of problem-solving heuristics on process and outcome measures have been investigated, as well as relationships among many performance variables. The general hypothesis of this study, that heuristic training can improve the problem-solving performance of advanced medical students functioning in a hypothesis-guided mode, has not been solidly supported by the findings; nevertheless, encouraging evidence is provided by trends with respect to group means on the diagnostic accuracy variable and the multivariate investigations.

11 / Conclusion

We have now arrived at the end of our long exploration of the thought processes of experienced physicians and medical students. For the reader who has followed us thus far, this chapter will recapitulate the major results and themes to aid long-term memory. These final pages also present enough about this work to enable a busy reader skimming the pages to decide rationally whether or not to read in further detail.

Scope of Work

This investigation deals with the psychology of medical reasoning and tries to connect medical reasoning with other areas of cognitive psychology. It seeks to explain the complex reasoning process in medicine in terms of simpler elements and through that understanding to help medical students and their teachers improve their reasoning and decision making. The focus of the study is largely on the processes of diagnostic reasoning, although questions of treatment selection and management are also addressed. We do not claim that to explain medicine as a rational cognitive process is a sufficient account of what clinicians do or how people find comfort and help from physicians. Much has been written about the significance of the doctor-patient relationship and the roles of affect and communication in patient satisfaction, compliance with treatment, and feelings of improved well-being. The human perspective is an important and necessary corrective for an overly technical view of medicine. However, we also believe that rationality is desirable and necessary in medicine, although it is by no means sufficient, and that it is therefore worthwhile to understand diagnostic reasoning.

Our approach to this problem has employed both observational and experimental studies. The former examined the reasoning of a group of experienced physicians; the latter tested several propositions derived from the observational studies on a number of independent groups of medical students. The tenor of the work is thus by turns naturalistic, it might even be said clinical, psychometric, and statistical. Some medical readers may feel that we have been too quantitatively oriented and have slighted important clinical points, while some educational researchers may be of the opinion that we have been too descriptive, phenomenological, and insufficiently quantitative. Both can probably point to pages in the work as evidence for these claims. Our stance is that we have tried to find a middle ground between the rigor of a laboratory investigation of the psychology of thinking, where artificial simplicity raises the problem of generalizability, and the complexity of the real world of clinical medicine, where the underlying processes may be obscured and where generalizability is also a problem. We have chosen to focus on a few simulated realities and to analyze them from a number of viewpoints. Our method has been eclectic, but intended to fit a set of complex practical tasks.

Our theorizing has been eclectic too. The major viewpoints about problem solving, judgment, and decision making that inform this work are summarized in the review of literature. Throughout our studies most attention has been given to the information-processing approach to cognition (Kleinmuntz, 1968; Newell and Simon, 1972). This approach aims to characterize the underlying thought processes by recording and analyzing the verbalizations of persons as they attempt to solve problems. The focus is on explaining human thinking in terms of basic psychological elements and principles. In this perspective recommendations for problem solving or decision making take the form of heuristic principles that are probably useful but do not guarantee an optimal solution, as algorithms do.

However, we have been interested also in the possibilities offered by mathematical representations of the problem-solving process (Slovic and Lichtenstein, 1971) and by the prescriptive approach of decision analysis (Lusted, 1968; Raiffa, 1968; Pauker, 1976). Both regression equations and decision analysis are concerned with how imperfect information ought to be optimally combined (Edwards, Lindman, and Phillips, 1965; Goldberg, 1970). Psychological research based on these models has shown that human beings often reach less than optimal solutions when complex probabilistic information must be integrated, but the research has not demonstrated that humans in fact use or try to use these prescriptive models in judgment and decision making (Green, 1968; Tversky and Kahneman, 1974). Nevertheless, since we are concerned with how medical reasoning can be improved, we have discussed portions of our data from these points of view.

In this chapter we shall review the major findings of the studies conducted under the aegis of the Medical Inquiry Project. We shall evaluate the advantages and disadvantages of the different research methods. We shall consider the implications of our findings and viewpoint for instruction and evaluation in medical education. And finally, we shall present a set of heuristics for medical problem solving that combines principles of cognitive psychology and decision analysis.

Findings

Criterial and Noncriterial Physicians

This research began with an effort to distinguish the reasoning strategies of two groups of experienced physicians, one recommended by their peers as good or criterial physicians, and a second group who were not so recommended, the noncriterial group. These two groups were studied with a variety of medical problems and personality scales. The medical problems included three cases in which simulated patients were employed, four modified patient-management problems (McGuire and Solomon, 1971), and four fixed-order problems in which the quantity and sequence of clinical data were out of the problem solver's control.

It was learned that the two groups of physicians could not be distinguished on any of the sets of problems. Chapter 4 discusses a number of reasons that could account for this finding—too few test items, poor test items, or lack of variability in the competence of the participating physicians. In our judgment the major reason is that physicians are not consistent in their performance on these tasks. Gordon, in his study of medical students' reasoning (Chapter 10), likewise noted substantial variability in performance by the same subject on different problems, with a concomitant difficulty in generalizing about a student's overall competence based on a limited number of cases.

In retrospect, this result does not seem so surprising, as it is consistent with a growing trend in cognitive psychology to reemphasize the role of memory, perceptual processes, and prior knowledge in solving complex problems, especially problems of concept attainment (Newell and Simon, 1967). Our research design—the use of a small number of problems to understand the reasoning processes of physicians at different levels of mastery—owes much to the research tactics of de Groot's (1965) classic study of reasoning in chess. Yet de Groot found that chess grand masters were not distinguished from weaker players in planning further ahead or thinking more deeply. The only differences he could identify were in memory and perception, a conclusion recently reaffirmed:

> Chess skill depends in large part upon a vast, organized long-term memory of specific information about chess board patterns . . . Hence, the overriding factor in chess skill is practice. The organization of the master's elaborate repertoire of information takes thousands of hours to build up, and the same is true of any skilled task . . . That is why *practice* is the major independent variable in the acquisition of skill (Chase and Simon, 1973, p. 279).

Similarly, Wason and Johnson-Laird (1972) conclude that rational thought cannot be understood by analysis of formal logical properties alone:

> For some considerable time we cherished the illusion that [using formal logic to construct psychological models of reasoning] was the way to proceed, and that only the structural characteristics of the problem mattered. Only gradually did we realize first that there was no existing formal calculus which correctly modelled our subjects' inferences, and second that no purely formal calculus would succeed. Content is crucial, and this suggests that any general theory of human reasoning must include an important semantic component (pp. 244-245).

Thus investigations of problem solving in chess, in logic, and in medicine are converging on the same conclusion. The differences between experts and weaker problem solvers are more to be found in the repertory of their experiences, organized in long-term memory, than in differences in the planning and problem-solving heuristics employed.

Following the failure to discriminate between criterial and noncriterial physicians, our attention turned to psychological processes associated with accurate and inaccurate diagnosis, identification of heuristics for effective problem solving, and the implications of our results for medical education.

Problem-Solving Processes

Although differences in the content of the memory store apparently distinguish stronger from weaker problem-solving performance, this does not imply that medical problem solving is dependent *solely* upon mastery of passively recalled content. Knowledge must be retrieved and organized. Medical problems typically require that additional data be gathered and evaluated. Ill-defined problems must be progressively better defined so that rational action can be taken. Alternative interpretations of probabilistic data must be generated and compared. These activities are summarized in a four-stage general model of medical inquiry that calls attention to cue acquisition, hypothesis generation, cue interpretation, and hypothesis evaluation. We shall now examine the relation of this model to two heuristics identified in other problem-solving research, forming a plan and means-end analysis.

Cue acquisition refers to the process of collecting data in clinical problem solving. Medical problems differ from many others traditionally used by psychologists to study problem solving, in that all the information needed to solve the medical problem is typically unavailable at the start. Consequently, medical problems are not usually solved by restructuring or drawing implications from available information, as are so many puzzles in the Gestalt tradition. Not only must one go beyond the information given by employing logical inference, but one must also gather data at certain specific points. Effective cue acquisition proceeds according to a plan that permits and facilitates selective data acquisition. Here we discern links to the work of Bruner, Goodnow, and Austin (1956); Polya (1957); Bartlett (1958); Getzels (1964); Shulman, Loupe, and Piper (1968); and Newell and Simon (1972).

Newell and Simon's information-processing theory of problem solving includes two fundamental propositions: (a) that the task environment, the problem, is represented internally as a problem space, and (b) that the structure of the problem space determines the information-processing activities to be used in the search for a solution in clinical medicine. As in other domains of problem solving, the potential size of the problem space is enormous. There are a vast number of elements (states of knowledge about the problem) that could be obtained, an exceedingly large number of potential operators (interview questions, physical-examination maneuvers, and laboratory tests) for obtaining them, and a considerable number of conditions that prior to any data collection could conceivably satisfy the question, "What is wrong with this patient?" Some way must be found to limit the size of the space to be searched.

Early generation of tentative diagnostic hypotheses is a major strategy used by clinicians to bound the regions of the potential problem space most likely to yield the solution. The subsequent workup is planned to permit testing or refinement of these early hypotheses. The open, ill-defined medical problem, "What is wrong with this patient?", is thereby transformed into a set of closed, better-defined problems; this simplifies matters considerably for the problem solver (Bartlett, 1958). Early hypothesis generation permits the use of a hypothetico-deductive method in which data are collected with a view to their usefulness in testing hypotheses. Some medical data are collected to resolve ambiguities and reach closure about problems or treatment alternatives. The method used to narrow diagnostic hypotheses or select a therapy is a form of means-end analysis in which specific clinical findings or clusters of findings serve as operators or moves to reduce the distance between the point where the problem solver is and where he would like to get.

Memory and Hypothesis Generation

Possible solutions to a diagnostic problem are retrieved from a physician's long-term memory store via an associative process that links cues to content stored in memory. Sprafka's study (Chapter 9) showed that medical students generated early hypotheses even when asked to withhold judgment. This strategy apparently has considerable natural force. The generation of early problem formulations was studied in detail by Allal (Chapters 7 and 8). She found that initial problem formulations are generated by association from a cue or cues to a list of competing formulations and by association from one formulation to one or more additional competing formulations. These competing formulations may be generated at one point in time based on the same set of cues, or at several points in time from different cues. The choice of method appears to depend more on the structure of the particular problem than on stylistic differences among physicians. In some cases an early hypothesis is progressively reformulated with increasing specificity. In others the working categories of the clinician appear to be quite specific from the outset.

Allal found that the generation of hypotheses was based more consistently on single salient cues than on combinations of cues, which indicated that more complex search strategies are adjuncts to a simpler process of associative retrieval from the memory store. Analysis of data obtained from high-fidelity simulations (Chapter 4) and fixed-order problems (Chapter 6) suggested that clusters of cues were more commonly used. The conflicting results may be caused by differences in research method. All our studies agree that hypotheses are generated from a very few cues at most, and that retrieval from memory is primarily an associative process and secondarily a process of selective search for best fits to the cluster. The searching and matching process is more consistently employed in the phase of hypothesis evaluation.

Several studies (Chapter 4 through 7) find a limit to the number of hypotheses generated by experienced physicians that is unrelated to their knowledge. The long-term store of medical knowledge of a physician with a reasonable amount of clinical experience is substantially larger than the number of hypotheses that can be evaluated simultaneously. Limitations of both the capacity of the human information-processing system and time play a role. The size of the set of hypotheses being explored at any point in time is usually around four or five and appears to have an upper bound of about six or seven. These estimates are entirely consistent with other estimates of memory capacity for complex material (Wortman, 1970; Simon, 1974).

Two strategies are available that facilitate the attainment of correct diagnostic classification in the face of limitations on the size of the problem space and variation in the content of the problem space across clinicians. First, a hypothesis can be replaced by a reformulation of the problem, one that may be functionally related to its predecessor. Second, hypotheses may be nested hierarchically so that storage capacity can be increased. In Chapter 7, Allal showed that however many problem formulations a physician generates, the maximum number of subspaces into which these formulations are grouped is consistent with the upper bound of the parameter that has been found to govern storage of information in working memory.

Cue Interpretation

In the problems studied, cues were interpreted by physicians as tending to confirm or disconfirm a hypothesis, or as noncontributory. Judgments on this scale were made spontaneously by experienced physicians (Chapter 3), and medical students can justify early problem formulations with this scheme of interpretation (Chapter 8). A seven-point weighting scheme, intended to identify pathognomonic cues, had no greater explanatory power in the cases analyzed in this report. A three-point weighting scheme can be shown to be a simplified approximation of one way of writing Bayes' theorem with multiple cues, if we assume conditional independence of all data (Neutra, 1976). This system of formal evaluation incorporates prior subjective probabilities in the list of hypotheses generated, but the quantification involved is so simple that its relation to Bayes' theorem has been unnoticed. The weighting scheme is also similar to regression equations in which only the signs of the coefficients, not their magnitudes, are important (Dawes and Corrigan, 1974).

Accuracy of cue interpretation was not early identified as a critical feature of medical problem solving, and so was assessed in only one of the three sets of medical problems used with experienced physicians. Accuracy of cue interpretation was found to be related to accuracy of diagnostic outcome and to be independent of thoroughness of cue acquisition. Thus, in contrast to some earlier schemes for scoring simulations and paper-and-pencil cases, we recommend that thoroughness of data collection and accuracy of cue interpretation be independently assessed.

The interpretation of cues in terms of hypotheses is a process that is not well understood, and additional studies of memory organization should be made. To speculate momentarily, the process may involve retrieval of lists of features from memory, each list being nested under a hypothesis, and then a comparison of the findings in a case with the expectancies implied by these lists. Accuracy of the lists obviously would be an important element in problem solving and clearly would be a matter dependent on memory and prior knowledge. One reason why physicians are inconsistent across cases may be that the adequacy of these lists for different hypotheses varies within a single individual as well as between physicians.

The decision process in medical reasoning, however, cannot be solely a process of template matching, in which the problem at hand is set against textbook descriptions, feature for feature. For one thing, passive template matching has been shown to be an insufficient account even of simpler perceptual processes (Lindsay and Norman, 1972). Second, since neither the physician nor the patient is indifferent to the diagnostic outcome, the process that governs it is likely to involve considerations of cost, benefit, and value as well as considerations of probabilistic matching.

Hypothesis Evaluation

The basis for choice among diagnostic alternatives is the topic of concern in hypothesis evaluation. Our studies explored two linear models for diagnostic judgment. The first chooses the hypothesis with a maximum of positive cues, while the second selects the hypothesis with the maximum difference between positive and negative cues. These models may not be appropriate for all diseases, since different diseases are diagnosed by different rules and requirements, but they appear to have broad usefulness.

Of great interest was the finding that the use of these formulas led to increased diagnostic accuracy in one case, an instance of bootstrapping. This finding suggested that many physicians had difficulty integrating a reasonably accurate set of cue weights into a decision, a conclusion consistent with the growing body of literature on problems of information integration, especially with probabilistic cues. Some of this literature has been reviewed in Chapter 2, where more is said about bootstrapping.

Gordon's research (Chapter 10) explored the effect of five experimental heuristics that were intended to facilitate more effective use of clinical information. He found that heuristic training or prompting did have some effect on the performance of subjects. In other words, *a conscious effort to employ useful heuristics does appear to help one adapt one's thinking to the demands of medical problems.* These effects might have been even clearer had a larger sample of cases been employed. Gordon also found that greater thoroughness in the history and physical examination are associated with increased costs, but not with greater diagnostic accuracy.

Concurrently with our studies, Gill and colleagues (1973) have provided independent evidence in support of the distinction between collecting data and evaluating findings properly by showing that a lack of thoroughness is not as important a cause of error in diagnosis as problems of integrating and combining information.

Methodological Issues

Comparison of Research Methods

The studies reported in this monograph have used a variety of methods for collecting data. They differ on two fundamental dimensions, the degree of fidelity to clinical reality and the freedom of the participant to determine the quantity and sequence of data collected. Simulations using actors to play the patient role offer the most fidelity to clinical reality by providing nonverbal cues as well as freedom in data selection. The stimulus films used in Allal's studies (Chapters 7 and 8) controlled the order of cue acquisition, as did the fixed-order problems of Chapter 6, but the films provided the voice, face, and gestures of the patient, while the materials used in Chapter 6 did not. Modified patient-management problems were used in the studies reported in Chapters 5, 9, and 10. They afford considerable latitude in quantity and sequence of data collection, although in both booklet and computerized formats there may be a sizable effect of suggestions for data collection from the printed materials. Visual data about the patient can include reproductions of slides, X rays, electrocardiograms, and the like, but physical findings, appearance, and manner of the patient are typically conveyed verbally and thus involve some verbal interpretation of visual stimuli. Patient-management problems may thus de-emphasize slightly the role of perceptual processes in data acquisition and emphasize the role of verbally mediated problem solving.

No one research method alone can adequately illuminate a process as complex as medical reasoning. Our choice of a variety of methods was deliberate. In the early planning stages of our studies, observations of physicians in outpatient settings were also made, but were found to be unsatisfactory for our purposes. Physicians in these settings were too busy to discuss what they were doing, and they were understandably reluctant to think aloud during a workup when a real patient was present. Also, since each physician saw different cases, it was impossible to standardize by observing various approaches to the same problem. Another disadvantage of the natural setting was that we were never sure if the data the physician reported he had obtained were correct or if some errors had been made. There seemed to be no way of knowing whether a physician had detected the information known to be in the case unless the case was programmed by the experimenters. Other work done by members of our research team (Kagan et al., 1967) implied that a transcription of the medical workup without thinking aloud or an equivalent method of tracing the physician's thought processes would be unsatisfactory.

These considerations all led to simulation formats as the

method of choice for studying medical thinking, but they did not settle the issue of how faithful to clinical reality a simulation ought to be, or what are the tradeoffs involved in different levels of task fidelity.

Any simulation is a representation of reality and its fidelity can vary. It is clearly possible to design simulations that represent fewer real-life circumstances of medical work than do high-fidelity simulations. Rimoldi's early test of diagnostic skills (1961), patient-management problems (McGuire and Solomon, 1971), sequential management problems (Berner, Hamilton, and Best, 1974), diagnostic management problems (Helfer and Slater, 1971), and computer-based simulations (Leaper et al., 1973) are some examples. These formats have distinct advantages in terms of cost of administration and preparation, time spent in staging and scoring each problem, and hence the breadth of the domain that can be sampled in a fixed time, a factor that in turn affects generalizability. But they have three weaknesses that, in our judgment, could only be overcome by a detailed study using higher-fidelity simulations.

The first and most serious weakness was the issue of what aspects of reality could be sacrificed to create a simulation. To eliminate, ignore, or alter the representation of certain aspects of medical reality on a rational basis, it is first necessary to know what aspects or features of the reality are critical. How can these be known without empirical study? Personal accounts of problem-solving procedure by respected and experienced physicians offer valuable leads for making this decision, but have the same problematic status as scientific statements that all anecdotal reports do: How representative are the events described? The lower-fidelity simulation techniques cited assumed that certain features were nonessential and eliminated them, particularly if they were inconvenient or expensive. It seemed, therefore, that there had not yet been assembled a data base sufficient to permit the rational identification of essential and nonessential features of a medical simulation or to permit specifying what was lost when a certain aspect was faded out.

The second difficulty with paper problems is the extent of cuing provided by simultaneous presentation of potential questions. In doing a history and physical examination, most experienced physicians consult a manual of procedures very little or not at all and usually receive suggestions about possible additional procedures only when ordering laboratory tests or when consulting with a colleague. Therefore, a simulation that offers extensive cuing by providing lists of potentially available information may be invalid for a physician, as it does not permit demonstration of actual data-gathering practices; however, it may still be valid for a student who has less experience in collecting data. Leaper and associates (1973) found substantial differences in physician performance in real life and in simulated situations. Goran, Williamson, and Gonnella (1973) have made similar observations. Both groups found that data collection under simulated conditions was more thorough than in actual clinical practice. This is understandable, since simulated data collection is less costly in terms of time, effort, discomfort, and risk to the patient, even if dollar costs are tallied. Putting physicians under time pressure, as in actual cases, might further reduce data collection. However, paper-and-pencil simulations are not necessarily invalidated. It may be possible to develop a satisfactory correction formula that relates the types of data collected under real and simulated conditions. Above all, the relation between omissions and quality of care should be determined by reference to health outcomes, not by simply asserting that economical data collection per se is poor care. As experienced clinicians can testify, thorough data collection that is not thoughtful is not good care either.

Paper-and-pencil or computer-based simulations do furnish a simulated interview setting, but one that is less real than the environment created by providing a person for the physician to interview. This lack implies additional advantages for the high-fidelity format. First, it has been argued rather widely that a key element that distinguishes good from average or poor clinical practice is the quality of interaction with the patient, as evidenced in how the physician modifies the sequence, pacing, and phrasing of questions, and in the rapport between physician and patient. Second, it has been sometimes claimed that the cognitive processes of a clinician are not truly evoked except in the presence of a real patient. This argument is actually quite far removed from the interactional emphasis of the first argument. Third, high-fidelity simulation is effective in eliciting cooperation from voluntary participants. Physicians were persuaded that we were seriously interested in studying their reasoning and were therefore more willing to cooperate with other parts of our experiments where the relation to clinical work was less obvious. The high-fidelity simulations lent credibility to the entire project. When voluntary participation of busy people is an issue, a strategy like this may be helpful. Moderate-fidelity formats have been used most widely with nonvolunteers, usually in educational evaluation.

From these considerations one might infer that high-fidelity simulation is always preferable, that the more faithful the simulation the better, and that naturalistic observation is best of all. Yet this is not our position, for there are serious problems with both naturalistic observation and high-fidelity simulation as research and evaluation techniques. One problem, paradoxically, is the sheer wealth of data provided. A research study, especially one broadly conceived, must eventually focus its inquiry. The programmed patients were originally to provide materials for analyzing both cognitive and interpersonal strategies. As matters turned out, there was so much material to assemble, analyze, and interpret that it was decided to concentrate on cognitive issues. Besides, since the actors all were college students in their early twenties, it could be argued that the data pertained only to the physicians' rapport and communication skills with that group, not patients in general. This point leads then to another difficulty with high-fidelity simulation, the question of generalization from a small sample of problems studied intensively.

Generalizability

The time required for a complete workup, including thinking aloud and videotape-stimulated recall, imposes severe constraints on the number of problems that can be used to assess an individual in an examining session of reasonable length. From the standpoint of test theory, each simulated problem may be viewed as a single test item. Even if patient-management problems and high-fidelity simulations are combined, the test has a maximum length of seven items. How much can one generalize from so short a test?

The research strategy of the descriptive studies in this book closely resembles that of de Groot's (1965) classic study of reasoning in chess masters. Both used small samples of problems and assumed that the problem-solving processes elucidated by intensive analysis of a small number of cases would be generalizable to a broader set of problems. Early in the implementation phase of this research, the design philosophy was criticized by Kenneth Hammond (personal communication, 1970) from a classic Brunswikian standpoint whose merit was at the time not fully appreciated. He argued that situations differ more than persons and that more would be learned by studying fewer individuals in a broader number of settings. To adopt this viewpoint and to remain committed to high-fidelity simulation creates a severe practical problem; as long as it takes from two to two and one-half hours to complete one high-fidelity simulation, it is unrealistic to expect any single physician to do more than three in the time he or she could spend in our laboratory. In general, given the difficulty of obtaining physicians able to participate in a study of this kind, it may be easier to obtain a larger group of subjects for a shorter time than a smaller group for more intensive study. Thus, the only feasible way to broaden the sample of problems attacked by each physician in a fixed and limited time is to reduce the fidelity of the simulation format.

The gains and losses of this tradeoff are clearer now than when the research was designed, for at the time generalizability was not identified as the prime validity problem. Content validity was, and we thought it would be best achieved by employing task environments that resembled the world of clinical work. We planned to handle the issue of generalizability of the results by also using lower-fidelity experimental materials and by testing certain propositions in a related series of experimental studies. In part our program succeeded and some general features of medical inquiry have been identified. But we are not able to generalize as forcefully as we had hoped because of problem specificity. There is considerable method variance between simulation formats, and an even more critical problem is the variation within a single format as a function of the content of the problem.

Some Educational Implications

The apparent conflict between content validity and generalizability in tests of clinical competence raises a very thorny issue for research and practice in medical education. Systematic sampling of performance with a number of patients may be recommended as preferable to intensive observation of a physician or a student with a single patient, real or simulated. In addition, it may be suggested that close attention be paid to identifying explicitly the components of skilled performance to be assessed. No evaluation technique or research program can answer all of the questions that may be asked. If the focus is on the physician as a gatherer and processor of clinical information, the consistencies observed in the observational studies of Chapters 4 to 6 and the experimental studies of Chapters 7 through 10 all suggest that paper-and-pencil tests can be designed that permit an examinee to display his thought processes adequately. These lower-fidelity formats do not permit assessing how well the physician relates to or communicates with patients or modifies his approach to deal with a particular patient's expectations or beliefs. The interpersonal and social aspects of medical practice can best be assessed by direct patient observation or by response to film clips of other physician-patient encounters.

Alternative Conceptual Approaches to Medical Inquiry

An information-processing approach to problem solving is the dominant theoretical perspective of the investigations of this project. Medical situations have been viewed as problems, and our studies have been conceptualized as the study of problem solving. We have tried throughout to relate our findings to psychological research in the field of problem solving, with special emphasis on the processes of formulating and testing solutions to a problem, on the constraints placed upon these processes by basic characteristics of the human information-processing system, and on the mechanisms used to adapt thinking to a variety of task demands. The methods used in most of our studies have also been in the spirit of this research paradigm: verbalizations of physicians or medical students while solving medical problems and subsequently reviewing their performance have been basic materials for analysis.

We arrived at this conceptualization and research approach from several directions. Our own interest in problem solving and reasoning was reinforced by the fact that the process-tracing paradigm for research on problem solving—the use of a limited number of subjects and problems with analysis of the sequence of verbalization—is a clinical method, in Piaget's sense: it seeks to capture not only what the problem solver did, but to explain why he did it. Then, too, the medical school environment in which the studies were conducted was and is one that emphasizes problem solving and the problem-oriented record. The nonmathematical character of process-tracing theories and research seemed to us to be a better approximation of how most clinicians approach their task than more formal mathematical approaches. Lastly, the process-tracing approach takes account of the sequential and selective aspects of cognition and is thus particularly suited for studying an activity like clinical reasoning, which is also sequential and selective (Hogarth, 1974).

Nevertheless, the terms *judgment* and *decision making* recur in this work. Although in some places they have been used almost interchangeably (partly in the interest of varying the style), we are aware that psychological research on judgment and on decision making employs very different paradigms. Had either paradigm dominated this research, the investigations would have a different appearance. Lusted's book (1968) conveys the tone of the decision-making approach applied to medicine. The review of the literature in Chapter 2 summarized much of the relevant nonmedical literature on these topics and identified some possible points of convergence among the approaches. Here it is appropriate to indicate some of the differences and to contrast the insights gained from a process-tracing approach with what the Bayesian approach and judgment theory (Slovic and Lichtenstein, 1971) could teach us.

Most of the investigations reported herein have concentrated on the problem of diagnostic classification, with secondary attention being paid to the issues of treatment selection and management. Consequently, the studies emphasized processes or heuristics associated with diagnostic accuracy more than they focused upon the costs, risks, and benefits of alternative actions. Some clinicians have criticized the work on precisely this score. In part, the emphasis reflects a view of diagnosis as concept attainment or concept recognition, a major theme of the psychology of thinking at least since *A Study of Thinking* by Bruner and his associates was published in 1956. But it also derives from the diagnostic model of medicine itself, a model that appears to fit the problems selected for study, since a common feature of all of them is a generally agreed-to course of treatment or management that follows the diagnostic process. Thus, "diagnosis first, then treatment" appears to be a useful model for many medical problems, though by no means all. It is not difficult to think of medical situations in which risky decisions must be made prior to definitive diagnosis, and where considerations of the expected value of alternative actions are at least as important as the probability distribution of various diagnoses. One's evaluation of our research may therefore be contingent upon one's prior conception of medicine—and there appear to be a number of defensible conceptions available. Indeed, we may speculate that different problems require different medical paradigms and that no single theoretical model is sufficient for so complex an activity as clinical medicine.

Many classic situations studied in the problem-solving paradigm are puzzles with but one correct solution. The problem solver has to prove a theorem in logic, or verify a syllogism, or draw a series of inferences, or identify a concept from a series of positive and negative instances. The search for the correct route through the logical maze bears some superficial resemblance to the decision analyst's search for an optimal strategy, but ordinarily it is quite different. Logical inference does not deal with probability and uncertainty; matters of utility and risk are usually irrelevant unless the problem solver has to pay for each move or for the time needed to reach a solution.

Thus, in addition to focusing on the sequence of operations leading to accurate solutions, the process-tracing approach tends to neglect the costs associated with error. In a problem used in a typical experiment, errors only delay solution by leading one down unproductive routes. They do not cost money and they do not harm others. Diagnostic reasoning that adheres excessively to this approach may overemphasize accuracy that can make no difference in treatment and be insensitive to cost-benefit considerations. Decision analysis, on the other hand, prescribes that actions should be selected on the basis of expected utility, calculated as a function of the probability of each outcome multiplied by its utility—a subjective but systematic weighting of costs, risks, and benefits. The word *prescribes* is important here, for it must be emphasized that decision analysis is a technique that advises how decisions under uncertainty ought to be made. It does not claim that people in fact make decisions accordingly; indeed if people were intuitive natural decision analysts, the technique would be largely superfluous.

In the discussion section of Chapter 4, it was suggested that the generation of diagnostic hypotheses is mediated by some combination of probability and utility. The diagnostic judgments studied in that chapter were largely accounted for by a preponderance-of-evidence rule which, as Lusted (1968) has shown, is equivalent to a probability statement. The role of expected value or utility in these judgments is unclear. How is the cost of a missed diagnosis incorporated into hypothesis evaluation? Are physicians striving for diagnostic accuracy without paying attention to the consequences of missing a diagnosis? That is very unlikely, if one listens to clinical conferences or consultations. There is reason to believe that when payoffs are biased by unequal probabilities, it is difficult to behave optimally—that is, as decision theory prescribes (Pitz and Downing, 1968). We may speculate that physicians in different practice settings have different strategies for coping with this problem, expressible as policies regarding the weights to be assigned to probability and utility, but to corroborate this thesis will require more thorough sampling of a physician's judgment than we have yet done and will take us into the topic of mathematical modeling.

The mathematical representation of human judgment by means of regression equations or other models (Einhorn, 1970; Slovic and Lichtenstein, 1971; Goldberg, 1971) began as an effort to describe and explain how humans process information, but it has become increasingly difficult to sustain that view. The models generally function as simultaneous processors of a large number of variables, while humans typically process such large data sets serially or in smaller packets. Consequently, judgment theory and mathematical modeling have not particularly illuminated the problems and issues raised by the cognitive perspective. However, capturing a judge's policy through a mathematical model has shown promise as a way of improving human judgment. It offers a means for increasing consistency and for taking optimal account of multiple cues (Goldberg, 1970; Dawes, 1971).

The process-tracing approach concentrates on offering a description and an explanation of how skilled humans solve problems, while mathematical models and decision analysis focus on recommending strategies for handling complex problems. Of course, the distinction between description and prescription is not hard and fast, for to the extent that any problem solver tries to behave in accordance with the norms of a particular approach, that approach becomes descriptive. For example, a problem solver could try to apply systematically heuristic principles derived from process-tracing studies, and to some extent then, a description becomes a prescription. These considerations are summarized in Table 11.1.

It might appear that decision analysis is unequivocally the conceptual framework of choice for the study and improvement of medical judgment. While we believe that this approach has many merits and should be pursued, it is not without limitations. First of all, decision analysis is a useful technique for evaluating alternatives, but it says little about how alternative solutions to a problem are generated. It is a theory of decision making without memory or knowledge. Second, it may be argued that complex clinical situations are so varied and individualized that a formal decision analysis might have to be performed repeatedly, since the partic-

Table 11.1   Comparison of three approaches to clinical decision making.

Approach	Aim	Data processed	Quantification
Process tracing	Descriptive and explanatory	Serially	Little
Regression or lens model	Descriptive and prescriptive	Simultaneously	Cue weights derived from multivariate (regression) analysis
Decision analysis	Prescriptive	Sequentially	Largely subjective estimates of probability and value

ulars of each case are different. This would put clinicians right back to the start—tailoring therapy to the particulars of each case. But what are the guiding heuristic principles that enable a clinician to proceed without such a formal analysis of each new case? How are the relevant variables in a new case identified? Psychological studies of decision making might profitably pursue the problem of how clinical decisions are made before moving to the prescriptive mode.

The unavailability of certain data necessary for decision analysis is an even more formidable obstacle. Without satisfactory estimates of the prior probability of long lists of diseases, of the probabilities of even longer lists of symptoms conditional on these diseases, and of the utility attached to each outcome, decision analysis becomes a conceptual framework rather than a detailed technology. Within this framework decision making is treated sequentially; one is advised to analyze a complex problem into independent components, estimating each separately before recombining. This is surely a useful heuristic for an information-processing system with a limited working memory! Still, the questionable adequacy of subjective estimates and the thorny question of estimating values render a thorough decision-analytic technology for medicine doubtful in the near term. Even without firm quantitative data, the tactics of decision analysis may be simplified into nonquantitative or semiquantitative heuristics very similar to those derivable from process-tracing studies.

Thus, we believe that in the foreseeable future useful work can be done with all three approaches, depending on one's purpose.

Implications for Medical Education

Curriculum: Content and Process

Contemporary medical education has been deeply concerned with curriculum revision. One new approach to curriculum construction uses the presenting problem as the chief organizing principle for materials and instruction, on the grounds that the common process underlying all medical work, regardless of specialty or organ system involved, is a rational approach to problem solving (Ways, Loftus, and Jones, 1973; Neufeld and Barrows, 1974).

Portions of our findings have been presented to groups of physicians in a number of contexts. The most startling and controversial aspects of our results have always been the finding of case specificity and the lack of intraindividual consistency over problems, with the accompanying implication that knowledge of content is more critical than mastery of a generic problem-solving process. For some medical educators, who have been attempting to build curriculum on the presumedly generic problem-solving process, this finding was discouraging if believed; if not, it had to be explained away in some fashion. In our opinion there is a general mental process common to all medical problem solving, and we have tried to outline it in the model of medical inquiry. However, the effectiveness with which this process is mobilized in any particular case depends on knowledge in a particular domain. The fact that all problems are approached by generating hypotheses and testing them implies that a general hypothetico-deductive method for problem solving is employed by all physicians. The observable differences in our results are caused more by content-related factors than by variations in method employed. Results with a group of less experienced physicians or with medical students might assign different magnitudes to these components.

It appears to us that the concept of a common process for solving any and all medical problems must be balanced by recognizing that effective problem solving depends also upon retrieval of relevant content from a well-organized store of long-term memories. The finding of case specificity does indeed raise a significant problem for curriculum planning in medical education, for it suggests that the extent of transfer from problem to problem is less than a case-oriented curriculum appears to require for justification.

We conclude that, beyond the fundamentals of the generic process, transfer is indeed limited; but we do not conclude that a case-oriented curriculum is inappropriate. On the contrary, the limitations on the extent of transfer may help us to understand why some medical students educated in a traditional preclinical curriculum that is the heritage of Flexner's 1910 report have difficulty adapting to the clinical approach; they find it hard to transfer scientific facts and principles to clinical applications because the classical curriculum does not offer enough early opportunities for practice. A case-oriented curriculum should ease this transition, but chiefly for problems studied in the preclinical years. A medical school curriculum built around clinical problems and case discussions in the preclinical years should therefore choose problems and cases carefully and deliberately. It cannot be assumed that any problem will do because all exemplify the problem-solving process. They do exemplify this process, but competence is also dependent upon knowledge of content. Our resolution of the content-process dichotomy is to emphasize both, to stress that content appears to transfer less than has been generally assumed, and to reformulate the process as a hypothetico-deductive method with heuristics suitable for probabilistic tasks.

Carefully selected problems are vehicles for building a store of memories (knowledge) as well as a set of formal strategies. With a problem-oriented curriculum a medical school might, therefore, be able to say something like this about its graduates: "At a minimum, students in our school have all encountered the following set of problems, both in preclinical exercises and in clinical clerkships. We warrant their competence to diagnose and treat these problems, and we warrant their understanding of the mechanisms involved in these problems, so far as these mechanisms are known. We warrant also their competence to diagnose certain other problems, but we have not provided them experience in managing these problems. We hope that they know and can do more than this, but we cannot warrant it." A list of selected medical problems would then follow. Although this statement of competence upon graduation may seem overly modest, it is entirely consistent with the finding of case specificity. It would have the additional virtue of telling a medical student what it is that he needs to know for graduation in terms of complaints or diseases he would be expected to diagnose and/or manage, and their underlying mechanisms.

Another explanation for the finding of case specificity is that it is a product of the educations of the physicians participating in the study and could be altered by a different approach to the organization of knowledge and learning. This argument can be neither proved nor refuted with the data available and rapidly moves into the area of large-scale longitudinal comparative evaluation of alternative medical curricula. In one sense the traditional medical curriculum has been explicitly aimed at learning broad scientific propositions and principles, precisely so that the physician could generalize across different cases. How this objective has been achieved or altered by the realities of clinical practice and postgraduate training in different settings is a problem that deserves a research monograph in its own right.

New Instructional Materials

We have suggested that there is evidence in our studies for the proposition that problem solving—the evaluation and integration of clinical data—is a skill that cannot proceed without a well-developed memory store. At the same time, information evaluation is not equivalent to storing and recalling facts from this store and is a skill that is acquired, like other skills, through practice. In this context the instructional potential of the materials developed for the studies reported in Chapters 8, 9, and 10 should be stressed. Additional stimulus films with appropriate feedback can be produced to provide students early in their training with opportunities to practice generation of multiple competing hypotheses on common problems. Film clips, slide-tape units, or paper-and-pencil simulations can help students structure their knowledge into clinically useful forms. Relatively simple problems and cases that would be useful in further experimental research on clinical judgment and decision making may also be appropriate instructional materials in the earlier phases of medical education, when isolated component skills are all that a student can be reasonably expected to practice or demonstrate. Film clips, paper cases, patient games, and computer-based simulations provide opportunities for students to consider and discuss the values and hazards of alternative diagnostic procedures and therapies without the time pressure inherent in an actual clinical setting.

Aiding the Decision Maker

A number of our studies have shown that the relation between thoroughness of data collection and accuracy of data interpretation is often modest. Instances have been presented in which diagnostic errors were caused not by failure to collect an appropriate item of data or to perform a recommended test, but by mistakes in appraising or combining large quantities of complex probabilistic information. Attention should be paid to teaching new physicians how to interpret their data as well as how to collect it. A research group at Leeds (Gill et al., 1973) has quite independently reached a similar conclusion.

A number of centers are pursuing the investigation of computer-assisted diagnosis. Although this trend may grow steadily, it appears that computer-mediated medicine is still in the future.

Some of our work with simple quantitative models of the judgmental process suggests that semiformal paper-and-pencil methods can also help to improve decision making and that clinicians need not wait until a terminal is installed in every consulting room. The research studies in this report, as well as those conducted in other centers, show convincingly that problems in clinical inference will not be solved solely by adding new sources of data to the clinician's armamentarium. Part of the problem already is drawing optimal inferences from large amounts of probabilistic data. A variety of strategies for systemizing this inference process are likely to be helpful, including regression analysis, discriminant function analysis, decision analysis, deliberate attention to effective problem-solving heuristics, and the routine use of flow charts and clinical algorithms (Tuddenham et al., 1969; Feinstein, 1974). We believe that the next generation of physicians will need greater familiarity with these techniques for handling increasingly large amounts of clinical information.

It is our opinion that computer-assisted instruction (CAI) focused on data interpretation as well as data collection might help physicians at all levels of training to improve their cognitive skills. Even though CAI will have very limited value in helping a student acquire a more effective approach to the patient, it could free clinicians to concentrate on the human side of medicine in their contacts with students. Some materials of the type we have in mind are already available through the Health Education Network, having been prepared at the Laboratory of Computer Science at the Massachusetts General Hospital (Laboratory of

Computer Science, 1976) and at the University of Illinois (McGuire and Solomon, 1971). Case specificity and intraindividual variability across tasks imply that additional materials are needed.

The inferential process identified in Chapter 4 consisted in assigning weights to data and combining these weights to reach defensible conclusions. Of the physicians studied none systematically employed Bayes' theorem or decision analysis in this task. Yet cue weights might be restated as the probability of a cue (sign, symptom, or finding), given a certain disease. There is evidence that formally combining subjective probabilities will not substantially increase accuracy over existing informal methods owing to the magnitude of error in these estimates (Leaper et al., 1972). Research to assemble objective probabilities for the more common and difficult problems has begun in a number of centers and might be expanded.

Meanwhile, curriculum planners in medical schools might begin to think about a place for instruction in probabilistic inference, decision making, and problem-solving heuristics. As decision makers, physicians must repeatedly make choices involving complex considerations of probability, cost, hazard, and benefit. Much of the psychological research on decision making reviewed earlier in this book, as well as work that has appeared since that review was completed, suggests that choices in complex situations are often based on simplifying heuristics that may not accurately reflect the overall values of the decision maker and his client or patient. Nevertheless, these heuristics are employed because the situation is extremely complex and sense must be made of it somehow. The tactics of decision analysis (Lusted, 1968; Raiffa, 1968; Fryback, 1974; Pauker, 1976) may be able to help us think more systematically about these problems.

Heuristics for Medical Students

Gordon (Chapter 10) found some evidence to support the proposition that systematic use of selected heuristics did have desirable effects on the problem-solving behavior of medical students. Since his study, analysis of other decision situations in medicine has led to formulation of additional heuristics and to revision of the original list.[1] Their effectiveness has not yet been

---

[1] This new list was developed by the senior author and his colleagues at the Center for the Analysis of Health Practices, Harvard School of Public Health, for a course in clinical decision analysis taught there in 1975–76.

experimentally verified, but they do offer testable guidelines for clinical information processing. The revised heuristics, given below, are a deliberate attempt to blend the insights of decision analysis and cognitive psychology and formulate a practical tool for students. They also extend the model of medical inquiry by specifically incorporating expected value as a decision criterion in hypothesis evaluation.

Generating a list of alternative hypotheses or actions:

(a) *Multiple competing hypotheses.* Think of a number of diagnostic possibilities compatible with the chief complaint and preliminary findings. Avoid making snap diagnoses. Key on "good" symptom clusters; organ-system links are helpful. Nesting overcomes limits of working memory.

(b) *Probability.* Consider the most common diagnoses first.

(c) *Utility.* Consider seriously those diagnoses for which effective therapies are available and in which failure to treat would be a serious omission. Try to keep separate your estimates of the probability of a disease and the cost of not treating it.

Gathering data:

(d) *Form a reasoned plan* for testing your hypotheses, one that reckons with probability and utility. Sequence laboratory tests to rule out first the most common diseases (probability), and next the diseases most needing treatment (utility).

Corollary 1: Diagnostic decisions should be related to treatment alternatives. There is no reason to pursue a differential among diagnoses that will make no difference in the action to be taken, and your data gathering should reflect this.

Corollary 2: There should be a reason for every datum gathered. For example, if a test result does not change your opinion about any of your diagnostic hypotheses, ask yourself why the test was ordered and what range of values could have changed your mind.

(e) *Branch and screen.* History taking and the physical examination should be branching procedures. Develop adequate screening tactics to help make overly detailed examinations unnecessary. For example, if a patient denies changes in weight, the physician can omit going down the branch that relates to certain endocrinopathies.

(f) *Cost-benefit calculation.* Consider the harm tests might do and their cost. Balance these against the information to be gained.

(g) *Precision.* Strive for the degree of reliability needed for the decision at hand. More is not necessary.

Aggregating data, evaluating hypotheses, and selecting a course of action:

(h) *Disconfirmatory evidence.* Actively seek out and evaluate evidence that tends to rule out any hypothesis or action alternative as well as the evidence that tends to confirm it. Be aware of the tendency to discount or disregard evidence likely to disconfirm your favorite alternative.

(i) *Multiple diagnoses.* Don't forget the possibility that a patient with multiple problems or complaints has more than one disease.

(1) The joint probability of two common diagnoses may well be greater than one rarer diagnosis.

(2) When failure to treat both hypothetical diagnoses might have disastrous results, and neither can be confirmed or ruled out, act as if both were established.

(j) *Bayes' theorem.* Revise probabilities after collecting data.

(1) In assessing the probability of a particular diagnosis, give special weight if it is common.

(2) If the clinical findings are relatively more likely in diagnosis A than in diagnosis B, revise your opinion in favor of A.

(3) If hard data are missing about how common a disease is, or about how likely particular symptoms are in it, make rough approximations. It is usually possible to weight each finding as at least tending to confirm, disconfirm, or not change one's prior belief.

(4) If you rank order diagnoses on the basis of the predominance of findings in their support, weighted as described in (3), this ranking will correspond roughly to a probability scale.

(k) *Probability and utility should guide action.* When a course of action is finally selected, consider both the probability of the diagnoses for which this action is appropriate and the benefits/penalties that would accrue. Combine these two considerations to estimate expected value and choose so as to maximize expected value.

Corollary 1: Consider clustering diagnoses that would be treated identically. This nesting effectively reduces the number of alternatives to be evaluated.

Corollary 2: Among the benefits and penalties of medical action, consider quality of life and morbidity as well as mortality.

Evaluation

Two major psychometric themes recur in these studies and have direct implications for the evaluation of clinical performance at all levels of training. Wherever we have turned, we have found that intraindividual consistencies across problems are modest at best. Physicians are far more variable in their performance across tasks than had been anticipated, so it is difficult to estimate how a clinician will perform on any one problem by extrapolating from performances on other problems. This variability was the basis for our failure to discriminate criterial from noncriterial physicians. It is apparently far easier to discriminate physicians of different levels of training than to discriminate competence among physicians with roughly comparable years of experience (Senior, 1974). In clinical evaluation, therefore, either the domain evaluated must be specified more narrowly than has been done previously, or the number of problems used in an assessment must be increased substantially. Clinical competence is not a unidimensional construct that can be assessed adequately with a limited number of test items.

Basing their action in part on a series of studies of the feasibility of a computer-based examination for recertification purposes (Hoffman, 1974; Senior, 1974), the American Board of Internal Medicine has recently enlarged the number of problems to be used in its certification examinations. This action is entirely consistent with the point of view developed in this report. Assessment of medical students in clerkships and of house officers should likewise be based on more extensive sampling of the objectives of the training experience.

Our studies have consistently shown that medical problem solving is a hypothetico-deductive activity in which early problem formulations partly guide subsequent data collection. The generation of multiple competing hypotheses is an almost universal feature of this problem solving. It may be useful to incorporate an assessment of hypothesis-generation activity into the overall evaluation. A number of systems for scoring paper-and-pencil or computer-based simulations have utilized cue acquisition as the major criterion of adequacy of process in the diagnostic workup. Yet several studies in this report have found only weak relations between thoroughness of data acquisition and accuracy of cue interpretation, although both variables play a part in diagnostic accuracy. Should our results be confirmed by further studies, they imply that the two variables ought to be assessed separately. Prototype evaluation instruments that employ this concept are now used in student evaluation at Michigan State University.

Future Research and Development

As we gaze into the future, two major concerns emerge: to apply what is already known about medical problem solving and decision making to clinical practice, and to increase our knowledge of these complex processes. In spite of a small but steady output of articles on medical decision making in the years since Lusted's book (for example, Schwartz et al., 1973; McNeil, Keeler, and Adelstein, 1975; Sisson, Schoomaker, and Ross, 1976; Pauker, 1976), a decision theoretic approach to medicine is still far from widely accepted. In this chapter we have tried to show some of the relationships between informal semiquantitative approaches that clinicians do use and the more rigorous, quantified, prescriptive approach of decision analysis. Perhaps this discussion will help to improve communications between clinical practitioners and advocates of decision analysis. It is still unclear how much additional power over ordinary practice would be gained by systematic application of decision analytic strategies. More research will have to be done to show the relative advantage of this innovation. It is not enough to show that computer-mediated diagnosis can duplicate a physician's decisions. The question is, rather, how much better off are the patients of physicians who use this approach in conceptualizing and analyzing medical decisions?

It is clear now, as perhaps it was not in 1968, that clinicians do not ordinarily use Bayes' theorem in reaching clinical decisions, but that some decision principles they do use are approximations to a more formal calculation of probability. The general logical method used is hypothetico-deductive. Creativity and inspiration appear to be less crucial than the organization of memory and the structure of the task. To flesh out these statements will require additional studies of how variations in the structure of the problem affect the actions taken by the physician. In-depth studies in the process-tracing tradition will encounter the difficult problem of generalizability. Larger-scale studies that make use of lower-fidelity simulation, in the regression or lens-model tradition, will have the difficulty of not capturing the cognitive processes of the decision maker but only modeling his output. A unified theory and research approach is not yet available. Until it is, both kinds of studies will help to advance knowledge. One might, for example, contemplate a series of process-tracing studies, linked with carefully designed computer simulations and paper-and-pencil vignettes, to explore more definitively some of the unanswered problems raised in this report:

(a) The relative weight assigned by experienced clinicians to considerations of probability and utility in evaluating diagnostic and treatment alternatives.

(b) The calibration of physicians' estimates of probability, as an extension of the calibration studies reviewed by Beach (1975) and Slovic, Fischoff, and Lichtenstein (1977).

(c) The effect of biased payoff matrices on clinical judgment.

(d) The effectiveness of decision models in increasing diagnostic accuracy and reducing costs. Fryback (1974) explored this topic, but it certainly merits further study.

(e) Intrapsychic, social, and task determinants of judgments of probability, hazard, and expected value in medicine.

We anticipate that, in general, the principles found to operate in human judgment in experimental settings will also obtain in clinical medicine, to the extent that they reflect characteristics of the human information processor. But research findings are also determined by the specific situation in which the adaptive human finds himself. That is why the psychological problem space largely reflects characteristics of the task environment, rather than personality variables, and why medical reasoning is case specific, rather than dominated by intraindividual consistencies. For this reason research into the effects of different tasks upon reasoning and decision processes is still much needed.

Closing Thoughts

The psychological principles that explain human problem solving and offer testable means for its improvement apply to the specific domain of medicine. Medical reasoning is particularly complex because the content to be mastered and the range of situations to be dealt with are so varied; however, like Simon (1969), we find that the complexity lies mainly in the environment and not in the operations that humans employ to understand and master it. Given the limited capacity of working memory, one is literally required to adopt a serial processing strategy, to select means carefully, and to represent the task environment as a problem space of limited size. Yet a system with these characteristics is capable of adapting to a broad range of exceedingly complex environments. In one sense, then, this view of medical problem solving is reductionistic, since the clinical process is seen as built up out of the complexity of medical content in conjunction with some heuristics that, once explained, are not mysterious and that are adapted both to our psychological limitations and to our environment. The adaptive capacity of this system is formidable indeed, precisely because it makes possible the flexible combination of a finite set of simpler elements.

Some may find this view of medical problem solving disquieting, as it de-emphasizes the importance of brilliant insight or creativity and stresses instead the importance of routinized programs for processing information. Most clinical problems, however, can be identified and resolved by the application of routinized means. The dramatic creative insight is rare, not commonplace. Furthermore, this dual perspective on human nature is itself a fundamental theme of human thought. Different temperaments emphasize either the uniqueness of the overall design or the common structure of the underlying elements of human activities and processes, in psychology as in biology.

Some may take exception to these research studies as focusing too much on a narrow class of medical problems, specific complaints that can be diagnosed, while so many clinical situations lack this property. We can only agree that problems still remain to be investigated. The resourceful researcher can find much to do and many difficult questions to tackle. Physicians especially may find the scope of these studies too narrow, since they must take the world as it is and try to find a course of constructive action. Theoretical sciences, on the other hand, inevitably attempt to narrow the scope of a particular inquiry in the interest of deeper understanding. One must then ask how relevant a particular investigation is to the world as it is. We have tried to combine descriptive and experimental analyses to improve our collective understanding of an important practical activity. We have not achieved all we set out to do, and we are keenly aware of the methodological limitations of these studies. Much remains to be done. Yet it is gratifying to have advanced as far as we have.

Appendixes
References
Index

Appendix A/ Sample page from PMP answer booklet

PROBLEM II: A SURGICAL ABDOMEN

Assume you are a young general practitioner, a member of the staff of your modern 300-bed community hospital. You are called by the intern at 10:30 P.M. to see a patient in the Emergency Room.

When you arrive, you find a forty-seven year old man who complains of abdominal pain and vomiting. Pain began 3 weeks ago; the patient took Bromo-Seltzer® with some relief. He continued to work until a week ago when he stopped working because of pain. After 2 days at home the pain began to improve, but began to vomit small amounts. Similar, though less severe, episodes of pain have occurred off and on the past three years.

What diagnostic possibilities are you considering at this point? List in order of priority:

_____

_____

_____

_____

_____

NOW CONTINUE WITH SECTION II-A

SECTION II-A

You would NOW (Choose ONLY ONE EACH time you are directed to this section):

- 6   Admit patient to hospital
- 7   Start treatment, reassure the patient, send him home and plan to see him at home early next morning
- 8   Obtain laboratory or X-ray examinations
- 9   Obtain more history from the patient
- 0   Examine the patient

SECTION II-B

You would NOW (Choose ONLY ONE):

- ___ 41   Obtain laboratory and X-ray studies
- ___ 42   Call the operating room and schedule the patient for immediate surgery
- ___ 43   Obtain further history from the patient
- ___ 44   Observe the patient closely for the next few hours
- ___ 45   Decide that admission to the hospital was not necessary after all; start treatment, send the patient home and plan to see him at home early next morning

Appendix B/ Instructions to selected subjects in investigation of early hypothesis generation

The following are the instructions read to the E-V group of medical students (those told to generate hypotheses early and verbalize), in addition to the common instructions given to all groups participating in the modified PMP experiment:

During this session you will be asked to solve three simulated clinical problems. Your task will be to arrive at a definitive diagnosis for each problem with the aid of the information available. The procedure used for solving all three problems is the same. As you can see from the sheet entitled Problem 1 which I have given you, a written introduction is given at the beginning of each problem. The introduction is followed by numbered options which you may request. These options give you information which will help you solve the problem, i.e. reach a definitive diagnosis. The options fall into the general categories of history, physical, laboratory and X-ray studies, and management. As you request the options, I will hand you the appropriate information printed on a card. Please request information *one* item at a time by stating the number of the item. As you request an option please list its number in the column labeled "Options" on the sheet provided.

As you work on the problem, I would like you to use any useful information you get to help you think of possible problem formulations. I encourage you to speculate somewhat and base formulations on relatively small amounts of information. Furthermore, if you wish to, use these formulations as guides in the selection of more information.

While you are doing the problem, I will interrupt you periodically and ask you to do two things. First, I will ask you to write down any problem formulations you may have thought of at that point. Secondly, I will ask you to quickly describe to me what caused you to entertain those formulations. For example, did a certain item of information cause you to think of a formulation; had you seen a case before which presented in this manner, and so on. Each time I ask you to list problem formulations, please list as many as you are thinking of up to five (5). If you have no formulations in mind, you need not list any. If you are still entertaining the same formulations you listed previously, you may simply list those same ones again. At the end of each problem, please state your definitive diagnosis for that problem.

You will be evaluated on the efficiency, thoroughness, and accuracy of your work. The accuracy score refers only to the definitive diagnosis. Efficiency and thoroughness refer to how much information you gather to reach a solution. These two scores are closely related. They tend to balance each other. A good performance is given by choosing that amount of information which results in an adequate workup. You should not try to solve the problem by choosing as few items as possible, nor should you request information which is useless to you or may be harmful to your patient.

I will keep this tape recorder going while you are working. Do not pay any attention to it. It is harmless. Now, are there any questions before we begin?

If you are ready, please read the introduction to Problem 1 aloud.

Appendix C/ Scoring of patient-management problems

An examinee completes a PMP by selecting items in an examination booklet, then obtaining information about his choices (the "answers" to his "questions") by removing an opaque overlay from an answer sheet or by rubbing the appropriate portion of a sheet that has been chemically treated with a special pen to reveal the response.

Each choice has been assigned a weight that indicates its value. These weights are assigned by a group of experts before the problem is administered. Strongly positive weights are given to those items which help most in diagnosis and management of the patient. Lesser positive weights are given to items that should be included in a thorough workup and conscientious management plan. Negative weights are assigned to items that should not be chosen (for example, because they may be costly to the patient) and zero weights are assigned to items that are noncontributory or are simply distractors.

Subjects are scored for overall competence in working up and managing a patient. A proficiency score and an efficiency score are calculated. A high proficiency score is obtained by choosing a reasonably large number of positively weighted items or by doing a thorough workup (diagnosis as well as management) of the patient. Distortions in performance as a result of cuing are greatly reduced by offering a large number of options and making it difficult for the subject to scan all available options at once.

PMP scores are calculated as follows:

$$\text{efficiency} = \frac{\Sigma H_s}{\Sigma H_s + \Sigma h_s},$$

$$\text{proficiency} = \frac{\text{weights of } H_s + \text{weights of } h_s}{\text{MAX}},$$

$$\text{errors of omission} = \frac{MAX - \Sigma \text{ weights of } H_s}{MAX},$$

$$\text{and errors of commission} = \frac{-\Sigma \text{weights of } h_s}{MAX},$$

where H_s = positively weighted items selected,
h_s = negative and zero weighted items selected,
and MAX = sum of all positive weights possible.

In addition to these four scores, the examinee receives a score for attack that rewards him for following an appropriate sequence of sections or penalizes him for doing certain sections out of order.

References

Allal, L. K. 1973. Training of medical students in a problem-solving skill: the generation of diagnostic problem formulations. Unpublished Ph.D. dissertation, Michigan State University.
Allender, J. S. 1969. A study of inquiry activity in elementary school children. *American Educational Research Journal 6*, 543–558.
Angoff, W. H. 1953. Test reliability and effective test length. *Psychometrika 18*, 1–4.
——— 1956. A note on the estimation of nonspurious correlations. *Psychometrika 21*, 295–297.
Bacon, F. 1962. Novum organum (original publication in Latin, 1620). Excerpted and retranslated in C. P. Curtis, Jr., and F. Greenslet, *The practical cogitator* (3rd ed.). Boston: Houghton Mifflin.
Balke, W. M., Hammond, K. R., and Meyer, G. D. 1973. An alternative approach to labor-management negotiations. *Administrative Science Quarterly 18*, 311–327.
Barron, F. 1967. *Creativity and personal freedom.* New York: Van Nostrand.
Barrows, H. S., and Abrahamson, S. 1964. The programmed patient: a technique for appraising student performance in clinical neurology. *Journal of Medical Education 39*, 802–805.
——— and Bennett, K. 1972. The diagnostic (problem solving) skill of the neurologist: experimental studies and their implications for neurological training. *Archives of Neurology 26*, 273–277.
Bartlett, F. D. 1958. *Thinking.* New York: Basic Books.
Beach, B. H. 1975. Expert judgment about uncertainty: Bayesian decision making in realistic settings. *Organizational Behavior and Human Performance 14*, 10–59.
Berner, E. S., Hamilton, L. A., and Best, W. R. 1974. A new approach to evaluating problem solving in medical students. *Journal of Medical Education 49*, 666–672.
Bieri, J., Atkins, A. L., Briar, S., Leaman, R. L., Miller, H., and Tripodi, T. 1966. *Clinical and social judgment.* New York: Wiley.
Bjorkman, M. 1972. Feedforward and feedback as determiners of knowl-

edge and policy: notes on a neglected issue. *Scandinavian Journal of Psychology 13*, 152–158.

Blatt, S. J., and Stein, M. I. 1959. Efficiency in problem solving. *Journal of Psychology 48*, 193–213.

Bourne, L. E., Jr. 1966. *Human conceptual behavior.* Boston: Allyn and Bacon.

────── and Dominowski, R. L. 1972. Thinking. *Annual Review of Psychology 23*, 105–130.

Brehmer, B. 1974. Hypotheses about relations between scaled variables in the learning of probabilistic inference tasks. *Organizational Behavior and Human Performance 11*, 1–27.

Bruner, J. S., Goodnow, J. J., and Austin, G. A. 1956. *A study of thinking.* New York: Wiley.

Brunswik, E. 1955. Representative design and probabilistic theory in a functional psychology. *Psychological Review 62*, 193–217.

────── 1956. *Perception and the representative design of psychological experiments* (2nd ed.). Berkeley, Calif.: University of California Press.

Chamberlin, T. C. 1965. The method of multiple working hypotheses (1890). Reprinted in *Science 148*, 754–759.

Chapman, L. J., and Chapman, J. P. 1967. Genesis of popular but erroneous psychodiagnostic observations. *Journal of Abnormal Psychology 72*, 193–204.

────── and Chapman, J. P. 1969. Illusory correlation as an obstacle to the use of valid psychodiagnostic signs. *Journal of Abnormal Psychology 74*, 271–280.

Chase, W., and Simon, H. A. 1973. The mind's eye in chess. In W. G. Chase (ed.), *Visual information processing.* New York: Academic Press.

Chernoff, H., and Moses, L. E. 1959. *Elementary decision theory.* New York: Wiley.

Claparède, E. 1934. La genèse de l'hypothèses. *Archives de psychologie 24*, 1–154.

Clarkson, G. P. E. 1962. *Portfolio selection: a simulation of trust investment.* Englewood Cliffs, N. J.: Prentice-Hall.

Collins, A. M., and Quillian, M. R. 1969. Retrieval time from semantic memory. *Journal of Verbal Learning and Verbal Behavior 8*, 240–247.

Cook, M. G., and Dixon, M. F. 1973. An analysis of the reliability of detection and diagnostic value of various pathological features in Crohn's disease and ulcerative colitis. *Gut 14*, 255–262.

Cope, O., and Zacharias, J. 1966. *Medical education reconsidered.* Philadelphia: Lippincott.

Cornfield, J., and Tukey, J. W. 1956. Average values of mean squares in factorials. *Annals of Mathematical Statistics 27*, 907–949.

Cox, D. R. 1958. *Planning of experiments.* New York: Wiley.

Cronbach, L. J. 1951. Coefficient alpha and the internal structure of tests. *Psychometrika 16*, 297–334.

Davis, G. A. 1973. *Psychology of problem solving: theory and practice.* New York: Basic Books.
Dawes, R. M. 1971. A case study of graduate admissions: application of three principles of human decision making. *American Psychologist* 26, 180–188.
―――― 1975. The mind, the model, and the task. In F. Restle, R. M. Shiffrin, J. J. Castellan, H. R. Lindman, and D. B. Pisoni (eds.), *Cognitive Theory* (vol. 1). New York: Halstead.
―――― and Corrigan, B. 1974. Linear models in decision making. *Psychological Bulletin 81,* 95–106.
de Dombal, F. T., and Horrocks, J. C. 1974. Computer aided diagnosis. Conclusions from an overall experience involving 4469 patients. In J. Anderson, and J. M. Forsythe (eds.), *Medinfo '74.* New York: American Elsevier/North Holland.
de Groot, A. D. 1965. *Thought and choice in chess.* The Hague: Mouton.
―――― 1966. Perception and memory versus thought: some old ideas and recent findings. In B. Kleinmuntz (ed.), *Problem solving: research, method and theory.* New York: Wiley.
Dewey, J. 1938. *Logic: the theory of inquiry.* New York: Holt.
―――― 1963. *Experience and education.* New York: Collier Books (originally published in 1938).
Dudley, H. A. F. 1970. The clinical task. *Lancet 2,* 1352–1354.
―――― 1971. Clinical method. *Lancet 1,* 35–37.
Duncker, K. 1945. On problem solving. *Psychological Monographs 58,* No. 270.
Ebel, R. L. 1951. Estimation of the reliability of ratings. *Psychometrika 16,* 407–424.
Edwards, W. 1954. The theory of decision making. *Psychological Bulletin 51,* 380–417.
―――― 1961. Behavioral decision theory. *Annual Review of Psychology 12,* 473–498.
―――― 1968. Conservatism in human information processing. In B. Kleinmuntz (ed.), *Formal representation of human judgment.* New York: Wiley.
―――― and Tversky, A. (eds.). 1967. *Decision making.* Baltimore: Penguin.
―――― Lindman, H., and Phillips, L. D. 1965. Emerging technologies for making decisions. Chapter 2 in *New directions in psychology.* New York: Holt, Rinehart, and Winston.
Einhorn, H. J. 1970. The use of nonlinear, noncompensatory models in decision making. *Psychological Bulletin 73,* 221–230.
―――― 1972. Expert measurement and mechanical combination. *Organizational Behavior and Human Performance 7,* 86–106.
Elstein, A. S., Kagan, N., Shulman, L. S., Jason, H., and Loupe, M. J. 1972. Methods and theory in the study of medical inquiry. *Journal of Medical Education 47,* 85–92.
Erdmann, J. B. 1964. *An appraisal of three scoring procedures as discrimi-*

nators between good and poor problem solvers (Loyola Psychometric Laboratory Publication no. 40). Chicago: Loyola Psychometric Laboratory.

Feinstein, A. R. 1973a. An analysis of diagnostic reasoning. I. The domains and disorders of clinical macrobiology. *Yale Journal of Biology and Medicine 46,* 212–232.

——— 1973b. An analysis of diagnostic reasoning. II. The strategy of intermediate decisions. *Yale Journal of Biology and Medicine 46,* 264–283.

——— 1974. An analysis of diagnostic reasoning. III. The construction of clinical algorithms. *Yale Journal of Biology and Medicine 47,* 5–32.

Flexner, A. 1910. *Medical education in the United States.* New York: Carnegie Foundation for the Advancement of Teaching.

Fryback, D. G. 1974. Use of radiologists' subjective probability estimates in a medical decision making problem. Ann Arbor, Mich.: Mathematical Psychology Program, University of Michigan.

Gagné, R. M. 1971. Instruction based on research in learning. *Engineering Education 61,* 519–523.

——— and Smith, E. C., Jr. 1962. A study of the effects of verbalization on problem solving. *Journal of Experimental Psychology 63,* 12–18.

Gettys, C. F., Kelly, C., and Peterson, C. R. 1973. The best-guess hypothesis in multistage inference. *Organizational Behavior and Human Performance 10,* 364–373.

Getzels, J. W. 1964. Creative thinking, problem solving and instruction. In E. R. Hilgard (ed.), *Theories of learning and instruction. 63rd Yearbook of the National Society for the Study of Education.* Chicago: University of Chicago Press.

Gill, P. W. , Leaper, D. J., Guillou, P. J., Staniland, J. R., Horrocks, J. C., and de Dombal, F. T. 1973. Observer variation in clinical diagnosis—a computer-aided assessment of its magnitude and importance in 552 patients with abdominal pain. *Methods of Information in Medicine 12,* 108–113.

Glaser, R., Damrin, D. E., and Gardner, F. M. 1954. The tab item: a technique for the measurement of proficiency in diagnostic problem solving tasks. *Educational and Psychological Measurement 14,* 283–293.

Goffman, E. 1959. *The presentation of self in everyday life.* Garden City, N. Y.: Doubleday.

Goldberg, L. R. 1968. Simple models or simple processes? Some research on clinical judgments. *American Psychologist 23,* 483–496.

——— 1970. Man versus model of man: a rationale, plus some evidence, for a method of improving on clinical inferences. *Psychological Bulletin 73,* 422–432.

——— 1971. Five models of clinical judgment: an empirical comparison between linear representations of the human inference process. *Organizational Behavior and Human Performance 6,* 458–479.

Goran, M. J., Williamson, J. W., and Gonnella, J. S. 1973. The validity of patient management problems. *Journal of Medical Education 48,* 171–177.
Gordon, M. J. 1973. Heuristic training for diagnostic problem solving among advanced medical students. Unpublished Ph.D. dissertation, Michigan State University.
Gough, H. G. 1957. *California Psychological Inventory.* Palo Alto, Calif.: Consulting Psychologists Press.
—— 1962. Clinical versus statistical prediction in psychology. In L. Postman (ed.), *Psychology in the making.* New York: Knopf.
—— Hall, W. B., and Harris, R. E. 1963. Admissions procedures as forecasters of performance in medical training. *Journal of Medical Education 38,* 983–998.
Green, B. F., Jr. 1968. Descriptions and explanations: a comment on papers by Hoffman and Edwards. In B. Kleinmuntz (ed.), *Formal representation of human judgment.* New York: Wiley.
Gregory, S., and Dawes, R. M. 1972. The linear analysis of sincerity. Paper presented at the Conference on Human Judgment, University of Colorado.
Grimm, R. H., Shimoni, K., Harlan, W. R., and Estes, E. H. 1975. Evaluation of patient-care protocols used by various providers. *New England Journal of Medicine 292,* 507–511.
Guilford, J. P. 1967. *The nature of human intelligence.* New York: McGraw-Hill.
Gustafson, D. H., Kestly, J. J., Greist, J. H., and Jensen, N. N. 1971. An initial evaluation of a subjective Bayesian diagnostic system. *Health Services Research 6,* 204–213.
Hammond, K. R. 1971. Computer graphics as an aid to learning. *Science 172,* 903–908.
—— and Summers, D. A. 1972. Cognitive control. *Psychological Review 79,* 58–67.
Harvey, A. M., Johns, R. J., Owens, A. H., and Ross, R. S. (eds.). 1972. *The principles and practice of medicine* (18th ed.). New York: Appleton-Century-Crofts.
Hayes, J. R. 1968. Strategies in judgmental research. In B. Kleinmuntz (ed.), *Formal representation of human judgment.* New York: Wiley.
Hays, W. L., and Winkler, R. L. 1970. *Statistics: probability, inference and decision.* New York: Holt.
Hebb, D. O. 1974. What psychology is all about. *American Psychologist 29,* 71–79.
Helfer, R. E., and Slater, C. H. 1971. Measuring the process of solving clinical diagnostic problems. *British Journal of Medical Education 5,* 48–52.
Hemphill, J. K., Griffiths, D. E., and Frederiksen, N. 1962. *Administrative performance and personality.* New York: Bureau of Publications, Teachers College, Columbia University.

Hoffman, P. J. 1960. The paramorphic representation of clinical judgment. *Psychological Bulletin 57,* 116–131.
——— 1974. Physicians appraise other physicians: improving the decisions of a medical specialty board. *Oregon Research Institute Research Bulletin 14,* no. 4.
——— Slovic, P., and Rorer, L. G. 1968. An analysis of variance model for the assessment of configural cue utilization in clinical judgment. *Psychological Bulletin 69,* 338–349.
Hogarth, R. M. 1974. Process tracing in clinical judgment. *Behavioral Science 19,* 298–313.
Holsti, O. R. 1969. *Content analysis for the social sciences and humanities.* Reading, Mass.: Addison-Wesley.
Holt, R. R. 1958. Clinical and statistical prediction: a reformulation and some new data. *Journal of Abnormal and Social Psychology 56,* 1–12.
Hoyt, C. J. 1941. Test reliability estimated by analysis of variance. *Psychometrika 6,* 153–160.
Jacquez, J. A. (ed.). 1964. *The diagnostic process.* Ann Arbor, Mich.: Malloy Lithographing.
John, E. R. 1957. Contributions to the study of the problem-solving process. *Psychological Monographs 71,* no. 447.
Johnson, D. M. 1955. *The psychology of thought and judgment.* New York: Harper & Row.
Kagan, N. 1973. Can technology help us toward reliability in influencing human interaction? *Educational Technology 13,* 44–51.
——— 1975. Influencing human interaction—eleven years with IPR. *Canadian Counsellor 9,* 74–97.
——— Krathwohl, D. R., Goldberg, A. D., and Campbell, R. 1967. *Studies in human interaction.* East Lansing, Mich.: Educational Publication Services, Michigan State University (ERIC Document Reproduction Service No. ED 017 946).
Kahneman, D., and Tversky, A. 1972. Subjective probability: a judgment of representativeness. *Cognitive Psychology 3,* 430–454.
——— and Tversky, A. 1973. On the psychology of prediction. *Psychological Review 80,* 237–251.
Kegel-Flom, P. 1975. Predicting supervisor, peer, and self ratings of intern performance. *Journal of Medical Education 50,* 812–815.
Kendell, R. E. 1975. *The role of diagnosis in psychiatry.* Oxford: Blackwell Scientific Publications.
Kessel, F. S. 1969. The philosophy of science as proclaimed and science as practiced: "identity" or "dualism"? *American Psychologist 24,* 999–1005.
Kleinmuntz, B. 1968. The processing of clinical information by man and machine. In B. Kleinmuntz (ed.), *Formal representation of human judgment.* New York: Wiley.
Knowles, J. H. (ed.). 1968. *Views of medical education and medical care.* Cambridge, Mass.: Harvard University Press.

Kuhn, T. S. 1970. *The structure of scientific revolutions* (2nd ed.). Chicago: University of Chicago Press.
Kumar, V. K. 1971. The structure of human memory and some educational implications. *Review of Educational Research 41,* 379–418.
Laboratory of Computer Science. 1976. *Medical education programs: user's manual.* Boston: Massachusetts General Hospital.
Leaper, D. J., Horrocks, J. C., Staniland, J. R., and de Dombal, F. T. 1972. Computer-assisted diagnosis of abdominal pain using "estimates" provided by clinicians. *British Medical Journal 2,* 350–354.
——— Gill, P. W., Staniland, J. R., Horrocks, J. C., and de Dombal, F. T. 1973. Clinical diagnostic process: an analysis. *British Medical Journal 3,* 569–574.
Lewy, A., and McGuire, C. H. 1966. A study of alternative approaches in estimating the reliability of unconventional tests. Paper read at the Annual Meeting of the American Educational Research Association.
Lindsay, P. H., and Norman, D. A. 1972. *Human information processing.* New York: Academic Press.
Luchins, A. S., and Luchins, E. H. 1950. New experimental attempts at preventing mechanization in problem solving. *Journal of General Psychology 42,* 279–297.
Lusted, L. B. 1968. *Introduction to medical decision making.* Springfield, Ill.: Thomas.
McCarthy, W. H., and Gonnella, J. S. 1967. The simulated patient management problem: a technique for evaluating and teaching clinical competence. *British Journal of Medical Education 1,* 348–352.
McGuire, C. H. 1970. A summary of the evidence regarding the technical characteristics of patient management problems. Special report prepared for the Committee on Examinations of the American Academy of Orthopedic Surgery.
——— and Babbott, D. 1967. Simulation technique in the measurement of problem solving skills. *Journal of Educational Measurement 4,* 1–10.
——— and Solomon, L. 1971. *Clinical simulations.* New York: Appleton-Century-Crofts.
McNeil, B. J., Keeler, E., and Adelstein, S. J. 1975. Primer on certain elements of medical decision making. *New England Journal of Medicine 293,* 211–215.
Maier, N. R. F. 1930. Reasoning in humans. I. On direction. *Journal of Comparative Psychology 10,* 115–143.
——— 1942. Mechanization in problem solving: the effects of Einstellung. *Psychological Monographs 54,* 1–15.
Mandler, G. A. 1967. Organization and memory. In K. W. Spence and J. T. Spence (eds.), *The psychology of learning and motivation* (vol. 1). New York: Academic Press.
Martin, D. W., and Gettys, C. F. 1969. Feedback and response mode in

performing a Bayesian decision task. *Journal of Applied Psychology* 53, 413–418.

Mead, G. H. 1934. *Mind, self and society.* Chicago: University of Chicago Press.

Medawar, P. B. 1969. *Induction and intuition in scientific thought.* London: Methuen.

Meehl, P. E. 1954. *Clinical versus statistical prediction.* Minneapolis, Minn.: University of Minnesota Press.

Neisser, U. 1968. The multiplicity of thought. In P. C. Wason and P. N. Johnson-Laird (eds.), *Thinking and reasoning.* Baltimore: Penguin Books.

Neufeld, V. R., and Barrows, H. A. 1974. The McMaster philosophy: an approach to medical education. *Journal of Medical Education* 49, 1040–1050.

Neutra, R. R. 1976. Lecture notes on Bayes' theorem with multiple tests and multiple diagnoses. Unpublished manuscript. (Available from Department of Preventive and Social Medicine, Harvard Medical School, 641 Huntington Avenue, Boston, Massachusetts 02115.)

Newell, A. 1966. On the analysis of human problem solving protocols. Rome: International Symposium on Mathematical and Computational Methods in the Social Sciences.

────── 1968. Judgment and its representation: an introduction. In B. Kleinmuntz (ed.), *Formal representation of human judgment.* New York: Wiley.

────── and Simon, H. A. 1967. Overview: memory and process in concept formation. In B. Kleinmuntz (ed.), *Concepts and the structure of memory.* New York: Wiley.

────── and Simon, H. A. 1972. *Human problem solving.* Englewood Cliffs, N. J.: Prentice-Hall.

────── Shaw, J. C., and Simon, H. A. 1958. Elements of a theory of human problem solving. *Psychological Review* 65, 151–166.

Norman, D. A. 1969. *Memory and attention: an introduction to human information processing.* New York: Wiley.

Nowick, R. 1976. Initial diagnostic impressions: judgment of probability and seriousness. Unpublished Master's thesis, Hebrew University of Jerusalem.

Omnibus Personality Inventory. 1968. New York: Psychological Corporation.

Oskamp, S. 1965. Overconfidence in case study judgments. *Journal of Consulting Psychology* 29, 261–265.

Pauker, S. G. 1976. Coronary artery surgery: the use of decision analysis. *Annals of Internal Medicine* 85, 8–18.

Pitz, G. F., and Downing, L. 1968. Optimal behavior in a decision-making task as a function of instructions and payoffs. *Journal of Experimental Psychology* 77, 249–257.

Polya, G. 1957. *How to solve it* (2nd ed.). Garden City, N. Y.: Doubleday, Anchor Books.

Popper, K. 1959. *The logic of scientific discovery.* New York: Basic Books.

Price, R. B., and Vlahcevic, Z. K. 1971. Logical principles in differential diagnosis. *Annals of Internal Medicine 75,* 89–95.

Radford, J. 1974. Reflections on introspection. *American Psychologist 29,* 245–250.

Raiffa, H. 1968. *Decision analysis: introductory lectures on choices under uncertainty.* Reading, Mass.: Addison-Wesley.

Rapoport, A., and Wallsten, T. S. 1972. Individual decision behavior. *Annual Review of Psychology 23,* 131–176.

Rappoport, L., and Summers, D. A. (eds.). 1973. *Human judgment and social interaction.* New York: Holt, Rinehart and Winston.

Rimoldi, H. J. A. 1955. A technique for the study of problem solving. *Educational and Psychological Measurement 15,* 450–461.

——— 1961. The test of diagnostic skills. *Journal of Medical Education 36,* 73–79.

——— 1963. *Evaluation and training of clinical diagnostic skills.* Chicago: Psychometric Laboratory, Loyola University (report no. 41).

——— Devane, J., and Haley, J. 1961. Characterization of processes. *Educational and Psychological Measurement 21,* 389–392.

Rokeach, M. 1960. *The open and closed mind.* New York: Basic Books.

Rubel, R. A. 1970. *Decision analysis and medical diagnosis and treatment.* Ann Arbor, Mich.: University Microfilms.

Sawyer, J. 1966. Measurement and prediction: clinical and statistical. *Psychological Bulletin 66,* 178–200.

Scheffé, H. 1959. *The analysis of variance.* New York: Wiley.

Schum, D. A., and Kelly, C. W. 1973. A problem in cascaded inference: determining the inferential impact of confirming and conflicting reports from several unreliable sources. *Organizational Behavior and Human Performance 10,* 404–423.

Schwartz, S. H., and Simon, R. I. 1972. Studying information processing and decision making in medical diagnosis. In H. Wesley (ed.), *Health research and the systems approach.* Detroit, Mich.: Wayne State University Press.

Schwartz, W. A., Gorry, G. A., Kassirer, J. P., and Essig, A. 1973. Decision analysis and clinical judgment. *American Journal of Medicine 55,* 459–472.

Senior, J. R. 1974. *The development and validation of a computer-based system for testing and teaching clinical competence.* Philadelphia: National Board of Medical Examiners and American Board of Internal Medicine.

Sherman, H., and Komaroff, A. L. 1974. *Ambulatory care project* (progress report no. 11A). Boston: Beth Israel Hospital.

Shulman, L. S. 1965. Seeking styles and individual differences in patterns of inquiry. *School Review 73,* 258–266.
────── Loupe, M. J., and Piper, R. M. 1968. *Studies of the inquiry process: inquiry patterns of students in teacher-training programs.* East Lansing, Mich.: Educational Publication Services, Michigan State University (ERIC Document Reproduction Service no. ED 028 157).
Shweder, R. A. 1975. How relevant is an individual difference theory of personality? *Journal of Personality 43,* 455–484.
Simon, H. A. 1969. *The sciences of the artificial.* Cambridge, Mass.: MIT Press.
────── 1974. How big is a chunk? *Science 183,* 482–488.
Sisson, J., Schoomaker, E., and Ross, J. 1976. Clinical decision analysis—the hazard of using additional data. *Journal of the American Medical Association 236,* 1259–1263.
Slovic, P. 1969. Analyzing the expert judge: a descriptive study of a stockbroker's decision processes. *Journal of Applied Psychology 53,* 255–263.
────── and Lichtenstein, S. 1971. Comparison of Bayesian and regression approaches to the study of information processing in judgment. *Organizational Behavior and Human Performance 6,* 649–744.
────── Fischoff, B., and Lichenstein, S. 1977. Behavioral decision theory. *Annual Review of Psychology 28,* 1–39.
────── Rorer, L. G., and Hoffman, P. J. 1971. Analyzing use of diagnostic signs. *Investigative Radiology 6,* 18–26.
Smedslund, J. 1963. The concept of correlation in adults. *Scandinavian Journal of Psychology 4,* 165–173.
Snapper, K., and Fryback, D. 1971. Inferences based on unreliable reports. *Journal of Experimental Psychology 87,* 401–404.
Sox, H. C., Sox, C. H., and Tompkins, R. K. 1973. The training of physicians' assistants. *New England Journal of Medicine 288,* 818–824.
Sprafka, S. A. 1973. The effect of hypothesis generation and verbalization on certain aspects of medical problem solving. Unpublished Ph.D. dissertation, Michigan State University.
Sutcliffe, J. P. 1972. On the role of "instructions to the subject" in psychological experiments. *American Psychologist 27,* 755–758.
Thomas, J. C. 1974. An analysis of behavior in the Hobbits-Orcs Problem. *Cognitive Psychology 6,* 257–269.
Thorndike, E. L. 1918. Fundamental theorems in judging men. *Journal of Applied Psychology 2,* 67–76.
Toulmin, S. 1961. *Foresight and understanding.* New York: Harper & Row.
Tuddenham, W. J., Houser, L. M., Tuddenham, P. S., Booth, R. E., Jr., and Matthews, S. 1969. Preliminary evaluation of effectiveness of logical flow charts in teaching roentgen diagnosis. *Radiology 93,* 17–24.

Tversky, A. 1972. Elimination by aspects: a theory of choice. *Psychological Review* 79, 281–299.
——— and Kahneman, D. 1971. Belief in the law of small numbers. *Psychological Bulletin* 76, 105–110.
——— and Kahneman, D. 1973. Availability: a heuristic for judging frequency and probability. *Cognitive Psychology* 5, 207–232.
——— and Kahneman, D. 1974. Judgment under uncertainty: heuristics and biases. *Science* 185, 1124–1131.
Twelker, P. A. 1971. Simulation and media. In P. J. Tansey (ed.), *Educational aspects of simulation*. New York: McGraw-Hill.
Wallace, H. A. 1923. What is in the corn judge's mind? *Journal of the American Society of Agronomy* 15, 300–304.
Warner, H. R., Toronto, A. F., Veasey, G., and Stephenson, R. 1961. A mathematical approach to medical diagnosis: application to congenital heart disease. *Journal of the American Medical Association* 177, 177–183.
Wason, P. C. 1968. 'On the failure to eliminate hypotheses . . .'—A second look. In P. C. Wason and P. N. Johnson-Laird (eds.), *Thinking and reasoning*. Baltimore: Penguin Books.
——— and Johnson-Laird, P. N. 1972. *Psychology of reasoning: structure and content*. Cambridge, Mass.: Harvard University Press.
Ways, P. O., Loftus, G., and Jones, J. M. 1973. Focal problem teaching in medical education. *Journal of Medical Education* 48, 565–571.
Weed, L. L. 1971. *Medical records, medical education and patient care*. Cleveland, Ohio: Case Western University Press.
Wiggins, N., and Wiggins, J. S. 1969. A typological analysis of male preferences for female body types. *Multivariate Behavioral Research* 4, 89–102.
Wortman, P. M. 1970. Cognitive utilization of probabilistic cues. *Behavioral Science* 15, 329–336.
——— 1972. Medical diagnosis: an information processing approach. *Computers and Biomedical Research* 5, 315–328.
——— and Kleinmuntz, B. 1972. The role of memory in information-processing models of problem solving. Unpublished manuscript (available from Paul M. Wortman, Northwestern University, Evanston, Illinois).

Index

Abrahamson, S., 12
Accuracy: of interpretation, 59, 75, 86, 88, 94, 114, 120, 280, 295, 299; of outcome, 60, 75, 93-94, 103, 108, 110, 242, 246, 249, 280; of formulation, 60, 110, 113, 144, 244. See also Diagnostic accuracy; Errors, diagnostic
Allal, L. K., 165, 203, 212, 278, 279, 282
Allender, J. S., 14
American Board of Internal Medicine, 119, 299
Associative processes, 188, 194, 195, 197-198, 278, 279
Austin, G. A., 17, 35, 277
Availability, 33, 44-45, 80, 115

Bacon, Francis, 35
Balke, W. M., 40
Barron, F., 112
Barrows, H. S., 12, 195
Bartlett, F. D., 21, 65, 277
Base rates, 31-32, 33, 80, 105
Bayes' theorem, 3, 24, 30-34, 41, 43, 44, 288; and probability, 30-31, 32-33, 98, 105, 280, 296, 298, 300; and prediction, 34, 43; and introspective data, 42. See also Decision analysis; Decision making
Beach, B. H., 301
Bennett, K., 12, 195
Bieri, J., 112
Binary tree structure, 15-16
Black-box tradition, 11
Bootstrapping, 29, 101, 281
Bourne, L. E., Jr., 10, 35
Brainstorming, 194

Brehmer, B., 45
Bruner, J. S., 17, 35, 277, 288
Brunswik, Egon, 36. See also Lens model

California Psychological Inventory, 112
Canadian College of Family Physicians, 120
Case specificity, 286, 292-294, 296, 301; and high-fidelity simulations, 85-86, 88-93, 112, 120; and PMPs, 146-147; and hypothesis-generation experiment, 235, 240, 242
Chapman, J. P., 34
Chapman, L. J., 34
Clarparède, E., 229
Clarkson, G. P. E., 12-13, 16
Closed systems, 65-66
Coding in fixed-order problems, 155-156
Cognitive complexity, 112
Common sense, 254
Complete problem solver, 11
Complexity scale, 112
Computer-assisted instruction (CAI), 295-296
Concept attainment, 17, 35, 276
Conservatism, 32, 228
Consistency: cue, 153, 160, 161-165, 166-167; internal, 237, 247, 250; scoring, 250; intraindividual, see intraindividual variability
Content, medical, 2, 86, 118, 235, 286, 292-293, 301
Control, 43
Cornfield, J., 203

Corrigan, B., 25, 29, 30, 45
Costs, diagnostic, 80, 289, 301; and heuristics, 8, 253, 256, 258, 260, 262, 266-269, 272, 281, 297, 298
Covariance, 210-211, 216-217, 219; analyses of, 214, 257-258, 261, 262
Cox, D. R., 262
Criterial versus noncriterial physicians, 275-276; selection, 5-6, 47; in high-fidelity simulations, 85, 86, 88-94, 116-120, 121; and fixed-order problems, 153-154, 160-161, 164, 166
Critical findings: in high-fidelity simulations, 58, 59, 81-83; in PMPs, 125, 132, 133, 146, 148, 149; in heuristics experiment, 256, 257, 258, 262, 265-266
Cronbach, L. J., 213
Cue acquisition, 277, 299; in high-fidelity simulations, 52, 53, 58, 66, 71, 80-86, 106-116; in PMPs, 123, 125, 132, 133, 138-139, 142, 143-144, 148, 149, 282; in fixed-order problems, 154-155; in problem-formulation experiments, 175, 200, 226; in hypothesis-generation experiment, 228, 235, 243-244, 249; and heuristics, 252, 258, 297-298. *See also* Thoroughness of cue acquisition
Cue-hypothesis matrix, 54-56, 60-61, 83, 98-99, 125
Cues, 31-32, 252; positive, 34-35, 53, 101, 102, 103, 114, 115, 150, 281; negative, 35, 53, 101, 102, 103, 114, 115, 150, 281; utilization, 37-38, 188, 195-197, 200, 214-215, 216-218; in high-fidelity simulations, 48, 51-56, 61, 62, 83, 98-116, 279; integration, 106, 108, 281, 294; noncontributory, 114; in PMPs, 125, 134, 141, 150; in fixed-order problems, 153, 154-155, 160, 161-165, 166-167, 279; consistency, 153, 160, 161-165, 166-167; in problem-formulation experiments, 181, 186-187, 188, 195-197, 200, 214-215, 216-218, 278-279; verbal, 196, 197; nonverbal, 196, 197, 226, 282; classification, 215, 216-217, 218; in heuristics experiment, 252; evaluation, 294. *See also* Critical findings; Cue acquisition; Interpretation, cue; Weighting cues

Curriculum, Medical, 292-294

Damrin, D. E., 17
Data, see Cues
Davis, G. A., 11
Dawes, R. M., 25, 27, 29, 30, 45, 112
Decision analysis, 30, 274, 289, 290-291, 300; and high-fidelity simulations, 105, 296; and heuristics, 297. *See also* Bayes' theorem
Decision making, 30-36
de Groot, A. D., 16, 17, 114, 276, 285
Determinism, 34
Diagnoses, 12, 18, 122, 228, 252, 298; computer assisted, 102, 295, 300; in PMPs, 127-128, 130-131, 137-139, 141-142, 147; in high-fidelity simulations, 147; multiple, 147-148, 298; of fixed-order problems, 153, 165; in hypothesis-generation experiment, 234
Diagnostic accuracy, 288, 299, 301; in heuristic experiment, 8, 256, 258, 262, 265, 269-270, 281; and base rates, 31-32, 80, 296; in high-fidelity simulations, 80, 101-105, 108, 109, 110, 114, 115, 120, 147; and bootstrapping, 101, 281; in PMPs, 128, 131, 138, 142, 144-145, 147; in hypothesis-generation experiment, 232, 234, 236, 238, 248. *See also* Errors, diagnostic
Diagnosticity, 31, 32
Dogmatism scale, 112
Dudley, H. A. F., 12, 228

Early hypothesis generation, 12, 229, 278; and training experiment, 7-8, 199-227; and high-fidelity simulations, 56, 64-65, 77-78, 83-84, 93, 115, 124; and PMPs, 142; and fixed-order problems, 155, 165-166; and problem-formulation experiment (physicians), 168-198; in hypothesis-generation experiment, 232, 238, 240-244, 248-249; and heuristics experiment, 255-256, 258, 262, 263, 265
Ecological validity, 37-38
Edwards, W., 24, 30, 32
Efficiency: in high-fidelity simulations, 58-59, 86, 108, 146; in PMPs, 126, 128,

132, 144, 146, 148-149, 150; in hypothesis-generation experiment, 232, 234, 236, 238, 247-248; in heuristics experiment, 256, 266, 271-272
Einhorn, H. J., 28, 35
Einstellung, 137, 144
Elimination by aspects, 106
Engel, G. L., 228
Episodic reviews, 49, 51, 61-62. *See also* Thinking aloud
Errors, diagnostic, 80, 106-111, 147-148, 151, 253, 269, 289; in interpretation, 60, 107, 115, 145, 268, 271, 295; in cue acquisition, 108, 109, 111, 115; in hypothesis generation, 115, 144-145, 147; of commission, 148, 149, 234; of omission, 149, 234. *See also* Accuracy
Evaluation of students, 299
Examination, computer based, 299
Explanation, 42, 43

Feedback, 168, 200-201, 206-207, 222, 225, 226-227, 294. *See also* Outcome feedback; Process feedback
Feedforward, 39
Feinstein, A. R., 68, 71, 79-80
Films, 282; in problem-formulation experiment (physicians), 8, 169-171, 181, 282; instructional, 8, 200, 201, 206-207, 208-210, 221-222, 225, 226, 282, 294
Fischhoff, B., 301
Fixed-order problems, 152-167, 279, 282
Flexibility scale, 112
Flexner, A., 293
Formulations, 61, 126, 169; accuracy, 60, 110, 113, 144, 244; physician experiment about, 168-198; hierarchical organization, 176, 177, 180-181, 184, 185-186; and multiple subspaces, 176-177, 181, 182-184, 187, 219-221, 279; functional relationships, 177, 181-182, 184, 188-190, 215, 216-217; associative processes, 188, 194, 195, 197-198, 278, 279; training experiment about, 199-227; and heuristics, 265. *See also* Hypotheses; Strategies, search
Franklin, B., 25, 30
Frederiksen, N., 14

Fryback, D. G., 301
Functionalism, probabilistic, 36

Gagné, R. M., 229, 230
Gardner, F. M., 17
Generality, 254
Generalizability, 4, 251, 274, 285-286, 300; and high-fidelity simulations, 88-93, 118, 286; in training experiment, 213; in hypothesis-generation experiment, 237; in heuristics experiment, 263, 275
Gettys, C. F., 44
Getzels, J. W., 277
Gill, P. W., 109, 281
Glaser, R., 17
Goldberg, L. R., 24, 27-28
Gonnella, J. S., 250, 284
Goodnow, J. J., 17, 35, 277
Goran, M. J., 250, 284
Gordon, M. J., 275, 281, 296
Gough, H. G., 27.
Green, B. F., Jr., 41
Griffiths, D. E., 14

Hammond, K. R., 29, 36, 39, 40, 118, 285
Hayes, J. R., 16
Health Education Network, 295-296
Hemphill, J. K., 14
Heuristics, 21, 105-106, 281, 293, 296-298, 302; experiment about, 8, 252-272, 281; and memory, 80, 276; and PMPs, 142-144; and fixed-order problems, 162, 164, 166-167; planning, 253, 276, 277; and diagnostic accuracy, 288; and decision analysis, 291
Hierarchies, general to specific, 15-16, 116, 176, 180-181, 185-186, 198
High-fidelity simulations, 11-12, 46-121, 279, 283-285, 286; and tab-item methods, 17; early hypothesis generation, 64-65, 77-78, 83-84, 93, 115, 124; and PMPs, 125, 145-148, 235, 250; and hypothesis-generation experiment, 248
Hoffman, P. J., 26, 27, 28, 119, 120
Holt, R. R., 27
Hypotheses, 21, 31, 35, 45, 169, 280; and

Hypotheses (continued)
  high-fidelity simulations, 51, 53-60, 75, 83, 84, 102, 105, 108; multiple, 53, 134, 148, 179-180, 294, 297, 299; serious, 98, 154, 160, 161-162, 166; in PMPs, 125, 134, 143, 148; competing, 148, 176-187 passim, 197, 219, 221, 253, 278, 294, 297, 299; in fixed-order problems, 154-155, 160, 161-167; about training model, 201-202; and hypothesis-generation experiment, 244-245; and heuristics experiment, 252-253. See also Formulations; Number of hypotheses; Problem formulations
Hypothesis evaluation, 277, 281, 297; and high-fidelity simulations, 66, 98-106, 108-109, 114-115, 116; and PMPs, 145; and heuristics experiment, 265. See also Judgment
Hypothesis generation, 45, 277; in PMPs, 8, 127, 129-130, 131-134, 135-137, 138-139, 140-141, 144-145, 147; and memory, 45, 75, 80, 84, 113, 116, 166, 180; and high-fidelity simulations, 66, 68, 85, 103, 109-111, 112, 113, 114, 116; experiment about, 228-251; and heuristics, 252. See also Early hypothesis generation; Number of hypotheses
Hypothesis specificity, 278; in high-fidelity simulations, 53, 64-65, 116; in fixed-order problems, 153, 164, 166; and heuristics, 253, 263-265
Hypothesis testing, 12, 16, 278, 297; and high-fidelity simulations, 79-80, 114, 120; and PMPs, 143, 149; and hypothesis-generation experiment, 235
Hypothetico-deductive method, 278, 292, 293, 300; and high-fidelity simulations, 79-80, 115; and hypothesis-generation experiment, 228-229, 244

Illusory correlation, 34-35
In-basket techniques, 12, 13-17
Incidence, 80, 193, 197
Inferences, 295, 296; statistical, 30; cascaded, 32; multistage, 32; logical, 112, 279, 289; negative, 253
Information-processing models, 20-21, 24-25, 32-33, 40-45, 175, 277; and thinking aloud, 13, 229, 274, 287; and lens model, 37; and hypothesis testing, 79; and decision analysis, 274, 291
Information search units, 51-53, 54-56, 58-59, 66, 81, 120
Inquiry, medical, 64-66
Instruction, see Training, medical
Instructions, experimental, 205-207, 229-234, 238-242, 247-250
Interactionism, symbolic, 36
Interpretation, cue, 277, 279-280; and high-fidelity simulations, 59, 60, 66, 75, 85, 86, 88, 94, 107-120 passim; accuracy, 59, 75, 86, 88, 94, 114, 120, 280, 295, 299; errors, 60, 107, 115, 145, 268, 271, 295; flexibility, 112; and PMPs, 133, 145; and heuristics experiment, 253, 268, 271
Intraindividual variability, 4, 292, 299, 301; in high-fidelity simulations, 85, 88, 112-113, 119, 275; in PMPs, 146-147, 150; in problem-formulation experiment (physicians), 183, 186; in heuristics experiment, 267, 275
Introspectionism, 15, 42-43. See also Thinking aloud

John, E. R., 17
Johnson, D. M., 22
Johnson-Laird, P. N., 112, 276
Judgment, 22-42, 281, 288, 301; regression models, 24, 41-45, 290; and high-fidelity simulations, 98-106, 108, 114-115, 289. See also Hypothesis evaluation

Kahneman, D., 32, 33, 44
Kendell, R. E., 12
Kleinmuntz, B., 15-16, 24-25, 44, 116, 185, 198

Leaper, D. J., 284
Lens model, 36-40, 42, 45, 98, 300
Lewy, A., 236
Lichtenstein, S., 26, 31, 42, 44, 301
Logic, 3, 112, 276, 289. See also Hypothetico-deductive method

Loupe, M. J., 277
Lusted, L. B., 80, 288, 289, 300

McGuire, C. H., 225, 229-230, 236
Management, of patient: in PMPs, 122, 125, 129, 134, 140, 144, 147; in high-fidelity simulations, 147; in hypothesis-generation experiment, 234. See also Patient-management problems
Mandler, G. A., 165, 183, 184, 220
Martin, D. W., 44
Means-end analysis, 21, 114, 277, 278
Meehl, P. E., 27
Memory, 4, 276, 277; short term (STM), 20, 84, 165, 166; long term (LTM), 20, 116, 164, 276, 278; and hypothesis generation, 45, 75, 80, 84, 113, 116, 166, 180; and high-fidelity simulations, 57, 75, 80, 88, 113, 116; working, 57, 113, 116, 183, 279, 291, 293, 301; and cue interpretation, 88, 280; and fixed-order problems, 153, 164, 165, 166; in problem-formulation experiments, 180, 183, 210, 278, 279
Mental representation, 188, 191-192, 197
Meyer, G. D., 40
Michigan State University, 47, 48, 171, 202, 230, 300
Minnesota Multiphasic Personality Inventory (MMPI), 15, 24-25
Misinterpretation, 60, 107, 109, 115, 145
Models: computer, 3; behavioral, 13; prior state, 13; formal, 23-24; task environment, 24; linear, 25, 28, 29-30, 38, 42, 45, 99, 104-105, 108, 109, 281; actuarial, 27-28, 30; clinical, 27-28, 30, 293; lens, 36-40, 42, 45, 98; training, 199-227. See also Bayes' theorem; Information-processing models; Regression equations; Simulations
Morgan, W. L., 228
Multiple-cue probability learning (MCPL), 38-39
Multistage inference, 32

National Board Examination, 230
Neisser, U., 15, 229
Newell, A., 16, 19-20, 21-23, 43-44, 175; and task environment, 24-25, 175; and cryptarithmetic problems, 65; and cue acquisition, 277
Novelty effect, 204-205
Nowick, R., 115
Number of hypotheses, 279; in high-fidelity simulations, 56-58, 84, 86, 93, 112, 115-116; in PMPs, 125, 126, 143; in fixed-order problems, 155, 160, 161-162, 166; and problem-formulation experiments, 182-183, 219-220; in hypothesis-generation experiment, 232, 238, 246, 248

Objectivity, 17, 51, 120
Omnibus Personality Inventory, 112
Open systems, 21, 65
Outcome feedback, 38, 39; in training experiment, 200-201, 203-204, 208, 218, 220, 221, 224, 225, 227
Outcomes, diagnostic, 228; in high-fidelity simulations, 57, 58, 60, 75, 93-94, 103, 108, 110; multiple, 58, 71, 147-148; accuracy, 60, 75, 93-94, 103, 108, 110, 242, 246, 249, 280; in problem-formulation experiment (physicians), 172-173, 182; and heuristics, 256
Overinterpretation, 60, 107

Parameter estimation, 16, 31
Pathophysiological process, 193-194
Patient-management problems (PMPs), 7, 18-19, 122-151, 282, 283; in hypothesis-generation experiment, 8, 230, 233-251, 282; no. 1, 126-128, 145, 148, 233; no. 2, 129-134, 144, 145, 148, 233; no. 3, 134-139, 144; no. 4, 139-142, 148-149, 233
Peer nomination, 6, 46-47
Personality variables, 112-113, 301. See also Intraindividual variability
Physicians in studies, 7, 46-47, 159, 165, 171, 250. See also Criterial versus noncriterial physicians
Piaget, J., 16, 287
Piper, R. M., 277
Planning, 253, 276, 277
PMPs, see Patient-management problems

Policy capturing, 28-29, 30, 41-42, 44.
   See also Regression equations; Variance, analyses of
Polya, G., 254, 277
Prediction, 27-28, 34, 43, 99-105
Preparation, and thought, 22, 23
Price, R. B., 228
Probabilistic Information Processing system (PIP), 32-33
Probability, 289, 291, 297, 298, 300, 301; subjective, 31, 32-33, 44-45, 80, 148, 280, 296; objective, 31, 296; and high-fidelity simulations, 98, 105, 115; and PMPs, 148
Problem formulations, 169, 218, 221, 234. See also Formulations; Hypotheses
Problem solver, complete, 11
Problem solving, 2-5, 11-22; instrument, 17
Problem spaces, 20-21, 116, 175-176, 277-278, 301, 302; in high-fidelity simulations, 66, 115, 116; in fixed-order problems, 165; and problem-formulation experiments, 175-176, 177, 220-221; functional, 176, 177; in hypothesis-generation experiment, 244, 248-249; in heuristics experiment, 264
Procedures, experimental, 47-50, 122-124, 172-173, 203-205, 230-233, 257-258
Process feedback, 38-42; in training experiment, 201, 204, 208-209, 218, 221, 224, 227
Process-tracing approach, 11-22, 41, 45, 287-292, 301; and thinking aloud, 12-13, 15, 42-43, 287; and scoring, 121; and generalizability, 300
Proficiency, 148, 149, 150, 234
Prudential (moral) algebra, 25, 30

Quantification, 44, 280

Rapoport, A., 31
Rappoport, L., 39
Recall: in high-fidelity simulations, 50, 51, 53, 56, 61-62; in problem-formulation experiment (physicians), 184-185, 186, 187, 188, 197
Reductionism, 302

Regression, statistical, 33
Regression coefficients, 45
Regression equations, 24, 41-45, 274, 290, 300; multiple, 26, 28, 29; and cue weighting, 29, 45, 280. See also Policy capturing; Variance, analyses of
Relevance, 31, 51, 121
Reliability: in tab-item methods, 17, 19, 236-238, 250-251; of PMPs, 19, 236-238, 250-251; of data, 31-32, 298; in high-fidelity simulations, 51, 120-121; and fixed-order problems, 155-156; in training experiment, 213; in heuristics experiment, 256-257, 272
Representativeness, 15, 33, 42, 44-45, 80
Reserve judgment approach, 199
Retrospective distortion, 61-62, 175, 250
Rimoldi, H. J. A., 17, 18, 112, 283
Risk, 194, 256, 257, 268, 269, 289
Rorer, L. G., 29
Routines, 52-53, 114, 116, 120, 192-194, 302
Rubel, R. A., 256
Ruling in, 106
Ruling out, 106, 194-195

Sawyer, J., 27-28
Schwartz, S. H., 44
Scoring, 45; in high-fidelity simulations, 50-60, 120-121; of PMPs, 124, 125-126, 142, 148-150, 250; in fixed-order problems, 156; in training experiment, 211-212, 222; in hypothesis-generation experiment, 233, 234, 236-237, 242-247; in heuristics experiment, 257, 262
Sequence in cue acquisition, 15-16, 53, 123-124, 225
Seriousness: of hypotheses, 98, 154, 160, 161-162, 166; of diseases, 193
Shulman, L. S., 14, 277
Simon, H. A., 19-20, 21-22, 43-44, 175; and parameter estimation, 16; and cryptarithmetic problems, 65; and task environment, 175, 301; and cue acquisition, 277
Simon, R. I., 44
Simulations, 11-19, 25, 46, 115, 282-285, 301; no. 1, 68-71, 100, 110, 148; no. 2, 71-75, 104, 108; no. 3, 75-77, 100, 108,

110; paper and pencil, 122, 284, 286-287, 294, 295; in training, 200, 201, 225-226. See also High-fidelity simulations; Patient-management problems
Slides, 226, 294
Slovic, P., 26, 31, 42, 44, 301
Smedslund, J., 34
Smith, E. C., Jr., 229, 230
Solomon, L., 225
Solutions, diagnostic, see Outcomes
Specificity, see Case specificity; Hypothesis specificity
Sprafka, S. A., 278
Spuriousness, 237
Stability, 190, 191-192, 195, 196
Stimulated recall, 50, 51, 53, 56, 61-62
Strategies, search, 4, 15-16, 188, 192-195, 197, 279; general to specific, 15-16, 116, 176, 180-181, 185-186, 198; routine, 192-194, 302; convergent, 194; divergent, 194
Students in studies, 202-203, 230, 247, 250, 254, 255
Summers, D. A., 39

Tab-item formats, 12, 17-19
Task environments, 5, 11-22, 24-25, 32, 277, 301, 302; and high-fidelity simulations, 150-151; and PMPs, 150-151; and problem-formulation experiment (physicians), 175, 181-182, 183-184. See also Problem spaces; Simulations
Task validity, see Validity
Thinking aloud, 228-230, 282, 287; in hypothesis-generation experiment, 8, 232, 238-242, 248, 250; and process-tracing approach, 12-13, 15, 42-43, 287; in high-fidelity simulations, 48-49, 50, 51, 53, 61-62, 99; in fixed-order problems, 153; in training, 201, 208-209
Thorndike, E. L., 30
Thoroughness of cue acquisition, 280, 284, 295, 299; in high-fidelity simulations, 81, 94, 108, 114, 120, 146; in PMPs, 125, 128, 132, 138, 139, 142, 144, 145, 146, 148; in hypothesis-generation experiment, 232, 234, 236, 238, 247-248; in heuristics experiment, 256, 260, 266, 267, 270, 271, 281
Toulmin, S., 43
Training, medical, 1-2, 7-8, 36, 199-227, 271-272, 281, 292-298
Treatability, 98
Tukey, J. W., 203
Turing's test, 13
Tversky, A., 32, 33, 44, 106
Twenty Questions formats, 12, 15-16

Underinterpretation, 60, 107
Understanding, 43
Utility: index, 18; and availability, 80; in hypotheses, 115, 297, 298, 301; and logic, 289; and decision analysis, 291
Utilization: of cues, 37-38, 188, 195-197, 200, 214-215, 216-218; of heuristics, 255

Validity: task, 3, 14-15, 17, 33, 34, 42, 44-45, 80, 250; ecological, 37-38; face, 46, 117, 118, 161; discriminant, 51, 121, 161; content, 118, 235, 286; concurrent, 235, 247
Variables, 6-7, 24, 25-26, 41, 42, 45; task, 4, 181-182, 183-184, 186, 188; in high-fidelity simulations, 56-60, 86; in PMPs, 125-126, 132, 143, 146; in fixed-order problems, 152, 153-155, 160, 166, 167; in problem-formulation experiment (physicians), 181-182, 183-184, 186, 188; in training experiment, 210-212, 214-217, 219; in hypothesis-generation experiment, 231-232, 242; in heuristics experiment, 260-262, 263. See also Intraindividual variability
Variance, analyses of, 28; and high-fidelity simulations, 86, 94; and fixed-order problems, 156, 166; in training experiment, 213; in hypothesis-generation experiment, 238; in heuristics experiment, 257-258, 261-262, 266. See also Policy capturing; Regression equations
Verbalization, see Thinking aloud
Vlahcevic, Z. K., 228

Wallace, H. A., 26
Wallsten, T. S., 31
Wason, P. C., 35, 112, 276
Weighting cues: and Bayes' theorem, 24, 31, 42, 280, 289; and regression equations, 24, 42, 45, 280; and prudential algebra, 25, 29-30; and policy capturing, 29-30, 41-42; and information-processing theories, 42-43; in high-fidelity simulations, 54, 58, 59, 60, 61, 83, 98-101, 102, 114, 296; in PMPs, 125, 141, 150; in problem-formulation experiment (physicians), 196; in hypothesis-generation experiment, 236-237; in heuristics experiment, 257
Williamson, J. W., 250, 284
Wortman, P. M., 15-16, 44, 165
Würzburg group, 16

Bei Fragen zur Produktsicherheit wenden Sie sich bitte an:
If you have any questions regarding product safety,
please contact:

Walter de Gruyter GmbH
Genthiner Straße 13
10785 Berlin
productsafety@degruyterbrill.com